# THE BRAIN
## towards an understanding

*by the same author*

Molecular Biology: A Structural Approach

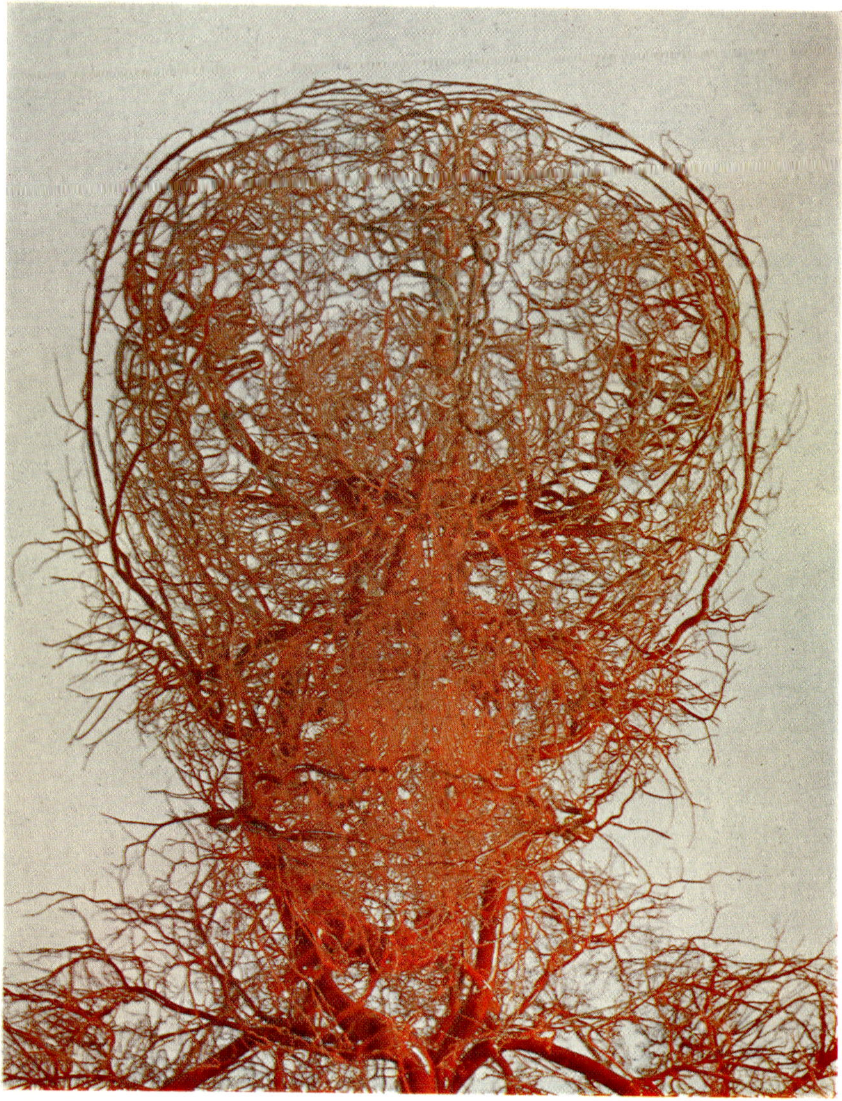

Cast of the arteries in the head of a still-born baby. The cast is seen from behind; the arteries supply both the brain and the face and surface of the skull. The adult brain, although only 2% of the body's weight, nevertheless receives about 15% of the cardiac output and uses roughly 20% of all the oxygen consumed by the body.
The cast was prepared by Dr D. Tompsett of the Royal College of Surgeons. The photograph is reproduced by courtesy of Dr Tompsett and the editor of the *Sunday Times*.

# THE BRAIN

*towards an understanding*

C. U. M. SMITH

FABER AND FABER
London

*First published in 1970*
*by Faber and Faber Limited*
*24 Russell Square London WC1*
*Printed in Great Britain by*
*Ebenezer Baylis & Son Ltd*
*The Trinity Press Worcester and London*


*SBN: 571 09170 9*

To My Father

*In Memoriam*

We can envisage this task (to understand the brain)
as an effort to put together an enormous jigsaw puzzle.

J. C. Eccles in *Brain and Conscious Experience*
Springer-Verlag, 1966, p. 50.

# Acknowledgments

As in previous books my main acknowledgments must be to the many gifted men and women whose researches have advanced scientific knowledge to its present position. Without their careful and long sustained endeavours our present understanding of the brain would be impossible.

More specifically I am most grateful to copyright holders for permission to reproduce photographs, drawings and extracts. These are acknowledged individually in the text. The photographs here reproduced from printed half-tone copy inevitably show a loss of detail and the quality of the results is not representative of the originals.

Finally I am once again greatly indebted to my wife for much help in typing, proofreading and in the preparation of the index.

# Contents

# Illustrations

## Plates



## Figures

## Tables

# Introduction

To understand the brain, its structure and its functioning, has been and still is one of mankind's greatest ambitions. For we should then have taken a giant step towards satisfying that ancient command: 'know thyself'.

Two thousand five hundred years ago, whilst the oracle at Delphi still prophesied the destiny of men, the first treatises on scientific medicine were being written on the other side of the Aegean Sea. In one of the most influential of these treatises we can still read today the following surprisingly modern passage: 'Men ought to know that from nothing else but the brain come joys, delights, laughter and sports, and sorrows, griefs, despondency and lamentations. And by this, in an especial manner, we acquire wisdom and knowledge, and see and hear, and know what are foul and what are fair, what are bad and what good, what are sweet and what unsavoury; some we perceive by habit and some we perceive by utility. . . . And by the same organ we become mad and delirious, and fears and terrors assail us, some by night and some by day, and dreams and untimely wanderings, and cares that are not suitable, and ignorance of present circumstances, desuetude and unskilfulness. All these things we endure from the brain'.[1]

Clearly Hippocrates, in that first dawn of scientific history, had grasped some of the significance of the wrinkled grey jelly within the arch of the skull. Today, two and a half millennia later, we should assign the brain an equal or even greater rôle in the physical basis of human life. It is hoped that this book will provide the numerate general reader and the beginning student of biological sciences some insight into our present-day understanding of the living brain.

A complete understanding of the human brain remains an achievement for the distant future. The combined activity of scientists in

[1] Hippocrates: *On the Sacred Disease,* translated by Francis Adams, Encyclopaedia Britannica Inc.

many different disciplines is, however, leading to a rapid increase in knowledge. This book is written in the hope of communicating these developing insights to a public outside the confines of the research laboratories. One of the more popular catchphrases of the present day has it that 'war is too important to be left to the generals'. This phrase might be adapted by saying that 'science is too important to be left to the scientists'. That, in other words, the *results* of scientific research are too important to be restricted to the scientific community. Nowhere is this more true than in the science of the brain.

Since at least the time of Descartes the aim of physiological research has been to 'reduce' the phenomena of life to physico-chemical terms. Thus when a physiologist speaks of 'understanding' the brain he means explaining its activity in the language of physics and chemistry. The brain scientist of today, like Descartes[1] in the seventeenth century, bases his work on the assumption that the brain is a piece of machinery, exceedingly subtle no doubt, but, nevertheless, machinery. Thus progress towards an understanding of the living brain means progress towards understanding how its activity emerges from the operation of the laws of physics and chemistry. The brain scientist, in short, stands towards the brain much as the electronics engineer stands towards the computer.

An understanding of the brain would imply knowing the answers to questions like 'What is memory?', 'What are dreams?', 'Why do we sleep?', 'How do we learn?', 'What are emotions?', 'Are our perceptions of the world around us true?', 'In what respects does our experience differ from that of the animals?'. It would be silly to pretend that anyone yet knows the final answers to these questions. Indeed the greatest of them all, 'What is consciousness and how far does it extend through the animal kingdom?' has hardly yet been dragged from the realm of philosophy to that of physiology. The honest brain scientist, like St Augustine of Hippo when faced with the analogous problem of the origin of human souls, must confess ignorance.

Another question which retains metaphysical overtones is the question about the truth of our perceptions. Philosophers from long before the time of Socrates right up to the twentieth century have incessantly argued this problem. It has been dressed up with the name of Epistemology. Of perhaps more biological interest, however, is

[1] Descartes, R., *L'homme*, Paris, 1664.

whether and how the perceptual worlds of animals differ from our own. Just as historians have learnt to project themselves imaginatively into the different *weltanschauungs* of the past so, perhaps, zoologists will one day be able to imaginatively reconstruct the way in which the world appears to the different animals.

Although the perceptual worlds of vertebrate animals must differ very greatly it seems possible that their emotions are all rather similar. We may perhaps guess this not only from observing their behaviour but also from the fact that emotive responses seem to be triggered in the most central and phylogenetically eldest parts of the brain. The seat of our most intimate 'self' seems to be located in the neuropil of the brain around the cerebral ventricles.[1] It is here, if it is anywhere, that we feel despondent or hopeful, angry or at peace. Destruction of these regions of the brain is more catastrophic by far than destruction of the much more recently evolved cerebral cortex. It is salutary to remember that these tracts formed during half a billion years of bitter struggle for existence are still today prompting our actions. The brain that nowadays controls the thermonuclear trigger was formed during Mesozoic wars and biased by Ordovician ordeals.

Other features of the brain's architecture raise other questions. What, for example, is the significance of all the sulci and convolutions which pucker its surface? In the early part of the nineteenth century Franz Josef Gall and Johann Spurzheim proposed that the various intellectual and moral faculties were localized in certain of these eminences. This theory, which became known as phrenology, achieved a considerable vogue in the nineteenth century. It was believed that hypertrophy or atrophy of these specific brain regions could be felt by palpation through the cranium and would thus give insight into the subject's mental potentialities and privations. Acquisitiveness, for example, was believed to be concentrated immediately in front of the ear, secretiveness above the ear and combativeness behind the ear. Although in this crude form phrenology is nowadays known to be false, Gall must be given credit for popularizing the

[1] It is interesting to notice that this idea would have seemed quite familiar to the eminent second-century physician Galen of Pergamon. In his book *On the opinions of Hippocrates and Plato* he writes '. . . If you press so much upon a (cerebral) ventricle that you wound it, immediately the living being will be without movement and sensation, without spirit and voice . . .' (Quoted in *The Human Brain and Spinal Cord* by Edwin Clarke and C. D. O'Malley, University of California Press, 1968, p. 16.)

idea that brain functions are localizable. It has since been established that certain regions of the cerebrum are indeed the seats of specific brain activities. These functions are not, however, intellectual, or moral faculties, but more basic processes such as speech, vision, hearing, etc.

Another basic aspect of the brain's architecture is its size. One often speaks of intellectual capacity and, possibly by a subconscious transference, supposes that this is in some way connected to cubic capacity. Lloyd George, who, by the way, took an interest in phrenology, is reported to have been aghast when first introduced to Neville Chamberlain because of the unusual smallness of the latter's head! In fact, brain size above a certain lower limit seems to have very little correlation with intellectual ability. Surveys of scholarship winners have shown that their skull capacities differ hardly at all from the general population.

Human brains, however, are all very big as brains go. The average adult brain weighs some 1350 gms. and consists of some 30,000,000,000 nerve cells. How big are the smallest brains in the animal kingdom? Many insects are capable of richly complex behaviour[1] yet their brains are of microscopic size. The blowfly's brain weighs some 0·84 mgms., and that of the African ant *Oligomyrex* is ten times smaller still. Such minuscule brains may contain only ten or twenty thousand nerve cells. This is a startling simplification compared with the giant human brain.

Perhaps it is as well that our brains possess such gigantic numbers of cells, however, for nerve cells do not reproduce themselves and die at the rate of over a thousand a day throughout adult life. Even so the brain of a nonagenarian may consist of only two-thirds the number of cells found in that of a twenty-year-old. It is an interesting speculation to consider why nerve cells do not reproduce themselves. Perhaps it is because the brain's experience, its memory, is held in the form of patterns of interconnected nerve cells. If this were the case the production of new nerve cells would very likely interfere with the pre-established organization and thus upset the memory.

The physical basis of memory is still, however, a very open question. Exciting recent researches have suggested that it may have a molecular basis (Chapter 15). Indeed the possibility of transferring specific memories from one individual to another by injecting the appropriate molecules has even been mooted. The technique used at present is to extract certain molecules from the brain of an experi-

[1] Dethier, V. G. (1964), 'Microscopic Brains', *Science*, *143*, 1138–1145.

enced animal and to inject them into the brain of a naïve animal. If this technique can be established and developed it is clear that some quite bizarre possibilities will present themselves. Instead of having to programme the brain by some twenty years of educational courses we may find ourselves able to programme it simply and relatively painlessly by a course of injections! Similarly we may be able to prevent the decay of memory by analogous chemical techniques.

Many other questions concerning the structure and function of the brain crowd in. Most of them are discussed in the ensuing pages. What, for example, is the physical nature of a nerve impulse? How fast can it travel? What sort of a cell is a nerve cell? How is the brain kept informed of environmental energy fluxes? Can behaviour be remote-controlled? Can memories be elicited by electrical simulation of the brain? What are the physical bases of psychedelic experience? To what extent does the brain resemble a computer?

In short, what sort of a machine is the brain and how does it work?

'Know thyself': but science has also a practical, social, motive. Francis Bacon distinguished between luciferous and lucriferous enquiries. Most science gets done out of a mixture of both motives. The least practical science, like the newest born baby, may, in time, come to have the most powerful effect on human life. The science of neurobiology is no exception.

Can we cure the brain's diseases? Surveys have shown that between 5% and 9% of the populations of the UK and the US will be hospitalized for mental illness at least once in their lifetime. This, of course, is a very large number of people. Not only are the consequences distressing for the patient and his relatives but the cost is distressingly high to the community in general. Mental illness is of very many different sorts and can be treated in many different ways. In some instances surgical techniques are effective. Perhaps the best known of these procedures is frontal leucotomy. It consists in cutting some of the tracts of fibres connecting the frontal lobes to the rest of the brain. This operation has an interesting history. It seems to have originated through the oversight of a road-maker, a certain Mr Phineas Gage. In 1848 he accidentally shot a four-foot iron bar clean through his head. Instead of quietly expiring Phineas Gage was soon back on his feet, walking to the hospital and joking about the hole in his head. It turned out that his left frontal lobe had been severely damaged but that his brain was otherwise intact. Indeed he survived his traumatic experience about twelve years. His mind was agile as ever and his memory was unimpaired, but he was otherwise a changed man. Instead of being conscientious he was feckless; care and forethought were replaced by slovenliness and unreliability. It was as though some inhibitory influence had been removed, as though some power of concentration had been eliminated. Nowadays frontal leucotomy is performed on patients suffering from pathological states of depressive anxiety. The depression is normally lifted as a result of the operation, but the patient's personality, like that of Phineas Gage, usually deteriorates.

Is it possible to construct artificial limbs controlled directly by the brain? Is it possible to construct artificial sense organs? The thalidomide tragedy has given a powerful impetus to the development of really dexterous artificial limbs. Some of the most interesting developments in this field have been artificial limbs controlled by electrical signals generated in the patient's own muscles. The amputee, for example, may in the future be able to operate the motor of his artificial limb by 'willing' certain muscles in his stump, or elsewhere, to move. Analogous to this on the input side has been the recent suggestion[1] that the implantation of arrays of electrodes in the visual cortex of the brain may, by appropriate activation, enable the blind to see simple patterns.

Can we prevent the falling off of mental powers with age? One aspect of this problem has already been touched on in what was said above about the possible molecular basis of memory. Preliminary experiments have indeed hinted that the injection of yeast RNA into ageing brains does have a small effect in halting the march of senility.

Can the computer engineer learn anything from the brain's design? In general the boot seems to have been on the other foot. Neurobiologists have hoped to achieve a better understanding of the living brain by studying the design principles of its electronic competitor. In fact, except in a very general way, the brain within our skulls does not seem to have a great deal in common with the computer. In some respects it is, of course, far inferior even to present-day computers. The speed and accuracy with which it is able to process logical operations is many orders of magnitude smaller. In other respects, however, most living brains easily outperform the computer. When they err, for example, they do not, in general, err so catastrophically. In its ability to recognize patterns, both visual and

[1] Brindley, G. S. and Lewin, S. (1968), 'The sensations produced by electrical stimulation of the visual cortex', *J. Physiol., 196*, 479–493.

auditory, the computer is just not in the same class as even quite primitive living brains. Perhaps it is here more than anywhere else that the computer designer may learn something from the animals.

Finally, can we perhaps mould the brain closer to the heart's desire? This is a dangerous question. Supposing the means were to be found: some might call the result conversion, others brain-washing. Indeed it has been suggested that the next step in the evolutionary process is the computer. 'Electronic' brains can perhaps be designed which are not only capable of producing improved designs for further computers but are also lacking the ingrained selfishness of human motivation.

The practical application of brain science, like the practical application of any science, is nevertheless a two-edged weapon. It can be employed for both good and evil. Let us, however, be optimists. Let us believe that it is better that decisions be taken for mankind by mankind rather than by the blind forces of a careless Nature.

No need to stress, therefore, that the science of the brain remains in a thermonuclear age a science of incisive importance: a science which, in Hippocrates' words, 'men ought to know'.

The preceding paragraphs give some indication of the questions which spring to mind when we speak of 'understanding' the brain. It is hoped that the present book, in attempting a semi-popular exposition of mid-twentieth-century brain science, indicates the direction in which the answers to at least some of these questions are nowadays believed to lie. The preceding paragraphs also indicate the extreme diversity of possible questions about the brain. No single book can hope to cope adequately with them all. Out of the many possible ways in which a book on the brain might be organized it was decided to follow a similar plan to that of the author's previous book: *Molecular Biology*.[1] Indeed the present volume is, in a sense, a sequel to the earlier book. The attempt in *Molecular Biology* was to show how an uninterrupted chain of cause and effect runs from atom, to molecule, to macromolecular assembly, to organelle, to cell; in the present book a similar approach is applied to the brain. Some levels of structural analysis in the brain are shown in Plates I and II.

In so far as the brain is composed of cells—nerve cells and neuroglial cells—the book on molecular biology provides a foundation; however the machinery of the living brain depends at root on the

[1] *Molecular Biology: a Structural Approach*, Faber & Faber, London, 1968.

fluxes of electrolyte solutions across lipoprotein membranes. This topic was not discussed in *Molecular Biology* and, in consequence, a separate foundation is laid in the present book. This foundation consists of a brief outline of membrane equilibria.

After this brief excursion into the realm of physical chemistry the account of the living brain mounts through a discussion of the components of living cells in general to an account of the structure of nerve cells and neuroglial cells in particular. From this basis it is possible to describe the physico-chemical nature of the nerve impulse, the mechanisms of impulse transmission from one neuron to the next, and the ways in which environmental energy is converted into nerve impulses by receptor cells.

Once the basic biophysics of the brain's componentry has been established it is possible to go on to a discussion of the ways in which the components work together to process sensory information and to co-ordinate behaviour. Again the policy of showing how complex forms and functions emerge from the interaction of simpler units has been adopted. Thus some of the beautifully simple nervous systems developed by invertebrate animals are discussed and used as steps in the argument.

By the time we reach Chapter 10, however, we can no longer put off a consideration of the highly intricate structure of the vertebrate, and, in particular, the mammalian brain. The account in Chapter 10 is developed from the evolutionary standpoint and shows, once again, how complex organic forms may not only be dissected into simpler constituents by the anatomist's scalpel, but have in fact evolved from simpler primordia during the history of the planet.

The mammalian brain, as we shall see, consists of at least thirty billion neurons and even more neuroglial cells. Are these neurons connected at random, as many have thought, or is there a precise genetically predetermined 'wiring diagram'? Some of the fascinating experimental work which is providing an answer to this fundamental question is discussed in Chapter 11.

In the next chapter the rôle of the brain stem in the motivation of human and animal behaviour is discussed. At this stage in the book we begin to recognize the footprint in the sands. It is our own. We begin to perceive that we are discussing not only the fluxes of ions across membranes and the organizational patterns of neurons but also the physical bases of our own personal experience. This must make us pause. We begin to approach what some philosophers have called

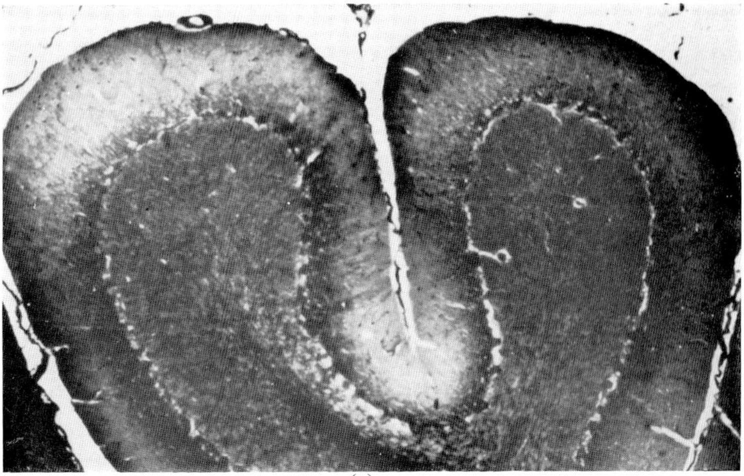

(a)

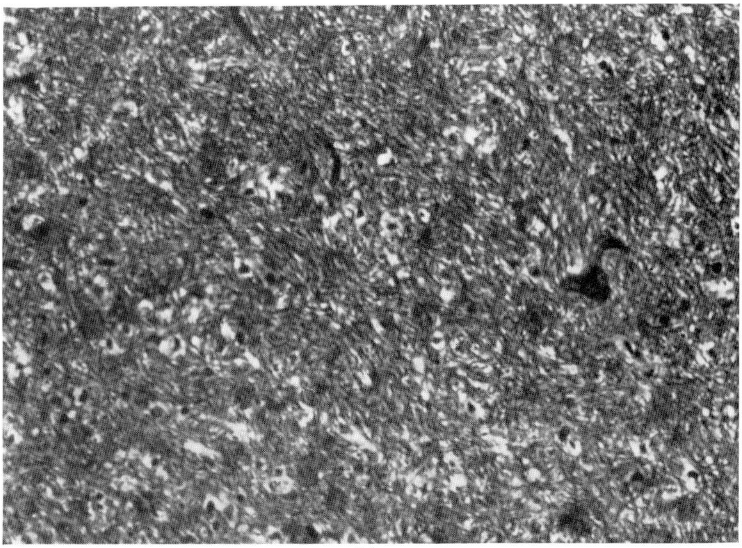

(b)

I. Levels of structural analysis (i)

(a) Section through a mammalian cerebellum ($\times$ 50). This photomicrograph shows the distinction between the cortical grey matter and the more central white matter in a portion of the cerebellum. At the junction of the two regions a layer of Purkinje cells may be seen.

(b) Higher powered micrograph of a portion of the white matter of the plate above. At this magnification ($\times$ 200) the white matter can be seen to be composed of a very complex web of intermeshing fibres.

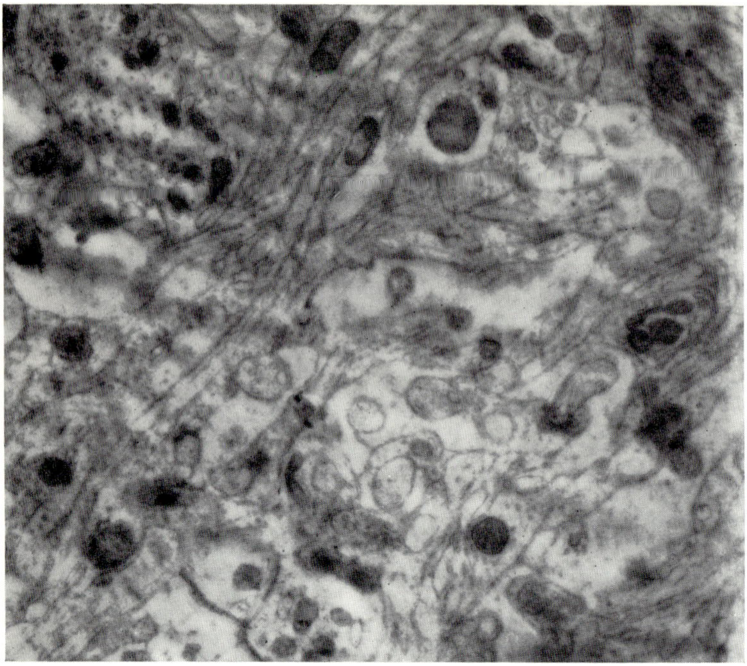

II Levels of structural analysis (ii)

(a) Electron micrograph of the white matter of the cerebellum ($\times$ 14,000). This plate shows that the electron microscope reveals the white matter to consist of a very intricate system of membrane-bounded compartments.

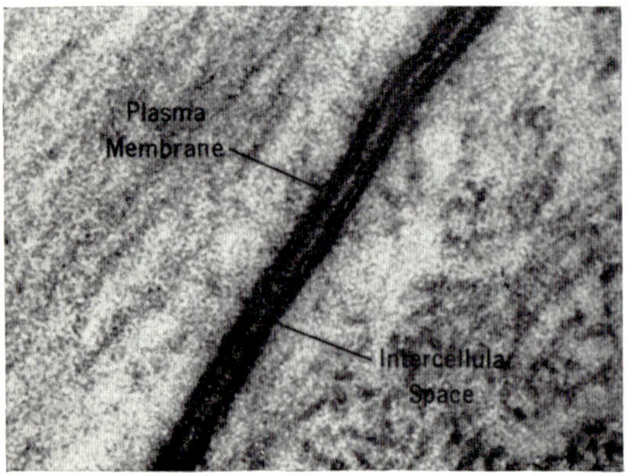


(b) This shows the cell membranes of two neuroglial cells of the annelid worm *Aphrodite.* The trilaminate structure of each membrane is clearly evident, as is the existence of a definite intercellular space filled with an amorphous material. Magnification 135,000 $\times$. (From Fawcett, D. W.: *The Cell: Its Organelles and Inclusions,* W. B. Saunders Co., Philadelphia, 1966.)

the 'World Knot'. The problem, to use the conventional formulation, of mind and matter.

In Chapter 13 the philosophical conundrum becomes more acute. Here we discuss the primate cerebral cortex. There are reasons to believe that it is the development of this tissue which is responsible for the emergence of the self-questioning intellect of mankind. It is at this level that matter first becomes fully aware of itself. The wheel has come full circle. In *Molecular Biology* we started out with atoms and the forces between atoms; in the final chapters of the present book we recognize ourselves. The force of this perception is, however, temporarily deflected by adopting, in these chapters, the policy of behaviourism. This is the policy of treating brains as just very complicated pieces of machinery designed (by evolutionary forces) to produce the behaviour observable in ourselves and others. Our questions are thus confined to queries about how the brain's machinery brings about this behaviour.

This policy is continued in Chapters 14, 15 and 16 where the topics of perception, memory and consciousness are discussed. In each case an attempt is made to identify the behaviour corresponding to the term and the neurological mechanisms held responsible for this behaviour outlined.

In Chapter 14 and, indeed, to some extent in Chapter 13, the idea of mapping assumes considerable importance. The basic idea of mapping seems to be that an abstract structure of relations embodied in one 'domain' of objects can be shown to hold between objects, usually of a different sort from the first set, in another 'domain'.[1] Thus, for example, a structure of relations may appear on the paper of a musical score, reappear in a sequence of vibrations of the strings of a pianoforte, be embodied once again in the pattern of variations in the width of a gramophone record's groove, obtain once more in the sequence of frequency modulations of a radio wave and so on. The domains of objects merely 'carry' the structure of relations: it is the latter which remains invariant and recognizable. Similarly with the neurophysiological account of perception. Structures of relations in the perceptual world are reproduced in the domain of physiological events in the brain. The mapping, however, is not always isomorphous. We shall see that features of importance to the life of the animal are emphasized and that unimportant aspects are minimized.

[1] See Nagel, E. and Newman, J. R., *Godel's Proof*, Routledge, London, 1958, Chapter 6.

The cerebral maps of the perceptual world are frequently more enduring than are, to advert back to our example, the ethereal vibrations of the wireless recital. In consequence we frequently see only what we have learnt to expect to see. This leads on to Chapter 15 where one of the most intriguing of all neurobiological problems is examined: the problem of memory. Much fascinating work has been done on this topic in recent years but the situation remains remarkably fluid. No firm answer to the question, 'What is the physical basis of memory?' has yet been obtained. Thus the last sections of this chapter are perforce frankly speculative.

With Chapter 16 we approach one of the most difficult topics in the physiology of living brains. What are the neurophysiological correlatives of consciousness? It has been said that the whole field of animal and human behaviour (except, perhaps, our own) can be studied and described without the aid of this concept. It is a superfluous construct and should, in consequence, be dropped from the scientific dictionary. However, if we define consciousness as attention or attentiveness we have a handle to grasp, a behavioural phenomenon to investigate. This is the approach adopted in this penultimate chapter. In the last section of this chapter we make one final move: we raise the discussion to the topic of self-consciousness. The method adopted here is to reverse the Freudian argument. Instead of attempting to mark off an 'unconscious mind' from consciousness, we mark off a special realm of consciousness—self-consciousness—from the more general realm of consciousness whose signature is attentiveness. This is done on behavioural grounds once more: obsessional neurotics and the majority of animals do not give any indication that they recognize the ends of their behaviours; to the extent that animals and humans are 'self-aware', however, their acts are marked by just this characteristic.

Finally, in Chapter 17, we turn to face the problem which has been nagging us throughout the last part of the book. If, as we have tried to show, the human brain is as much a part of the physical universe as the sticks, the stones or the stars, then 'Who', to put once again the immemorial query, 'are we?' It is certainly not supposed that a riddle which has perplexed thinkers for millennia can be solved in the final chapter of a book on neurobiology. However it is hoped that the rough-and-ready efforts towards an understanding exhibited in this chapter indicate the general area in which one biologist thinks the solution might lie.

It is clear from the foregoing resumé that our developing understanding of the brain is firmly based on a prior knowledge of the sciences of physics and chemistry. It is, however, only in quite recent times that the necessary tools, both intellectual and laboratory, have been forged so that the 'cutting edge' of physical science can be applied to the 'ravell'd knot' within our skulls. It is only in the second half of the twentieth century that the brilliant prospect of a cerebral mechanics worthy to rank beside the celestial mechanics developed in the seventeenth century becomes real. And this mechanics, as was emphasized above, is likely to be just as revolutionary in its consequences as was the Copernican theory first propounded some four hundred years ago.

There are no ghosts in the brain's machinery, no unmoved movers. It is all a matter of physics and chemistry. In the same way that an understanding of celestial mechanics depends on a prior knowledge of mathematics and physics, so an understanding of the burgeoning brain science of our times depends on a prior knowledge of the thermodynamics of ions, membranes and aqueous solutions. It is from an understanding of events at this level that the dawning comprehension of the entire system stems. It is only from this background that the nature of the nerve impulse, synaptic transmission and sensory transduction can be understood. And it is a combination of these phenomena which makes the ongoing activity of our brains.

It follows that the reader completely ignorant of the elements of physics and chemistry may find the initial chapters somewhat tedious. Persevere. A dawning understanding of the most intricate piece of matter in the known universe can hardly be achieved without effort. The treatment in these early chapters has been simplified so far as is consonant with accuracy; the general reader, moreover, will find most of the key terms explained in the glossary.

The essential ideas in these initial chapters are the concepts of chemical and electrochemical potentials. These terms are applied to neutral and electrically charged chemical substances respectively. Like the analogous electrical and gravitational potentials they may be taken, *for our purposes*, to indicate the direction in which a substance will move when freed from constraints. They are, in other words, measures of energy possessed by chemical substances by virtue of their position in a chemical system. Just as a current of electricity will move along a conductor from a region of high electrical potential to a region of low electrical potential, and just as a weight some distance above the ground (relatively high gravitational potential) will move (fall) to ground level (relatively low gravitational potential), so chemical substances in solution will move from positions of high to positions of low chemical potential.

It will become apparent, as the argument of the book develops, that these ideas are fundamental to much neurophysiological theory. It will become apparent that the controlled flux of charged ions across membranes is the essence of the electrical activity which characterizes the living brain. For the computer within our skulls is largely composed of an electrolyte solution divided into innumerable compartments by lipoprotein membranes. It is a computer no electronics engineer would recognize. Indeed it has been likened to 'two handfuls of porridge'. Yet from this porridgy computer have emerged the mathematical systems of Willard Gibbs, the poetry of Shakespeare and the inductive generalizations of Charles Darwin. Without doubt it is a computer we all should try to understand.

# CHAPTER ONE

# Fluxes of Material across Membranes

## 1.1 Thermodynamics

Let us begin at the beginning. Science nowadays offers an explanatory continuum stretching from the subatomic particle to the brain of man. Without doubt there are still lacunae in this continuum: important lacunae. But they rapidly diminish in size. In general there seems no good reason to believe that the spate of scientific research will meet insuperable problems; there seems no good reason to doubt that a complete description of the observable world is possible. A description, moreover, which shows how all the parts hold together in a unitary scheme; how complex forms like organisms and brains have evolved from simpler elements. How, indeed, the properties of these highly organized structures may be 'explained' in terms of the simpler units of which they are built.[1] This being so we have, if we wish to understand the present-day scientific view of the living brain, to begin far away from the sciences of biology and neurobiology.

We have to begin, in fact, by reviewing some aspects of the science of thermodynamics. This is one of the most fundamental of the physical sciences. Its axioms stand partly in the field of logic and partly in the field of observational science. Controversion of the second law, for example, would imply not only that our basic perceptions of the physical world were mistaken but also the strange logic of asserting that the most probable state was at the same time not the most probable state. It would imply not only that we might some day see the kettle start to boil on an unlit stove and that the stove would become yet cooler in order to provide the energy necessary for the boiling, but also that populations of molecules

[1] See Oppenheim, P. and Putnam, H., 'Unity of Science as a Working Hypothesis' in *Minnesota Studies in the Philosophy of Science*, Vol. 2, Minnesota Press, 1958, pp. 3–36.

would be *likely* to spontaneously sort themselves into *unlikely* groups.

Thermodynamics studies the interrelations and interactions of matter and energy. It is basic to all considerations of the dynamic aspect of things. Its formulations mark the bounds of what is physically possible. Thermodynamics, we have said, is concerned with energetics; indeed it is sometimes known *as* energetics. In a quite general sense, therefore, as well as for its practical utility, it is fitting to initiate a discussion of living brains which, in their human manifestation, are the foci of so much activity, by an outline of some relevant parts of this science.

### 1.2 'The world as a molecular chaos'

The phrase which heads this section was used by Sir Cyril Hinshelwood to introduce the subject matter of his book *The Structure of Physical Chemistry*.[1] The phrase is also appropriate in the present context. We shall find as we develop our theory of the brain that the workings of neurons and thus of brains are based firmly on the anarchic conditions prevailing in the submicroscopic world.

It is interesting to notice that the unceasing turmoil characteristic of the world of the almost infinitely small had been observed, millennia ago, by the peoples of classical antiquity. Aristotle, in his discussion of that self-moved mover, the soul, remarks that a common analogy for it in his day and before were the motes to be observed in a shaft of sunlight. 'The motes,' he writes,[2] 'are always seen to be in motion, even when the air is completely still.'

A more up-to-date index of microscopic and submicroscopic motion is provided by the phenomenon known as Brownian motion. If we examine through a microscope a small particle suspended in some fluid we shall find that it is in constant motion. Some of this irregular jigging hither and thither is probably due to convection currents in the surrounding fluid, but most of the erratic movement is due to the particle being bombarded on all sides by yet smaller, submicroscopic, particles. The submicroscopic world thus reveals itself as an animated, discordant crowd scene whose individuals incessantly hurry hither and thither.

[1] C. N. Hinshelwood, *The Structure of Physical Chemistry*, Oxford University Press, 1951.

[2] Aristotle, *De Anima*, 404a, 17, translated by J. A. Smith, Encyclopaedia Britannica Inc.

It follows that randomness is the signature of this submicroscopic scene. Let us now look a little more closely at this notion. Surprisingly it is basic to all the apparently ordered structures of the visible world. A little thought, moreover, shows us that far from being surprised that this is the case, we should be very surprised if it were not.

Let us suppose, for example, that our submicroscopic particles are represented by billiard balls. Let us further imagine that some of these balls are painted white and some are painted black. Let us put fifty black balls and fifty white balls into a bag and shake vigorously. We should be most astonished, on opening the bag, to find all the white balls on one side of the bag and all the black balls on the other. Indeed, we should feel compelled to look for an explanation. If, however, on opening the bag we were to see the billiard balls evenly distributed we should not be surprised. This would be what we expected and we would feel no further explanation necessary.

Take another example. Suppose we put a number of dice in the bag instead of billiard balls. After shaking (it will be remembered that motion is characteristic of the atomic world) we should be most suspicious if, on opening up, we found all the dice with six spots facing upwards. Indeed we might well conclude that the dice were loaded. Once again we feel that there is only one 'natural' result—randomness, mixed-upness—any other arrangement requires explanation.

## 1.3 Osmosis

Now how does all this tie up with the workings of living brains? It turns out that the brain at root depends for its living activity on the passage of materials across membranes. Let us, therefore, consider next some of the characteristics of such movements.

To make a start let us take an example well known to biologists: osmosis. Fig. 1.1 shows a common arrangement for demonstrating this phenomenon. A parchment membrane is stretched tautly over the mouth of a thistle funnel. Within the funnel is an aqueous solution of sodium chloride (NaCl). The funnel is immersed in a tank of distilled water. It is found that the funnel appears to imbibe water so that a column mounts the tube to a height 'h', or, if the tube is shorter than 'h', spurts out of the top. Now what force is at work to sustain a column of water in the tube? At root it is the force generated by the random movement of water molecules in the

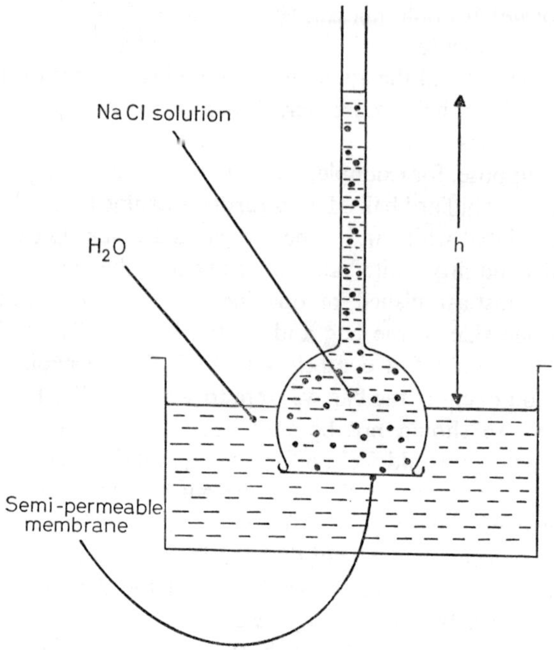


1.1 Osmosis

system. The parchment acts as a semi-permeable membrane (SPM) which allows, in this case, the passage of water molecules but not of sodium or chloride ions. The discimination is probably simply a matter of size. Hydrated sodium and chloride ions have larger radii than water molecules and hence are unable to pass through openings which are adequate for water molecules. This idea is schematized in Fig. 1.2.

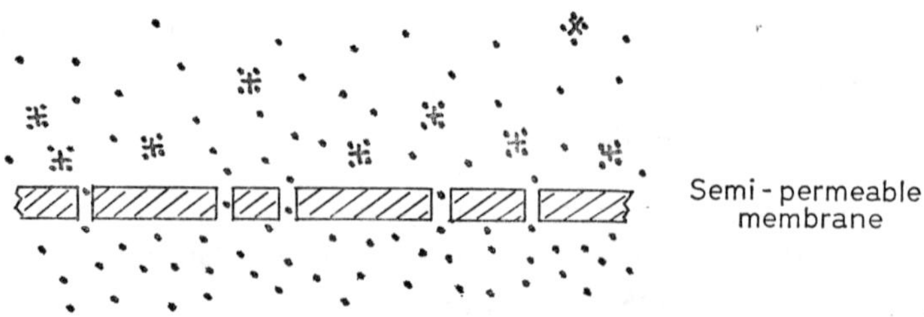


1.2 The physical basis of osmosis. Water molecules are represented by dots, hydrated ions by crosses surrounded by water molecules.

Fig. 1.2 shows that water molecules will pass through the membrane in both directions. However there are obviously more water molecules in a given volume of pure distilled water than in an equivalent volume of salt solution. Clearly some of the space in the latter solution is occupied by sodium and chloride ions. It follows that more water molecules will approach the SPM from the side of the pure solvent than from the side of the solution. Hence there will be an overall movement of water through the SPM into the thistle funnel.

Water molecules will continue to pass through the SPM into the thistle funnel until an appropriate back pressure, due to the column of water in the tube above the thistle funnel, builds up. In molecular terms this means that the molecules of water within the thistle funnel are moving at greater velocities than those outside the funnel. Hence a position of equilibrium is reached in which the number of water molecules passing from the inside of the funnel to the outside exactly matches the number passing in the opposite direction. The greater number of molecules approaching the membrane from the outside is balanced by the fact that the smaller number approaching from the inside is approaching at greater velocities. Thus the numbers effecting a passage are equivalent in both directions.

## 1.4 The idea of a chemical potential

So far in our discussion we have dealt with matters largely at the qualitative level. It is important, however, if we wish to gain a firm and precise grasp of the processes at work, to initiate a quantitative approach. In the last section we described how water passes through an SPM into a thistle funnel until a position of equilibrium is reached. Another example which brings out much the same points is found in the haemolytic action of some salt solutions on suspensions of red blood cells. For these purposes a red blood cell may be considered as a flexible semi-permeable membrane surrounding a haemoglobin-containing solution whose ionic strength is roughly equivalent to that of 0·9% NaCl. If the erythrocyte is placed in a solution of 0·7% NaCl water will pass into the cell diluting its contents. An equilibrium position is eventually reached wherein a combination of factors including dilution and back pressure due to the elasticity of the boundary membrane ensures that the outflow of water molecules equals the inflow. If the red blood cell is placed in 0·3% NaCl, on the other hand, water enters the cell to such an extent that the boundary membrane stretches and then breaks. Haemolysis is said to have occurred.

This example serves to emphasize the conclusions implicit in the previous section. The equilibrium position is not reached merely by a dilution of the internal medium to a point at which the number of water molecules per unit volume is identical on both sides of the semi-permeable membrane. The situation is considerably more complicated than this. Many factors may influence the overall flux of water or, for that matter, any other chemical molecule, across a membrane. It is thus important to have some label which we can attach to molecules in such situations which will tell us in which direction the flux occurs.

We are all of us nowadays familiar with the basic features of electricity and electric currents. We have been brought up in the convention that electric currents flow along conductors connecting two points at different electric potentials. A current flows from a point with a high potential to one with a low potential. Similarly we are all even more familiar with gravitational forces. It is customary to allude to a mass raised some distance above the ground as being at a higher gravitational potential than one actually on the ground. This merely means that if we remove the support from the highly placed weight we are in no doubt as to which way it will move. Thus it should come as no surprise to learn that there is such a thing as a *chemical potential*, conventionally symbolized by $\mu$.

In the examples we have been considering we can assign one value to the chemical potential of water on one side of the membrane and another on the other side. It follows that water molecules will move across the membrane from the side on which $\mu_{H_2O}$ is higher to the side on which it is lower. This overall movement will continue until $\mu_{H_2O}$ on the inside equals $\mu_{H_2O}$ on the outside. When this condition is attained just as many water molecules will be passing in one direction as in the other. It follows that no overall movement of water will be observable. Hence we may write the condition for equilibrium across the membrane in the following way:

$$\mu^{i}_{H_2O} = \mu^{o}_{H_2O} \qquad \ldots\ldots (1.1)$$

The superscripts 'i' and 'o' in this formulation signify 'inside' and 'outside'. We may, next, generalize this equation so that it refers to any chemical species, A, distributed between any two phases[1]—$\alpha$ and $\beta$. This generalized equation may be written as follows:

$$\mu_A^\alpha = \mu_A^\beta \qquad \ldots\ldots (1.2)$$

## 1.5 Towards the definition of a chemical potential

Now this is all very well in its way but what exactly are these convenient chemical potentials? How can we observe and, more important still, measure them?

To answer the first question first we can say that a chemical potential is a form of potential energy. It is in other words a quantity of energy associated with a chemical species 'A' in virtue of its being part of a system. In just the same way gravitational potential energy is associated with a particular body because that body stands in a particular relation to another mass—usually the Earth. When the body is freed from its constraints it 'falls' to the ground and its potential energy is converted into various forms of kinetic energy. This kinetic energy may, at least in theory, be collected and measured. In much the same way the energy liberated when our chemical species 'A' moves from a region of high potential, say phase $\alpha$, to a region of low potential, say phase $\beta$, may also, in theory, be collected and measured. Thus if *n* molecules, or ions, of 'A' move from phase $\alpha$ to phase $\beta$ we may define the energy liberated as

$$(\mu_A^\alpha - \mu_A^\beta)n \quad \text{units of energy}$$

It follows that, knowing *n*, the quantity $(\mu_A^\alpha - \mu_A^\beta)$ is, in principle, measurable.

In order to simplify matters it is usual to work in *moles* rather than '*n* molecules'. A mole, it will be recalled, is Avogadro's number ($6.02252 \times 10^{23}$) of molecules. This is the number of molecules contained in 1 gm. molecule of any chemical substance. Using this convention $(\mu_A^\alpha - \mu_A^\beta)$ ergs is the quantity of energy evolved when one mole of 'A' moves from phase $\alpha$ to phase $\beta$.

In this way we can at least observe and determine, in principle, the *difference* in chemical potential of the same substance 'A' in two different phases. It would, however, be very useful to be able to define a chemical potential in terms of other chemical parameters

[1] A phase may be defined as any homogeneous body.

such as temperature and concentration. Adverting back to the gravitational analogy, we are well accustomed to defining the gravitational potential of an object in terms of its mass and distance from the surface of the Earth. It would be most convenient to have a similar type of expression for a chemical potential.

The best means of arriving at this desirable goal seems to be via that most classic example of classical thermodynamics: the isothermal expansion of a gas against a piston.

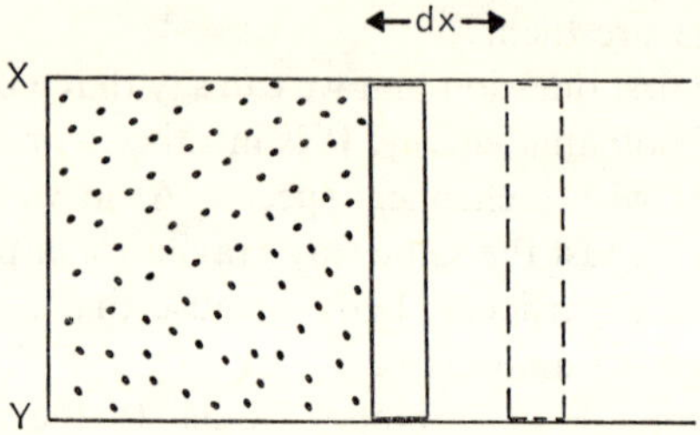


1.3 The isothermal expansion of a gas against a piston.

Fig. 1.3 shows a piston pressing against a volume of a perfect gas in a cylinder. It will be remembered that the molecules of a perfect gas are, by definition, completely independent of each other. There are no attractive or repulsive forces between them; when they collide they rebound from each other with perfect elasticity. In addition the walls of the cylinder and the edges of the piston which are to be employed in this thought experiment are so impossibly smooth that no frictional forces develop. Now let us try to imagine what happens when a constant gentle heat is applied to the bottom of the cylinder (X–Y).

Suppose first that the heat is very gentle indeed, in fact infinitely gentle. In consequence the gas only expands by an infinitely small amount. The piston moves back an infinitely small distance. Let us call this minute distance $dx$.

Now the work done in pushing the piston back a distance $dx$ is readily calculable if the area of the piston's face is known. Let us designate this area $A$ cm$^2$. Before the expansion begins the gas molecules bombarding the piston's face exert a collective force, or pressure, which we may symbolize as $P$ gms/cm$^2$. It follows that taken over the whole area of the piston's face this force adds up to $P \times A$ dynes. Next let us recall from elementary physics that work,

$W$, is said to be done by a force when its point of application moves along the line of action of the force. In our example an infinitesimal displacement, $dx$, occurs and hence an infinitesimal amount of work $dW$ is done. This minute quantity is given by equation 1.3.

$$dW = PAdx \qquad \ldots\ldots (1.3)$$

At this point we notice that $Adx$ is in fact a volume, $V$, albeit an infinitely small one. Hence we may rewrite 1.3 in the following way:

$$dW = PdV \qquad \ldots\ldots (1.4)$$

In this analysis of our thought experiment we have, so far, been dealing with infinitesimals and these, by definition, are too small to be measured. In order to bring matters into our observational world we have, therefore, to convert the infinitesimals into finite quantities. This is done by the mathematical technique of integration. It is supposed that the finite, observable, expansion of the gas occurs in a series of infinitesimal jumps, each symbolized by $dV$. If all these infinitely small expansions are added together we arrive at the observable expansion $\Delta V$. It is this process of adding up the infinitesimals that is called integration. $\Delta V$ is clearly the difference between the final volume, $V_2$, and the initial volume, $V_1$. It is also clear that if an infinitesimal quantity of work, $dW$, is associated with each $dV$, then a finite quantity of work, $W$, must be associated with the finite expansion $\Delta V$. Let us, therefore, attempt to integrate equation 1.4.

$$\int_0^W dW = \int_{V_1}^{V_2} PdV$$

$$\text{i.e., } W = \int_{V_1}^{V_2} PdV \qquad \ldots\ldots (1.5)$$

It turns out that whilst the left-hand side of equation 1.4 is readily integrable, the right-hand side is, as it stands, recalcitrant. It is necessary to search for some means of expressing $P$ as a function of $V$. Fortunately we do not have to search very far. In fact we do not have to look further than the familiar gas equation:

$$PV = RT,$$

$$\text{or } P = \frac{RT}{V} \qquad \ldots\ldots (1.6)$$

In equation 1.6 $R$ is a constant (the gas constant) and $T$, the temperature, is also in the case we are considering a constant (it will be remembered that the gas in the cylinder expands isothermally, that is at a constant temperature). Let us therefore substitute equation 1.6 into 1.5;

$$W = \int_{V_1}^{V_2} \frac{RT}{V} dV = RT \int_{V_1}^{V_2} \frac{dV}{V} \qquad \ldots\ldots (1.7)$$

Now equation 1·7 is very easy to integrate. Every schoolboy mathematician will recognize that:

$$\begin{aligned} W &= RT\,(\ln V_2 - \ln V_1) \\ &= RT \ln \frac{V_2}{V_1} \qquad \ldots\ldots (1.8) \end{aligned}$$

So far, so good. We now have an expression[1] which allows us to calculate the work done by a gas expanding isothermally. Let us now return and consider what light all this throws on our confrontation with chemical potentials.

Let us suppose that in Fig. 1.3 the end of the cylinder, X—Y, is a permeable membrane separating two phases $\alpha$ and $\beta$. Let us further suppose that the interior of the cylinder is filled with phase $\beta$. Now imagine that a chemical species, $A$, is dissolved in phase $\alpha$ and is able to pass through the membrane into the cylinder. As in our previous discussion we can assume that the chemical potential of $A$ is greater in phase $\alpha$ than in phase $\beta$. It follows that $A$ will pass through the membrane X—Y into phase $\beta$ until a condition of equilibrium is obtained. Now let us remember the very special conditions of our imaginary experiment. The movement of the piston in the cylinder is retarded by no frictional forces: it slips back perfectly freely. Hence there will be no back-pressure and $A$ will pass into the cylinder until the concentrations on both sides of the membrane are equal. Furthermore, just as the gentle heat applied to X—Y in our previous discussion remained constant, so we must suppose that the concentration of $A$ in $\alpha$ remains the same. In other words we must suppose that phase $\alpha$ is infinitely large so that the passage of a small amount of $A$ into phase $\beta$ has no effect on its concentration in $\alpha$. Alternatively we may imagine that $A$ is being continually added to phase $\alpha$.

[1] In equation 1.8 'ln' is a conventional abbreviation for 'natural logarithm'. To convert to normal logarithms it is necessary to multiply by 2·303.

Next let us recall that in the earlier part of the argument we defined the difference between two chemical potentials in terms of energy. Energy is, of course, the potentiality for doing work. A body possesses a certain quantity of energy when it is able to do a certain quantity of work. Thus we see the possibility of combining our two 'thought experiments' into one powerful synthesis. In short we can substitute the chemical potential difference $(\mu_A^\alpha - \mu_A^\beta)$ for $W$ in equation 1.8:

$$(\mu_A^\alpha - \mu_A^\beta) = RT \ln \frac{V_2}{V_1} \qquad \ldots\ldots (1.9)$$

The next step is to notice that we have assumed all along that the quantity of *solvent* in phase $\alpha$ and phase $\beta$ does not change during the experiment. It is only the solute, *A*, which migrates. Hence the volume of phase $\beta$ is directly proportional to the amount of solute it contains. In other words we see that the volume of phase $\beta$ varies in direct proportion to the concentration of *A*.

Let us symbolize the concentration of *A* in phase $\alpha$ at the beginning of the experiment as $c_A^\alpha$, and the concentration of *A* in phase $\beta$ at the outset as $c_A^\beta$. At the end of the experiment we saw that the concentration of *A* in phase $\beta$ is equal to its initial concentration in phase $\alpha$. We can therefore write down the following proportionalities:

$$V_1 \propto c_A^\beta, \qquad V_2 \propto c_A^\alpha$$

Substitution of these proportionalities into equation 1.9 gives

$$\mu_A^\alpha - \mu_A^\beta = RT \ln \frac{c_A^\alpha}{c_A^\beta} \qquad \ldots\ldots (1.10)$$

All the quantities on the right-hand side of equation 1.10 are easily measurable. However, it is still only a *difference* in chemical potentials which is defined. We have yet to determine what might be meant by a chemical potential on its own.

It turns out that the absolute value of a chemical potential is entirely arbitrary. Like the value of the force of gravity it depends on the acceptance of a completely *ad hoc* standard. In order to explain what this arbitrary standard is we have first to discuss the concept of a *mole fraction.*

So far in this chapter we have been using the familiar concept of the concentration, *c*, of a solute in a solvent. We have now to become a little more precise and to make use of a parameter which refers not only to the solvent but also to any other solute which may be present.

This parameter, the *mole fraction*, may be defined in the following way: the mole fraction ($x_A$) of a substance, *A*, is the fraction of the phase composed of that substance. Clearly when a phase consists of the pure substance alone then the mole fraction, $x_A$, is equal to unity.

Now it is the chemical potential of the pure substance that thermodynamicists take as the arbitrary standard against which to measure the potential of the same substance in solution. This standard chemical potential is symbolized as $\mu_A^o$. Bearing in mind that the $x_A$ corresponding to $\mu_A^o$ is unity we may substitute in equation 1.10 in the following way:

$$\mu_A^\alpha - \mu_A^o = RT \ln \frac{x_A^\alpha}{x_A^o}$$

$$= RT \ln x_A^\alpha$$

$$\text{or,} \quad \mu_A^\alpha = \mu_A^o + RT \ln x_A^\alpha \qquad \ldots\ldots (1.11)$$

Thus, in equation 1.11, we finally reach the conclusion of our argument. We have defined the meaning of a chemical potential. In the next chapters it will become clear how important and fundamental this concept is to the workings of neurons and brains.

# CHAPTER TWO

# Ions and Bioelectric Potentials

## 2.1 The electric force

In Chapter 1 we discussed some of the phenomena resulting from the invisible dance of submicroscopic particles. We saw that this fundamental property of molecules and atoms led to a maximum randomization or 'mixed-upness'. We saw, moreover, that this over-arching trend towards randomization motivates the flux of materials across membranes. Finally we saw how thermodynamicists have developed parameters which determine the direction and rate of these fluxes.

In this chapter we turn our attention to another fundamental physical force. A force, moreover, of a lineage equally as ancient and distinguished as the diffusional forces of the last chapter. Thales in the fifth century B.C. is reported by Aristotle to have believed that the lodestone, because it could move iron, was consequently endowed with life and soul. Thales is also credited with a knowledge of and interest in the electrostatic phenomena observable after a piece of amber has been rubbed. It is these electrical forces with which we shall be primarily concerned in this chapter.

## 2.2 Definitions of units

The basic equation (2.1) in this branch of physics shows that the force developed between two charged particles situated in empty space is inversely proportional to the distance between them:

$$F \propto \frac{q_1 \times q_2}{r^2} \qquad \ldots\ldots (2.1)$$

In 2.1 $q_1$ and $q_2$ are the magnitudes of the two charges under consideration and $r$ is the distance between them. The electrostatic force ($F$) developed between the two charges may be either repulsive or attractive. If $q_1$ and $q_2$ are oppositely charged it is found that the force is one of attraction; on the other hand if $q_1$ and $q_2$ are charged in the same sense then a repulsion develops between them.

Now it was stressed that 2.1 only applies to charged particles situated in empty space. This, of course, is never the case in situations of biological interest. The space separating the particles is invariably filled with some medium. It is found that the existence of a medium between two charges always blunts the electrostatic force. Hence a factor, $D$, the dielectric constant, is introduced into the denominator of 2.1. This factor is always greater than unity and varies from one medium to another. Hence we may rewrite 2.1 as follows:

$$F = \frac{q_1 \times q_2}{D \times r^2} \qquad \text{.....} \ (2.2)$$

Having introduced the notions of electrostatic forces and electrostatic charges it is next necessary to define their magnitudes. This is quite easy to do. We merely place two equally charged bodies 1 cm. apart in a vacuum. When the force between the two bodies is observed to be one dyne we define the charge carried on each as a unit electrostatic charge.

It can be shown that the electrostatic charge carried by any body is always an exact multiple of an elementary charge, $e$. This charge is associated with a subatomic particle and is positive ($+ e$) when the particle is a proton and negative ($- e$) when it is an electron. This fundamental unit of electrostatic charge is found to be equal to $4{\cdot}803 \times 10^{-10}$ of the electrostatic units defined in the previous paragraph.

### 2.3 Electrovalent (ionic) bonds and ions

The electrostatic force is the force which binds atoms together to form molecules. It is thus basic to the structure of much of the world around us. Chemists have shown that there are two principal types of chemical bond. Both are ultimately based on the electrostatic force. A covalent bond is formed when two or more atoms hold electrons in common. An electrovalent, or ionic, bond develops when an electron is donated from one atom to another. Covalent bonds are basic to most of the molecules of which the body is fabricated;[1]

[1] See: *Molecular Biology: a Structural Approach*, Faber & Faber, 1968.

electrovalent bonds are of first-rate importance in many biophysical and biochemical activities. Not the least important of these activities are those underlying the functioning of nerves and brains.

A very familiar example of a compound whose atoms are held together by electrovalent bonds is afforded by common salt—NaCl. Sodium possesses one electron in its valency shell whilst chlorine possesses seven. If sodium is to achieve a stable octet of electrons in its outermost shell it needs must lose its valency electron. Chlorine, on the other hand, requires an extra electron to complete its valency octet. Clearly, therefore, these valency requirements can be met if the sodium and chlorine atoms respectively donate and accept electrons when they meet.

Fig. 2.1 shows that the donation of sodium's electron to chlorine nicely satisfies the requirements of both atoms. The electron transference, however, leaves sodium positively and chlorine negatively charged. The resulting electrostatic attraction holds the crystals of common salt together. The two charged bodies can no longer be called atoms of chlorine and sodium for, because of the alterations

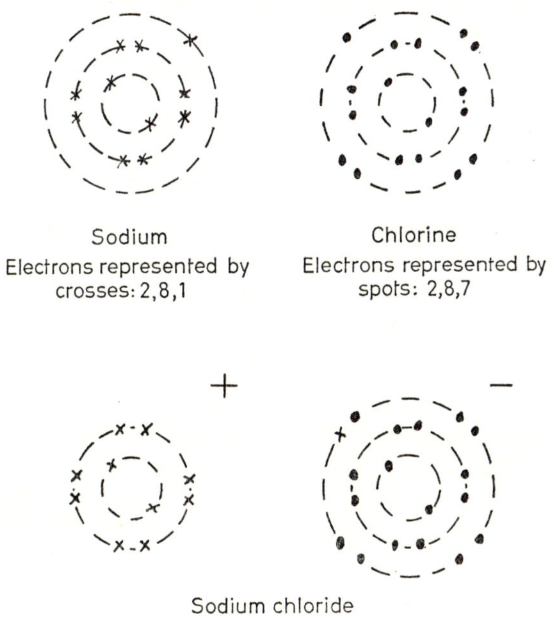


2.1 The formation of sodium chloride.

in their valency shells, they no longer show the familiar chemical characteristics of these two elements. Instead, owing to their properties in solution, they are called *ions*.

### 2.4 Electrolyte solutions

It is the properties of ions in solution which are, in fact, of most significance to the neurophysiologist. Whereas covalently bound molecules show very little solubility in water the opposite is the case with ionic compounds. Sodium chloride, it need not be stressed, dissolves very readily in aqueous solvents whilst an entirely covalent compound like, for example, olive oil shows little if any solubility. The opposite is, of course, the case with organic solvents like, say, benzene. In these solvents covalently bound molecules easily dissolve whereas electrovalently bound substances remain insoluble.

The solubility of different substances in different solvents is a very large subject and this is certainly not the place to go into it in detail. Solutions, according to thermodynamicists, may be defined as perfectly homogeneous mixtures. They are, in fact, molecular mixtures. The molecules of solute rub shoulders in a very intimate fashion with the molecules of solvent. It follows, in very general terms, that solutions are most easily formed when solvent and solute are similar types of molecule.

Now water, although a covalent molecule, is nevertheless electrically polarized. This is because the oxygen atom is highly electronegative and tends to pull the electrons which it shares with the two hydrogens far over into its sphere of influence. In consequence the oxygen 'end' of the molecule is negatively charged compared with the hydrogen 'end'. This important feature of the water molecule is shown schematically in Fig. 2.2.

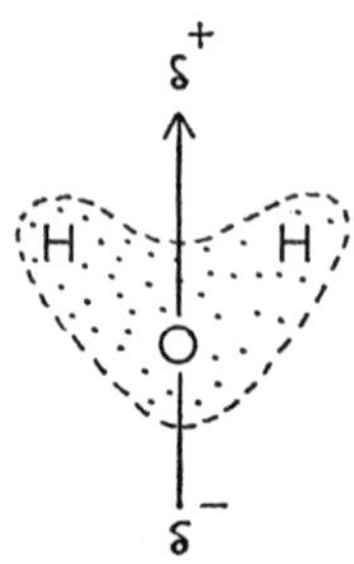


2.2 The electrical polarity of the water molecule.

This electrical polarity of the water molecule renders it somewhat similar to ionic compounds which, as we have just seen, are also electrically polarized. Thus we would expect from the rule of thumb set out above that water and ionic substances form solutions. In fact the solution of a salt such as sodium chloride in water is an even more intimate mixing than has been suggested so far.

There is good evidence to show that water molecules actually insert themselves between the sodium and chloride ions and thus neutralize, to some extent, their attraction for each other. This action is shown in Fig. 2.3.

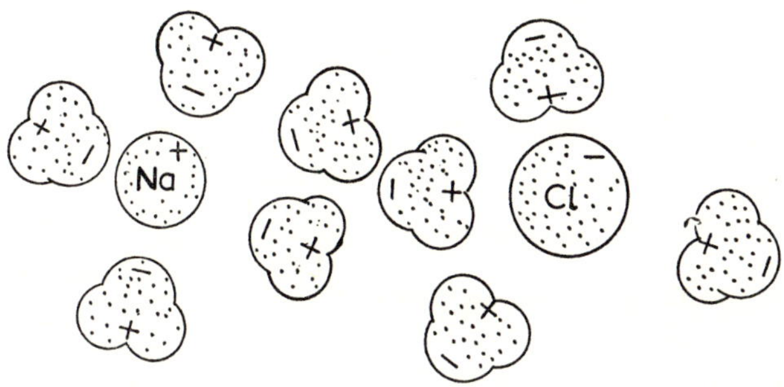


2.3 Water molecules cluster around sodium and chloride ions thus keeping them in solution. From *Molecular Biology*, Faber and Faber, 1968.

In this way the two ions are kept apart from each other: kept afloat, if you like, on 'rafts' of water molecules. In non-polar solvents, where this flotation does not occur, the $Na^+$ and $Cl^-$ ions 'gravitate' towards each other under the influence of the electrostatic force and consequently crystallize out of solution.

This clustering of water molecules around ions not only keeps oppositely charged ions apart but also, because the electric field associated with the water molecules is directed in the opposite direction to that of the ion itself (Fig. 2.3), reduces the electrostatic attraction. Water is thus said to have a high dielectric constant. It will be remembered that this constant appears as one of the denominators in equation 2.2.

Finally it is found that differentions have characteristically different number of water molecules clustered around them. This determines the effective size of an ion in aqueous solution. A list of the hydrated radii of ions of physiological significance appears in Table 2.1. We shall find in Chapters 5 and 6 that these radii are of considerable importance in neurophysiology.

TABLE 2.1

Hydrated and non-hydrated radii of ions of physiological importance.

| *Ion* | *Non-hydrated radius* (Å) | *Hydrated radius* (Å) | *Molecules of water carried* |
|---|---|---|---|
| $K^+$ | 1·33 | 3·8 | 5·4 |
| $Na^+$ | 0·98 | 5·6 | 8·0 |
| $Ca^{2+}$ | 1·06 | 9·6 | 16·6 |
| $Mg^{2+}$ | 0·78 | 10·8 | 22·2 |
| $Cl^-$ | 1·80 | 3·6 | 4·0 |

## 2.5 The electrostatic charge on an ion

Ions, we have emphasized, are able to move apart from each other in aqueous solution and wander off in all directions; indeed the word *ion* like the word planet derives from a classical root meaning 'wanderer'. Unlike the molecular species of Chapter 1, however, ions bear electric charges. We noticed above that the electric charge associated with an electron ($e^-$) was $4{\cdot}803 \times 10^{-10}$ electrostatic units (e.s.u.). It follows that the chloride ion of our example bears a charge of this magnitude and sign, whilst the sodium ion bears a charge of the same magnitude but opposite sign.

Now when we discussed the concept of a chemical potential in Chapter 1 we saw that it was conventional to work in moles (gm. molecules). Similarly the chemist interested in the movement of ions works in terms of gm. ions. The atomic weight of sodium is, for example, 22·98; it follows that the gm. ion of sodium weighs 22·98 gms. Similarly 35·46 gms constitutes the gm. ion of chloride.

Next let us remember (p. 43) that the number of molecules making up a mole of any substance is constant and equal to Avogadro's number ($N$). In precisely the same way a gm. ion of any substance is always built of exactly $N$ ions. It follows that a gm. ion of any univalent ion always bears the same charge: $N \times 4{\cdot}803 \times 10^{-10}$ e.s.u. This quantity of electricity is defined as the *Faraday* ($F$) and is equal to 96,500 coulombs.

Not all ions, of course, are univalent. Many are divalent, for example $Ca^{2+}$, $Mg^{2+}$, $SO_4^{2-}$. Others, for example $PO_4^{3-}$, are trivalent. Clearly these ions will carry twice or three times the quantity of electrostatic charge carried by a univalent ion.

We have now established a background from which it is possible to develop further some of the concepts derived in Chapter 1.

### 2.6 The nature of electrochemical potentials

It will be remembered that the main argument of Chapter 1 was directed towards finding an expression for a chemical potential. It will be recalled that this concept was finally defined in equation 1.11 as follows:

$$\mu_A^\alpha = \mu_A^o + RT \ln x_A^\alpha \qquad \ldots\ldots (1.11)$$

Equation 1.11 defines the chemical potential of a neutral substance, *A*, in a phase, α. The only forces involved are diffusional forces. In the case of ions, however, electrical forces must also be considered. These forces are additional to the diffusional forces affecting neutral molecules. It is clear that a term to take account of this additional force must be added to the right-hand side of equation 1.11.

Let us suppose that the phase α has an electrical potential symbolized as $\psi^\alpha$. It follows that this potential will exert a force on any charged body, such as an ion, *I*, located in the phase. The force exerted is proportional to the magnitude of the charge carried by the ion multiplied by $\psi^\alpha$. By convention the charge on an ion is symbolized as $z$. Thus $z = 1$ when the ion is, like $Na^+$, a univalent cation and $z = -1$ when the ion is a univalent anion, like $Cl^-$. Thus we can easily write an expression for the electric force, *P*, to which the ion is exposed in phase α.

$$P = z_I \psi^\alpha \qquad \ldots\ldots (2.3)$$

Now we emphasized in the previous section that it is of little practical interest to consider the forces on single particles, be they molecules or ions. It will be recalled that it is standard practice to work in terms of gm. molecules (moles) and gm. ions. It will also be recalled that a gm. ion of any univalent ion bears a quantity of electrostatic charge exactly equal to one Faraday (*F*). Thus we may conclude that the electric force on a gm.ion of an ion *I* in phase α is given by:

$$P = z_I F \psi^\alpha \qquad \ldots\ldots (2.4)$$

Now this force, *P*, is, as we noted above, additional to the non-electric forces which, as we saw in Chapter 1, act on uncharged solutes. Therefore to form an expression for the *electrochemical* potential ($\bar{\mu}$) of an ion, *I*, in phase $\alpha$ it must be added to the right-hand side of equation 1.11:

$$\bar{\mu}_I^\alpha = \mu_I^o + RT \ln x_I^\alpha + z_I F \psi^\alpha \qquad \ldots\ldots (2.5)$$

In equation 2.5 we have a complete expression for the electrochemical potential of an ion, *I*, in a phase, $\alpha$. We can now go on to consider how such an ion might be expected to distribute itself across a permeable membrane separating two phases $\alpha$ and $\beta$. Such a situation is basic to our understanding of the working of neurons where ions distribute themselves across the neuronal membrane between the interior and exterior of the cell.

## 2.7 Derivation of the Nernst equation

Fig. 2.4 shows the physical situation we are about to discuss.

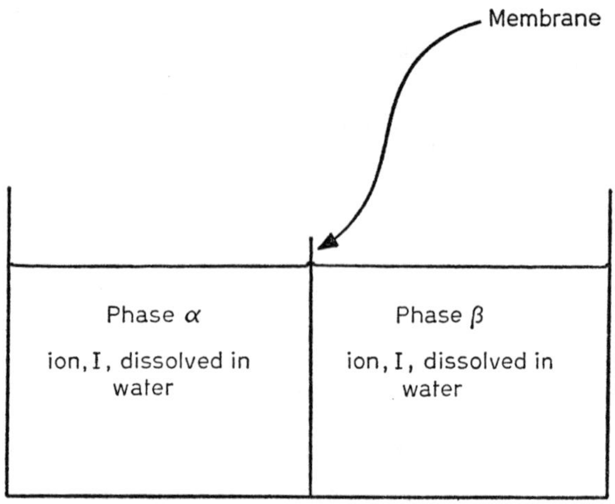


2.4 The physical situation basic to the development of electrochemical potentials.

The figure shows two phases $\alpha$ and $\beta$ separated by a membrane permeable to the ion, *I*. In general the electrical potential of phase $\alpha$ will differ from that of phase $\beta$. Similarly the mole fraction, $x_I$, of *I* in phase $\alpha$ will not be equal to its mole fraction in phase $\beta$. We have, therefore, both electrical and diffusional forces acting on *I* causing it to move from $\alpha$ to $\beta$, or vice versa. We want to know the balance of these forces so that we can predict in which direction *I* will in fact move.

In order to do this we make use of one of the important ideas discussed in Chapter 1. It will be remembered (equation 1.2) that a chemical substance achieves dynamic equilibrium across a permeable membrane when its chemical potentials on either side are identical. Exactly the same reasoning applies to ionic substances. When the electrochemical potential of *I* is the same on both sides of a membrane no further large-scale movement will occur. Just as many ions will pass through the membrane in one direction as will, in the same time, pass through in the reverse direction. This condition for dynamic equilibrium may be expressed in symbols as follows:

$$\bar{\mu}_I^\alpha = \bar{\mu}_I^\beta \qquad \ldots\ldots (2.6)$$

With the help of equation 2.5 we can expand equation 2.6 as follows:

$$\mu_I^o + RT \ln x_I^\alpha + z_I F\psi^\alpha = \mu_I^o + RT \ln x_I^\beta + z_I F\psi^\beta \ \ldots\ldots (2.7)$$

Clearly the term $\mu_I^o$ may be eliminated from both sides of 2.7 so that we have:

$$RT \ln x_I{}^\alpha + z_I F\psi^\alpha = RT \ln x_I{}^\beta + z_I F\psi^\beta$$

which, on rearrangement, may be written as:

$$z_I F(\psi^\alpha - \psi^\beta) = RT(\ln x_I{}^\beta - \ln x_I{}^\alpha)$$

$$\text{or,}\quad \psi^\alpha - \psi^\beta = \frac{RT}{z_I F} \ln \frac{x_I{}^\beta}{x_I{}^\alpha} \qquad \ldots\ldots (2.8)$$

Finally, let us note that the term $(\psi^\alpha - \psi^\beta)$ on the left-hand side of 2.8 represents the difference between the electrical potentials of the two phases $\alpha$ and $\beta$. Clearly this potential difference must be located across the membrane separating the two phases. Conventionally it is symbolized by *E*, or *V*. Hence we may rewrite equation 2.8 more simply as follows:

$$V = \frac{RT}{z_1 F} \ln \frac{x_1{}^\beta}{x_1{}^\alpha} \qquad \ldots\ldots (2.9)$$

We shall find as we go on that equation 2.9 is of great importance in neurophysiology. It is called the *Nernst equation* and, as we have stressed, relates the transmembrane distribution of ions to the transmembrane potential. It is important to remember that the equation is only valid when the membrane is freely permeable to the ion under consideration. When this is the case large-scale movement of the ion population across the membrane occurs until a position of dynamic equilibrium is reached. This position, symbolized by equation 2.9, is such that the diffusional forces consequent upon a difference in the mole fraction of the ion in the two phases are exactly counterbalanced by the electrostatic force due to the potential difference between the two phases.

### 2.8 Membrane equilibria and bioelectric potentials

The Nernst equation shows that when a diffusible ion is asymmetrically distributed across a membrane a transmembrane potential results. Let us now consider a very common cause of such ionic asymmetry and thus of electrical potential differences across cell membranes.

At root the cause of the uneven distributions we are about to consider lies in the presence within cells of large, indiffusible, ions. The presence of these ions distorts the distribution of all the others.

The cell membrane, as we shall see in Chapter 3, is very thin and is built of lipids and proteins. For the present purpose it may be likened to a sieve with very minute holes. Only the smallest ions, for example $K^+$ and $Cl^-$ (see Table 2.1), are able to squeeze through these holes. Larger molecules and ions are retained.

Now the protoplasm of cells contains, of course, many large ions. Notable amongst these are the proteins and amino-acids. The extracellular fluid outside the cell will contain far fewer, if any, of these massive ions.

Let us consider the case where a solution of potassium proteinate (KPr) within a cell is separated by a membrane from a solution of potassium chloride (KCl) outside. This situation is schematized in Fig. 2.5.

In Fig. 2.5 '*i*' and '*o*' stand for inside (intracellular) and outside (extracellular) respectively. The vertical line represents the membrane: permeable to $K^+$ and $Cl^-$, but not to $Pr^-$. Finally we suppose that there are '*a*' moles of KPr within the cell and '*b*' moles of KCl immediately outside.

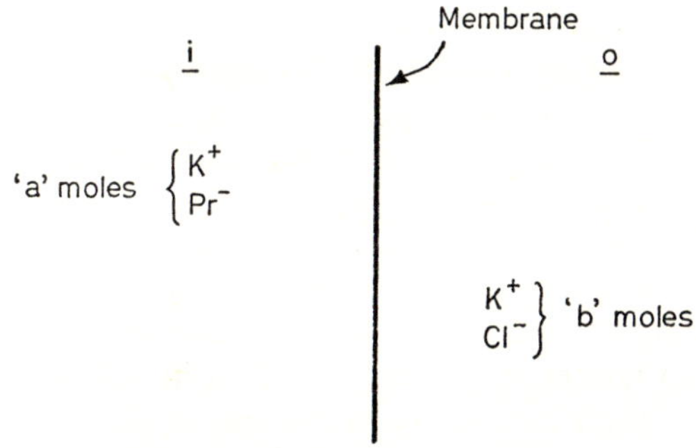


2.5 Gibbs-Donnan equilibrium: initial state.

Now, as we have been emphasizing all along, the ions and molecules in the submicroscopic world are in a state of turmoil, continuously moving in all directions. It follows that ions small enough to pass through the membrane will do so until a state of dynamic equilibrium is achieved. However because $Pr^-$ is, by definition, unable to get through the membrane an equivalent amount of cation ($K^+$) is kept within the cell by the electrostatic force. This consideration does not apply to the $K^+$ and $Cl^-$ in the extracellular space. Both these ions are able to traverse the membrane. Let us suppose, therefore, that '*x*' moles of KCl do in fact diffuse through the membrane. This movement is depicted in Fig. 2.6.

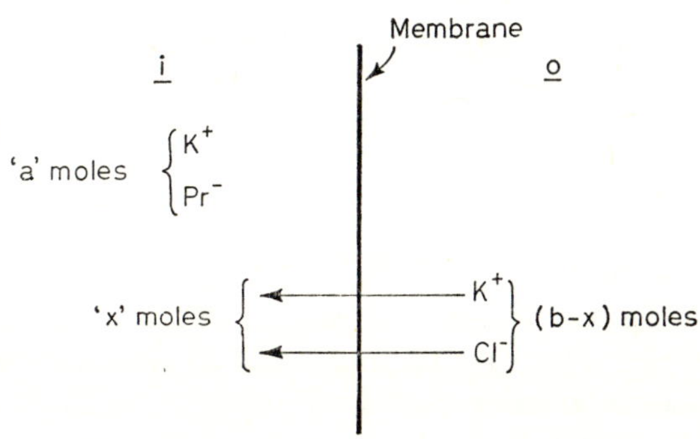


2.6 Gibbs-Donnan equilibrium: final state.

Now what is the value of '*x*' in this formulation? In other words how much KCl traverses the membrane before a condition of dynamic equilibrium is attained? In order to answer this question we have to consider what is meant by 'dynamic equilibrium' in the context of Fig. 2.6.

It is not difficult to see that an overall movement of diffusible ions will continue until the number of ions approaching the membrane from the outside is exactly balanced by the number approaching from the inside in any given time. Until, in other words, the electrochemical potentials of the diffusible ions within and without are identical. This condition, it will be remembered, is expressed for a single ion by equation 2.6. When this condition obtains, although the flux of diffusible ions across the membrane will continue in both directions, no further large-scale, overall, drift will occur. In other words the diffusible ions will be in dynamic equilibrium.

In the physico-chemical situation depicted in Fig. 2.6 there are two sets of diffusible ions. The condition for equilibrium is thus given by the following equation:

$$\mu_K^i \times \mu_{Cl}^i = \mu_K^o \times \mu_{Cl}^o \qquad \ldots\ldots (2.10)$$

In biological systems we may, to a first approximation, substitute concentrations for chemical potentials. When this is done we have:

$$(a + x) \times (x) = (b - x) \times (b - x) \qquad \ldots\ldots (2.11)$$

One thing is immediately obvious in equation 2.11. It is that as '*x*' is by definition a positive integer (a + x) is necessarily greater than (x). In other words,[1]

$$[K^+]_i > [Cl^-]_i \qquad \ldots\ldots (2.12)$$

A little thought will also show that if 2.11 is valid then it follows that,

$$(a + x) > (b - x) \text{ and } (x) < (b - x) \qquad \ldots\ldots (2.13)$$

In other words,

$$[K^+]_i > [K^+]_o, \text{ and } [Cl^-]_i < [Cl^-]_o$$

Thus we see that the existence of an indiffusible ion on one side of a membrane affects the distribution of all the diffusible ions. If the quantities of diffusible ions are substituted in the Nernst equation it is clear that we shall obtain a value for *V*, the electrical potential across the membrane:

$$V = \frac{RT}{F} \ln \frac{[K]_o}{[K]_i} = \frac{RT}{-F} \ln \frac{[Cl]_o}{[Cl]_i} \qquad \ldots\ldots (2.14)$$

[1] The concentration in moles, or gm. ions, of a substance is symbolized by writing the formula of that substance within square brackets.

In general, of course, the ionic situation in biological tissues is far more complicated than that depicted in Fig. 2.5 or 2.6. Quite a number of different diffusible and indiffusible ions are present. Although, as we shall see, the Nernst equation gives a good approximation to the observed value of $V$, for more accurate work a more complex formulation is necessary. This more complicated expression is due to Goldman and is in consequence termed the Goldman equation. For our purposes, however, the Nernst equation will prove adequate.

### 2.9 A liquid state computer

In this chapter and in Chapter 1 an attempt has been made to lay a physico-chemical foundation for a study of the brain's machinery. It is already clear that considerations of the movement of ions in a watery medium are a far cry from the computer engineer's concern with the movements of electrons in metallic conductors and semiconductors. In the same way it will become clear as we proceed that the structure and workings of the living brain are in many ways radically different from those of electronic computers. As different, in effect, as a team of six horses is from a six horse-power engine.

CHAPTER THREE

# Proteins, Nucleic Acids, and Biomembranes

## 3.1 Components of the living cell

So far in our discussion we have focused on some essential aspects of the inorganic world. We have seen that this world is pervaded by an incessant submicroscopic movement. Only at absolute zero ($-273°$ C) does this frenetic dance cease. We have already noticed (p. 38) that this fact had impressed the thinkers of classical antiquity; indeed they drew from it the conclusion that the whole world was alive. Today we recognize that the dance of the motes in a shaft of sunlight is due to minute air currents and other microscopic causes. Nevertheless we would be inclined to agree with their main thesis: there is no gulf fixed between animate and inanimate creation. The great discoveries of modern biology leave no doubt that the 'living' has evolved from the 'non-living'. A continuous chain of forms connects an organism as complex as man with a crystal as simple as that of common salt. Where the line is drawn between animate and inanimate, between organic and inorganic, is entirely arbitrary. This must give us furiously to think of the mind's place in nature.

For practical purposes, however, it is, of course, usual to distinguish the quick from the dead: the living from the non-living. Usually, too, this arbitrary line is drawn at the level of the cell. This may be conveniently defined as the simplest entity capable of independent life. This independence is founded upon an ability to reproduce its own kind in isolation. In other words cells, by definition, possess a genetic apparatus consisting of nucleic acids and proteinaceous enzymes. Partly in order to prevent the components of this vital apparatus diffusing away into the surrounding environment cells are bounded by a distinct membrane. This boundary membrane also has the vitally important task of regulating the ingress and egress of materials. In nerve cells, as we have already hinted, the membrane has other, vastly important, properties.

In this chapter we shall glance briefly at these quintessential components of living cells. The nervous system, like all other parts of the human body, is composed of cells. In later chapters we shall see how the cell components described below play important roles in the functioning of the brain.

### 3.2 Proteins and nucleic acids

The central characteristic of a living organism is its ability to reproduce itself. Given this property, and assuming that the reproduction is not always exact, it is possible to see how the vast congeries of organic forms at present populating the planet could have evolved. No forces other than those recognized by physics and chemistry need be invoked. In the fullness of time Darwinian natural selection has achieved the human brain.

As is nowadays well known, biologists have shown, in the last decade, that this all-important self-replicative ability depends on the interaction of proteins and nucleic acids. The explosive development of the subject known as molecular biology has revolutionized thinking in genetics and sent shock waves through the whole of biomedical science. These shock waves have reached the field of neurobiology and have strongly influenced thinking on, for example, the physical basis of memory.

Electronic computers have been disparaged as 'information crunchers'; the same epithet might be applied to the living brain. For it operates on the information communicated to it from the sense organs so that the animal behaves in some appropriate fashion. It is thus very interesting and suggestive to find that one of the central concerns in the science of molecular biology is also a concern with information. In this case the information is not, of course, derived from sense organs but is obtained by the trial and error methods of natural selection working on a genetic system. Molecular biologists have shown that the information obtained in this way is stored in 'informational macromolecules'.

Informational macromolecules are heteropolymers. In other words the units, or monomers, of which the polymer is composed are not all the same. Two principal types of heteropolymer are developed by living organisms: nucleic acids and proteins. Nucleic acids are built of monomers called nucleotides whilst the monomers of which proteins are built are amino-acids. Two types of nucleic acid are distinguished: DNA in the nucleus and RNA in the cytoplasm. Four different nucleotides can be detected in DNA. They differ only in the nature of their basic groups which may be either adenine (A), or cytosine (C), or guanine (G), or thymine (T). RNA is similarly composed of a long chain of nucleotides which, again, are in general of four different types depending on their base: adenine (A), guanine (G), uracil (U) and thymine (T). Proteins, on the other hand, have a rather more complicated structure being composed of twenty different types of amino-acid.

One of the basic insights achieved by molecular biologists is that the hereditary information is inscribed on these biological heteropolymers as unique and specific sequences of their monomeric units. In an analogous way information is stored in written languages as sequences of letters, spaces and punctuation marks.

Another basic insight is that it is possible to translate from one macromolecular language into the other. So far as is at present known this translation is in one direction only. Cells can translate the information stored in the nucleotide sequences of their nucleic acids into the amino-acid sequences of proteins but not vice versa.

A third fundamental tenet of molecular biology is that the amino-acid sequences of a protein determine its often complicated three-dimensional shape. This configuration, in turn, determines the biological activity of the protein. As all enzymes are proteins it will be appreciated that this biological activity is often of very great importance.

The means whereby genetic information stored in the nucleotide sequence of the cell's nucleic acid is translated into the amino-acid sequences of the cell's proteins has been the object of much brilliant research. The outcome of this work may be summarized in a phrase which has been called the 'central dogma' of molecular biology: 'DNA makes RNA and RNA makes protein.'

Let us examine in a little more detail what is meant by this phrase. First let us note that there is nowadays much evidence to show that the hereditary information is stored in DNA in the form of a triplet code. This means that triplets of nucleotides specify particular amino-acids. GCU, for example, specifies alanine; UAC specifies tyrosine. Now this information is, as we have stressed, built into the structure of DNA and this molecule is, in higher cells, largely restricted to the nucleus. Yet proteins are synthesized in the cytoplasm, often at some distance from the nucleus. Thus some means of transmitting the genetic information across the cell is necessary.

This is where RNA comes in. We have seen that the 'central dogma' states that DNA makes RNA. In fact a special type of RNA —messenger-RNA (mRNA)—is synthesized alongside the nuclear DNA and carries its imprint to the sites of protein synthesis in the cytoplasm. These synthetic sites take the form of small granules known as ribosomes. In metazoan cells ribosomes are often found to be attached to membranes of the endoplasmic reticulum. This is especially the case in cells which are very active in protein synthesis. It is interesting to note that amongst these cells are numbered many nerve cells (p. 182).

The arrival of mRNA at a ribosome is not, however, the end of the story. At this point another type of RNA plays a vital rôle. This is transfer-RNA (tRNA). There are at least twenty different types of tRNA molecule: at least one specific to each type of amino-acid. It is found that amino-acids in the cytoplasm become attached to the appropriate tRNA molecule. It is also found that at the other end of the tRNA molecule is a triplet of nucleotides. This triplet of nucleotides is designed to fit one, and only one, nucleotide triplet in the mRNA molecule.

Thus we begin to see how the translation from one molecular language to the other is accomplished. Fig. 3.1 shows that tRNA molecules align themselves on the mRNA tape in accordance with the imprint carried out from the DNA master copy. The amino-acids attached to the other ends of the tRNA molecules are, in consequence, also aligned in a specific sequence. A sequence, moreover, determined by the nucleotide sequence of the DNA molecule.

Fig. 3.1 (b) shows that the ribosome can accommodate two tRNA molecules. *Which* two molecules are accommodated is, of course, determined by the mRNA template. Once the two tRNAs are in position the attached amino-acids can link together. When this occurs the left-hand tRNA molecule becomes detached and falls away from the ribosome to recycle. The ribosome then moves one mRNA triplet to the right. This implies that the right-hand tRNA-amino-acid complex moves across to the left-hand side of the ribosome. This frees the right-hand side for another tRNA-amino-acid complex. When this arrives the sequence of events is repeated. In this

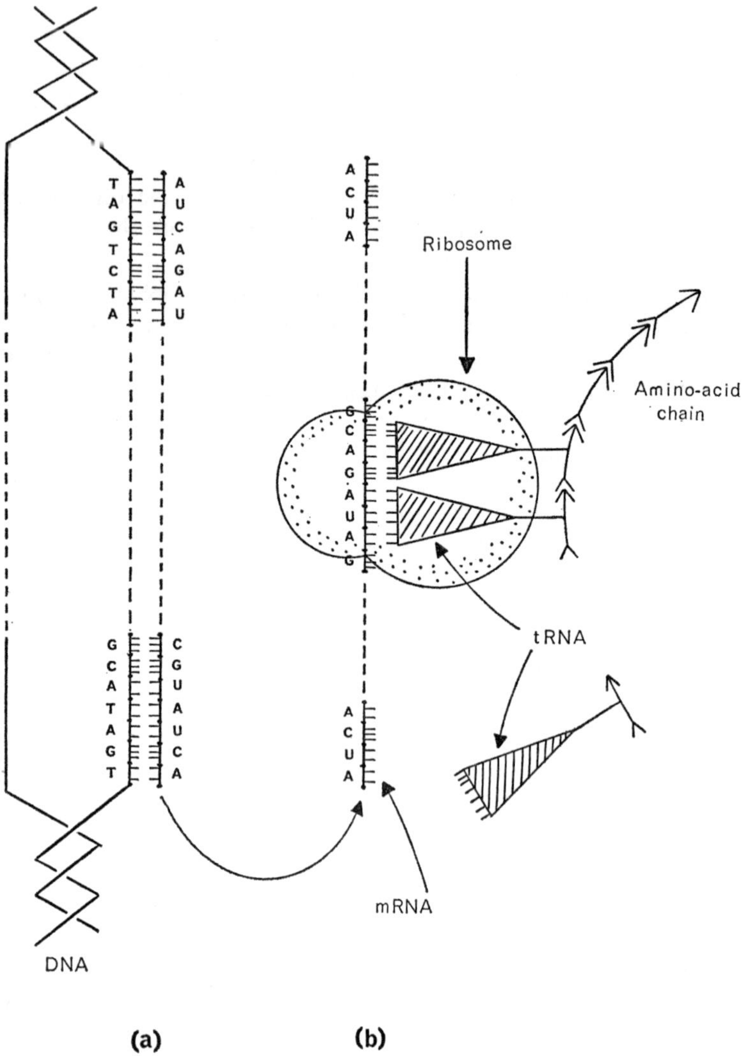


3.1 Schematic diagram to show the essential aspects of protein synthesis. In (a) an mRNA chain is shown being synthesized alongside a DNA template. When the synthesis is complete the mRNA drops away and passes to the ribosomes (b). Here it acts as a 'master tape' determining the sequence of amino-acids in the protein being synthesized. The 'left-hand' tRNA site referred to in the text is drawn at the top in the diagram.

way a long chain of amino-acids joined in a specific order begins to grow from the 'top' of the ribosome. When the amino-acid chain is complete a special triplet on the mRNA tape causes it to drop away from the ribosome. Thermodynamic forces are then believed to ensure that the amino-acid chain assumes a particular three-dimensional conformation.

### 3.3 Switching genes on and off

There is much evidence to show that the DNA complement of all the cells of an organism, even highly specialized cells, still possesses all the information required to specify the form and function of the entire organism. This is a very striking fact. It means that the DNA complement of cells as specialized as neurons still carries all the information necessary to programme the production of, say, insulin, haemoglobin and pepsin, or to specify the characteristic morphology of a kidney, liver or intestinal cell. It must also mean that this programming potential is normally 'switched off'. The study of the means whereby genes are 'switched' on and off forms one of the most fascinating chapters of molecular biology. It is quite possible, moreover, that this topic is of considerable relevance to neurobiology.

First let us specify what we mean by the term 'gene'. In most cases we can say that a gene is a section of the cell's DNA responsible for programming the production of a single polypeptide or protein. We shall see below that some genes—operator genes—escape this definition. These genes initiate the activity of other genes.

Modern understanding of the mechanisms responsible for switching genes on and off is summarized in Fig. 3.2.

The figure shows a length of DNA consisting of three genes. The structural gene (S) is able to programme the cell's ribosomes, via $mRNA_2$, to synthesize an enzymatic or structural protein, P. This programming activity, that is the synthesis of an mRNA strand alongside the structural gene, is initiated by the operator gene (O). However the operator gene's activity is itself controlled by yet another gene—the regulator gene (R). This gene, as Fig. 3.2. shows, is able to programme the synthesis of a largish globular protein, Rp. This protein is specifically designed to inhibit the initiatory activity of the operator gene. In this way the regulator gene keeps this particular structural gene 'switched off'.

However the protein produced at the regulator gene's command is

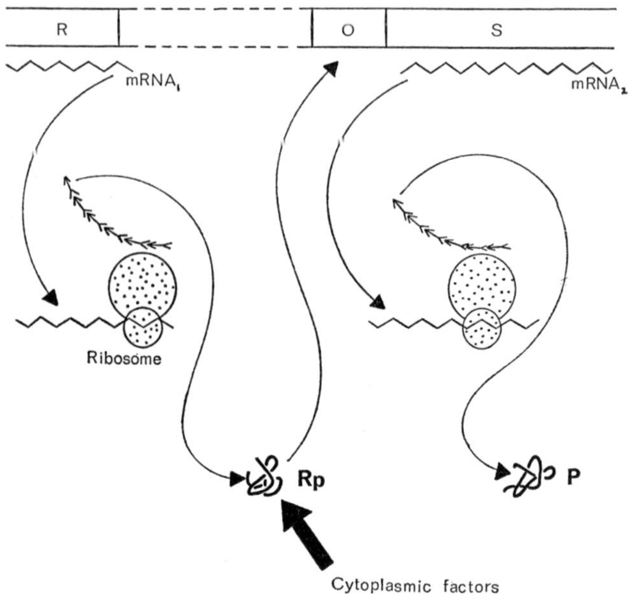


3.2 Control of the expression of a structural gene. R = regulator gene, O = operator gene, S = structural gene, Rp = repressor protein, P = protein whose synthesis is programmed by the structural gene.

exposed to the influence of the cytoplasmic environment. These influences may well alter its three-dimensional configuration so that it can no longer do its job. The structural gene is, in consequence, released from inhibition—technically it is said to be derepressed. It follows, in turn, that its particular protein, P, is manufactured by the ribosomes. Vice versa it is known that in some cases the regulator gene programmes an inactive repressor protein. In this case cytoplasmic influences may affect the inactive repressor converting it into an active form. In consequence the operator gene is inhibited and the structural gene is switched off.

These genetic mechanisms have been largely worked out in bacserial systems. There is however no reason to suppose that they do not also operate in the cells of higher organisms. Indeed there is much suggestive evidence to indicate that they do.[1] From the point of view of neurobiology the most significant feature is that they

[1] For a brief outline of this evidence see *Molecular Biology: a Structural Approach*, Faber and Faber, 1968.

operate through the cell's cytoplasm. It is also significant that the cytoplasmic control appears to be exerted by changing the three-dimensional configuration of a large globular protein. It is well known that the three-dimensional structure of globular proteins is critically dependent on their ionic environment. Now we shall see in the next chapters that the propagation of nerve impulses, one of the central features of the brain's machinery, is based on ionic fluxes. We may *speculate*, it is not yet possible to do more, that these ionic fluxes are sufficient to cause changes in the conformation of repressor proteins in the neuronal cytoplasm. In other words *it may be* that neuronal activity has become linked during animal evolution with the cell's system of genetic switching. This possibility is, as we shall see in Chapter 15, of particular interest in connection with the problem of cerebral memory.

The development of a molecular neurobiology along these lines is, however, still largely a task for the future. The parts played by proteins and nucleic acids in the life of the brain are still hotly debated. There can, however, be no doubt that the machinery of the brain depends very intimately on the properties of nerve cell membranes. Thus our next task must be to look at some of the general characteristics of biological membranes.

### 3.4 Biomembranes

It may never be possible to discover how the first boundary membrane formed. It seems certain, however, that it, like all present-day biological membranes, depended primarily on the physico-chemical properties of certain lipid molecules.

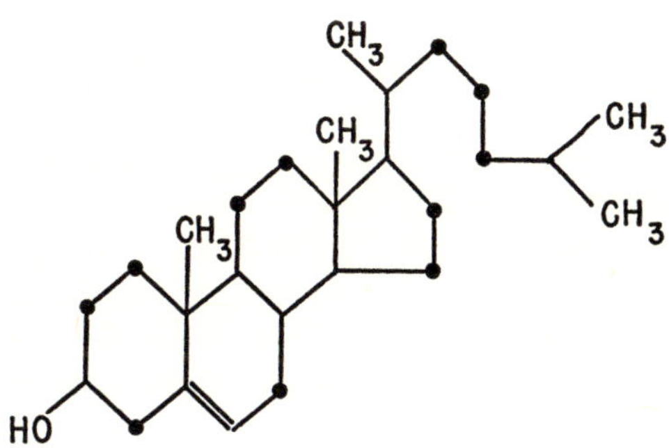


3.3 Structural formula of cholesterol. $CH_2$ groups are represented by dots.

Lipids are a heterogeneous group of molecules which hold little in common except a very marked insolubility in water. Two principal types of lipid are of importance in the architecture of biological membranes: sterols and phospholipids. The most important sterol is cholesterol whose structural formula is shown in Fig. 3.3.

Several different types of phospholipid play an important part in the structure of biological membranes. In general they have the structure shown in Fig. 3.4.

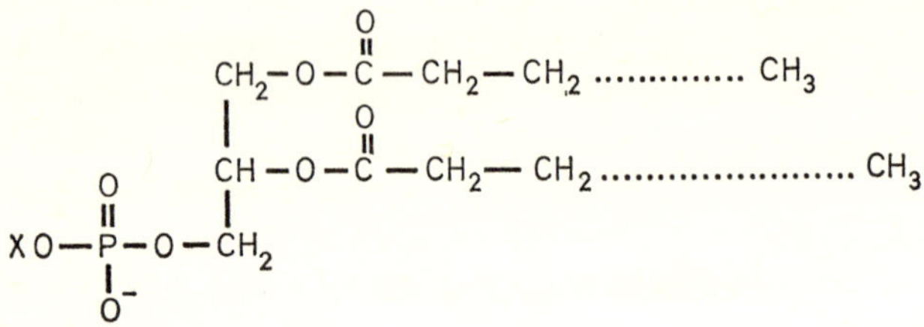


3.4 General formula of a phospholipid. See text for further explanation.

The molecule shown in Fig. 3.4 consists of two rather different parts. On the right-hand side of the figure are two long hydrocarbon chains. There may be more than twenty carbon atoms in these chains. Because the atoms constituting the hydrocarbon chains are joined together by covalent bonds, and because there are no hydrogen-bonding possibilities, this part of the molecule is completely insoluble in water. In this respect phospholipids are typical lipids. On the left-hand side of the figure, however, there is a phosphate group and a variable group symbolized by 'X'. Both these groups are ionizable and hence in aqueous solution bear electrostatic charges. It follows from our discussion in Chapter 2 that this end of the molecule *is* soluble in water. Thus phospholipids have dual solubility characteristics. One end of the molecule, the hydrocarbon chain end, is completely insoluble in water; the other end, the phosphate end, is completely soluble. This feature is, as we shall see, of fundamental importance in the design of biological membranes.

Before going any further let us pause to consider briefly the nature of the variable group 'X'. Table 3.1 shows that this group may vary from a simple hydrogen atom to the quite complicated nitrogen-containing groups of ethanolamine, serine and choline. All these groups are to a greater or lesser extent electrostatically charged and hence are able to insert themselves into an aqueous phase.

TABLE 3.1

Phospholipids

| *Name* | *X* (the variable group) |
|---|---|
| Phosphatidic acid | $-H$ |
| Phosphatidyl choline (lecithin) | $-CH_2-CH_2-\overset{+}{N}(CH_3)_3$ |
| Phosphatidyl ethanolamine (cephalin) | $-CH_2-CH_2-\overset{+}{N}H_3$ |
| Phosphatidyl serine | $-CH_2-CH(\overset{+}{N}H_3)-COO^-$ |

Now let us see how the solubility properties of phospholipid molecules cause certain types of multimolecular organization. It is clear from our discussion above that phospholipid molecules are bound to orientate themselves at air/water or oil/water interfaces in a regular manner. The hydrophilic (water-loving) ends of the molecules will insert themselves into the water whilst the hydrophobic (water-hating) hydrocarbon ends will project into the air or oil. Such sheets of phospholipid molecules are called monomolecular layers, or, alternatively, monolayers.

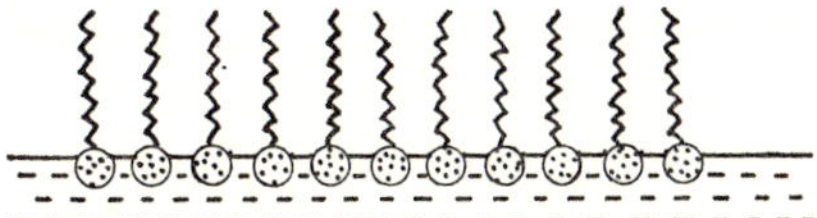

3.5 Monomolecular layer of phospholipid molecules. The charged ends of the molecules are represented by stippled circles and the hydrophobic hydrocarbon chains by zigzag lines. From *Molecular Biology*, Faber and Faber, 1968.

Another form of multimolecular organization readily assumed by phospholipid molecules is the micelle or droplet. Phospholipid micelles automatically form in the bulk of an aqueous or oil phase. The physico-chemical basis of this formation is shown in Fig. 3.6. In an aqueous phase phospholipids form minute spheres with their hydrophilic ends facing outwards and their hydrophobic tails inwards. Vice versa in an organic phase such as, for example, olive oil phospholipid micelles are formed with their hydrophilic ends tucked in towards the centre and their hydrophobic hydrocarbon chains projecting outwards.

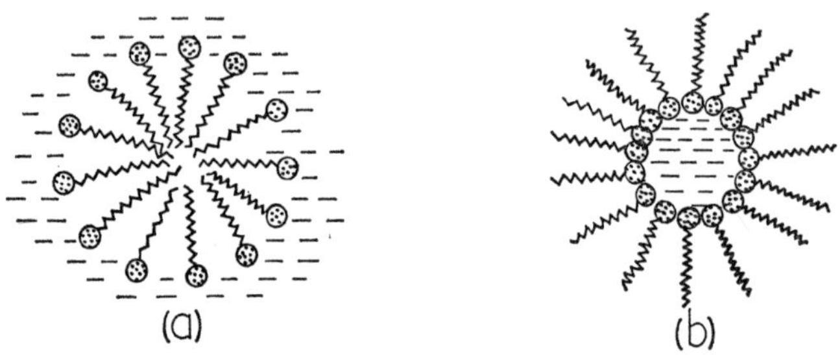


3.6 Phospholipid micelles. Phospholipids form micelles of two main types depending on the nature of the surrounding phase. If the phase is an aqueous solution then the hydrophilic ends of the phospholipids face outward, (a). If, on the other hand, the surrounding phase is non-polar, like benzene, then the hydrophobic tails face outward, (b). Note that in most biological situations non-polar phases are contaminated with at least small quantities of water. It is this water which is drawn at the centre of the micelle (b).

Now neither of the types of multimolecular organization schematized in Figs. 3.5 and 3.6 could on its own act as a biological membrane. The monolayer shown in Fig. 3.5 cannot, by definition, separate two aqueous phases from each other. Yet this, of course, is the function of cellular membranes. The extracellular and intracellular phases are invariably aqueous solutions. However it is not difficult to imagine how phospholipids might form such a membrane.

All we have to suppose is that the phospholipids instead of forming a monolayer organize themselves into a bilayer. If the bilayer is formed with the hydrophilic heads of the phospholipid facing outwards (Fig. 3.7) the membrane could well separate two aqueous phases.

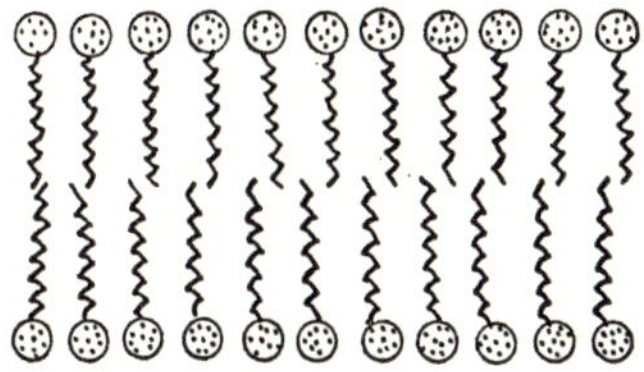

3.7. A bimolecular layer (bilayer) of phospholipid molecules.

We have arrived at the organization depicted in Fig. 3.7 merely by a consideration of the solubility characteristics of phospholipid molecules. However it is not difficult to establish the reality of this structure. Artificial, or model, bilayers can be formed by painting a solution of phospholipids across a small hole in a perspex partition separating two aqueous solutions (Fig. 3.8). The solvent in which the lipids are dissolved quickly disperses into the aqueous solution and leaves some of the phospholipids aggregated together over the hole where they form a very thin membrane (Fig. 3.8 (b) ). It is possible to show by an optical technique that this membrane is only two phospholipid molecules thick.

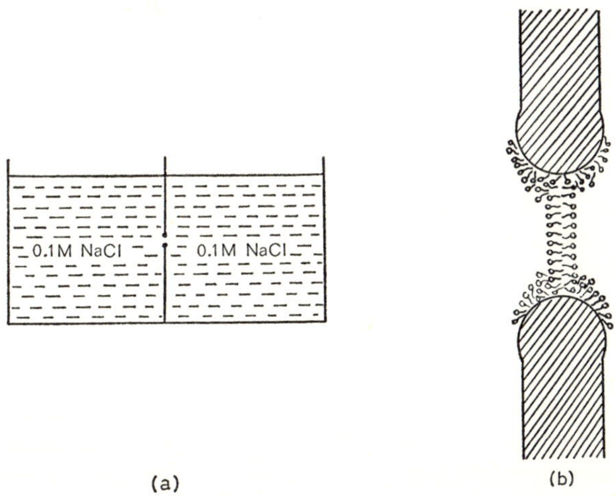


3.8 Formation of an artificial phospholipid bilayer. A solution of phospholipids is painted across the aperture shown in (a); after the solvent has diffused away into the NaCl solution a bilayer of phospholipids is left across the aperture, shown enlarged in (b). After Mueller, P., Rudin, D. O., Ti Tien, H. and Wescott, W. C. (1963), 'Methods for the formation of single bimolecular lipid membranes in aqueous solution', *J. Phys. Chem.*, *67*, 534–535.

The fact that phospholipids can form bilayer membranes separating two aqueous phases does not, of course, prove that they also have this function in the living cell. However there is much evidence today to show that the cores of biological membranes do indeed have this structure.

It has long been known that biomembranes contain large amounts of protein. Indeed the majority of biological membranes are constituted of roughly equal amounts of protein and lipid. In addition smaller quantities of carbohydrate are believed to be present. These non-lipid molecules are believed to be attached to both surfaces of the phospholipid bilayer. This concept of the architecture of biological membranes is schematized in Fig. 3.9.

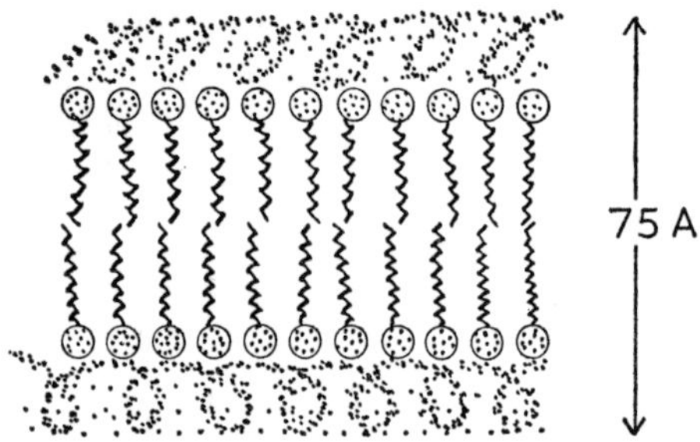


3.9 The classical concept of the molecular architecture of biological membranes. Cholesterol, which is present in some membranes, has been omitted. The stippled spirals represent protein. From *Molecular Biology*, Faber and Faber, 1968.

This idea of membrane structure is borne out by electron microscopy. In fact the image of a biological membrane varies somewhat with different methods of specimen preparation. In most cases a trilaminate or 'sandwich' type of structure can be seen. It is believed that the electron stain, osmium tetroxide for example, becomes attached to the charged ends of the phospholipid molecules and, perhaps, to the amino-acid side chains of the protein. In contrast the hydrocarbon chains of the phospholipids do not take up any stain and are thus responsible for the translucent layer in the centre of the membrane. This trilaminate membrane structure can be seen in several of the plates in this book—for example, Plates II (b) and VI.

Other electron microscopists, using different methods of specimen preparation, have presented evidence for the existence of a micellar structure in some biological membranes. Instead of being extended in a more or less continuous two-dimensional sheet the phospholipids are believed by these workers to form a large number of minute globules or micelles. We saw in Fig. 3.6 that this is another possibility for the multimolecular organization of phospholipids. Fig. 3.10 depicts the type of architecture a micellar membrane might have.

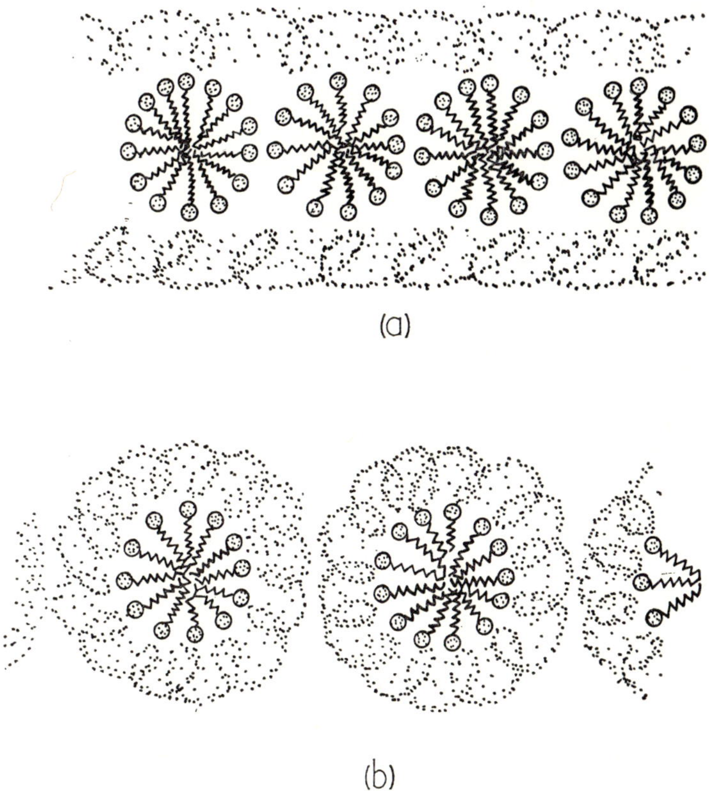


3.10 Two possible designs for a micellar membrane. From *Molecular Biology*, Faber and Faber, 1968.

It is probable that the structure of most biological membranes is highly labile. It follows that it is not improbable that the same membrane may at some periods assume the form of a bimolecular sheet and at others the form of a micellar array.

An alternative structure, halfway between the bimolecular sheet and micellar type membranes, has been proposed by some investigators. These workers suggest that the lipid bilayer we have described may act as a scaffolding to which are affixed arrays of globular proteins. Now globular proteins have many biological activities. All enzymes, for instance, are globular proteins, antibodies are globular proteins, etc. If membranes are indeed arrays of globular proteins then they are likely to have many functions in addition to acting as the structural scaffolding of cells. In the case of the nervous system such a concept of membranous architecture would go far towards explaining the extraordinary chemoaffinities between neurons which we discuss in Chapter 11. Moreover, if these two-dimensional macromolecular arrays can be adapted to act as memory stores we can also begin to see an explanation for their vast proliferation in central nervous systems. Fernandez-Moran has pointed out[1] that if all the membranes intricately folded within the human skull were flattened out they would cover the surface of the entire planet.

[1] Fernandez-Moran, F., 'Membrane Structure in Nerve Cells', p. 299, in *The Neurosciences, A Survey for Synthesis*, Rockefeller University Press, New York, 1968.

## CHAPTER FOUR

# Cells of the Nervous System

### 4.1 The nervous system consists of cells

There are good reasons for believing that the 'unit of life' is the cell. Certainly the bodies of the larger animals and plants are subdivided into cells. It is easy to see that this is the case if the skin, the gut or the blood is examined under the microscope. But it is not so easy to see that this is the case with the central nervous system.

Perhaps this is not altogether surprising. The tissue of the central nervous system is enormously complex. Until the early years of this century many reputable investigators preferred to regard this organ as a great syncytial mass lacking sharp subdivision and delimitation into separate cells. Although this concept has lingered on it is nowadays very much a minority view. The great majority of workers nowadays believe the central nervous system to be built of cells in the same way as other parts of the body. These cells are of two major types. First are the nerve cells, or neurons. These carry out all the characteristic activities of the nervous system: the conduction of nerve messages, the processing of sensory information, the computation and signalling of appropriate behavioural responses, etc. Second are the neuroglial, or glial, cells. These cells, although they greatly outnumber neurons in vertebrate nervous systems, are believed to play a much more passive rôle. They are believed to give structural support to nerve cells, and perhaps to have some part in their nutrition.

### 4.2 The morphologies of neurons

'When the animal body reaches some degree of multicellular complexity, special cells assume the express office of connecting together other cells. Such cells, since their function is to stretch from one cell to another, are usually elongated; they form protoplasmic threads and they interconnect by conducting nervous impulses'.[1]

[1] Sherrington, C. S. (1906), *The Integrative Activity of the Nervous System*, Cambridge, p. 5.

Thus Sir Charles Sherrington introduces the nerve cell. Neurons, unlike other cells, are characterized by one or more lengthy processes. These run out from a metabolically very active cell body (= cyton, perikaryon). Along these processes messages are transmitted. We shall see in Chapter 5 that the messages are transmitted in the form of action potentials. It is found that action potentials proceed, normally, in only one direction along the nerve cell process. This direction is called the *orthodromic* direction. It is possible in certain experiments to induce action potentials to travel in the opposite direction to normal. This direction is called the *antidromic* direction.

Many different types of neuron have been distinguished in animal central nervous systems. Some of these will be mentioned in later chapters. These different kinds of neuron may be classified in various ways. One important classification is based on shape—morphology. Fig. 4.1 shows some of the more important general types of morphology that vertebrate neurons and neurosensory cells may assume.

The figure shows that in all cases certain physiological specializations can be detected. One pole of the cell—the dendritic or receptor zone—is sensitive to extracellular influences of various kinds. The opposite pole is capable of secreting minute amounts of chemical substance. Between these two poles lie the axon and the nerve cell body. The axon is a very specialized process able to conduct action potentials rapidly and without decrement. Its characteristics will be discussed in some detail in Chapter 5.

On the left-hand side of Fig. 4.1 a neurosensory cell is depicted. This is probably the most primitive type of conductile cell. It is, for example, developed in the most lowly of metazoan phyla—the Coelenterata. In the simple body of *Hydra*, for instance, neurosensory cells responding to some environmental stimulus—mechanical pressure, perhaps, or chemical substances—signal directly to the appropriate effector organ. Neurosensory cells, however, are certainly not confined to the most primitive of animal phyla. They are developed in all species of animal up to and including man. In mammals neurosensory cells are to be found in the nasal mucosa and in many internal organs and muscles. They will be discussed more fully in Chapter 7.

It is easy to see that, in a sense, all nerve cells are highly specialized neurosensory cells. For all neurons must be able to transduce stimuli occurring at their dendritic zones into action potentials along their

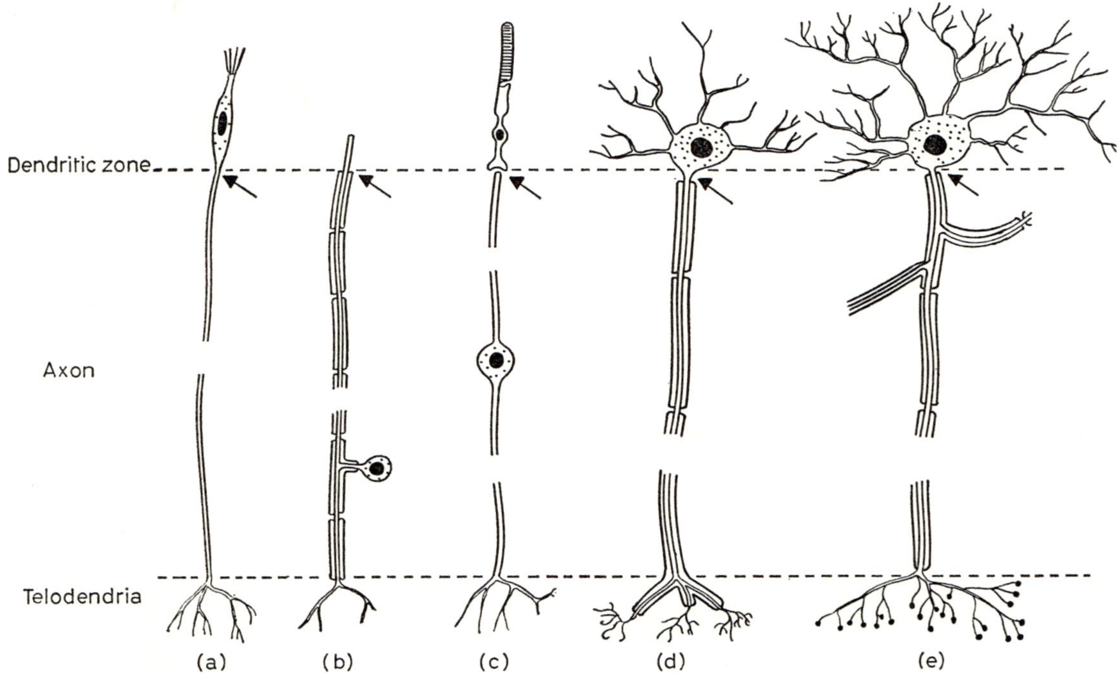


4.1 Morphologies of some vertebrate neurons and neurosensory cells. (a) Olfactory neurosensory cell, (b) somaesthetic neurosensory cell, (c) bipolar neuron, (d) multipolar motor neuron, (e) interneuron. For further explanation see text. After Bodian, D. (1962), 'The generalised vertebrate neuron', *Science*, *137*, 323–326.

axons. In nearly all cases these stimuli are of a chemical nature. Thus we might regard neurons as highly specialized chemosensitive neurosensory cells.

Another type of neurosensory cell is shown in Fig. 4.1 (b). This type of cell is developed in many vertebrates including the mammals. It is stimulated by temperature change or mechanical distortion of its dendritic zone. The axon carries information concerning these variables into the central nervous system. It will be noticed that the perikaryon of this type of neurosensory cell is no longer adjacent to the dendritic zone. In fact the perikarya of these cells are housed in ganglia adjoining the spinal cord. It will also be noticed that the cell is so organized that only one process springs from the perikaryon. In consequence this type of cell is said to be unipolar.

The cell shown in Fig. 4.1 (c) is a 'genuine' neuron, not a neurosensory cell. Because it has two processes emerging from its perikaryon it is called a bipolar cell. Neurons of this type are to be found, for example, in the retina of the eye (section 8.4). In this position they are associated with specialized photoreceptor cells—the rods and cones—which, when they are illuminated, secrete a small quantity of a transmitter substance on to the neuron's dendritic zone. This initiates an action potential in the bipolar cell's axon. More will be said of the biophysics of this initiation in Chapter 6.

The action potential is not believed to be initiated in the dendritic zone itself. Instead it is thought that an adequate stimulation of the dendritic zone leads to the generation of an action potential at the axon hillock (marked by an arrow in Fig. 4.1). This will be considered in more detail in Chapter 6.

Perhaps the most intensively studied of all neurons is that shown in Fig. 4.1 (d). This is a motor neuron, or motoneuron, of the spinal cord. The figure shows that a large number of processes spring from the perikaryon. In consequence the cell is said to be multipolar. The majority of these processes are short and branched. These are called dendrites. One process is long and, except at its termination, unbranched. This is the axon. The axon runs out from the spinal cord to the body's musculature which it controls.

Finally, in Fig. 4.1 (e), an interneuron is represented. Except that its axon is sometimes branched its morphology is very similar to that of a motor neuron. Interneurons are mostly confined within the central nervous system. Thus whereas the telodendria of motor neurons terminate on an effector organ—a muscle or gland—the

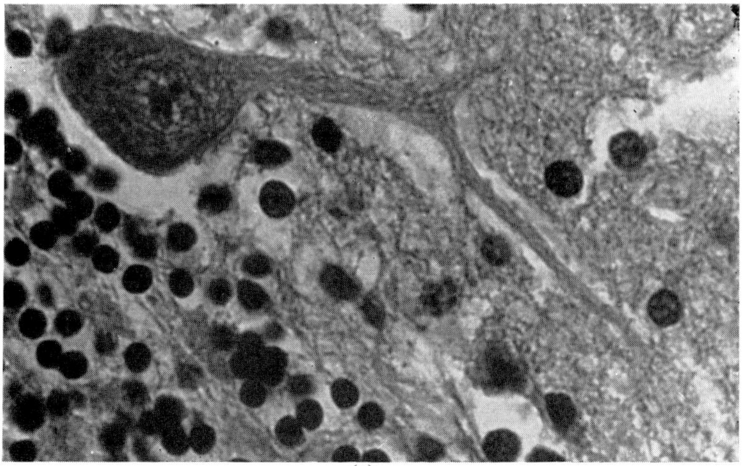

(a)

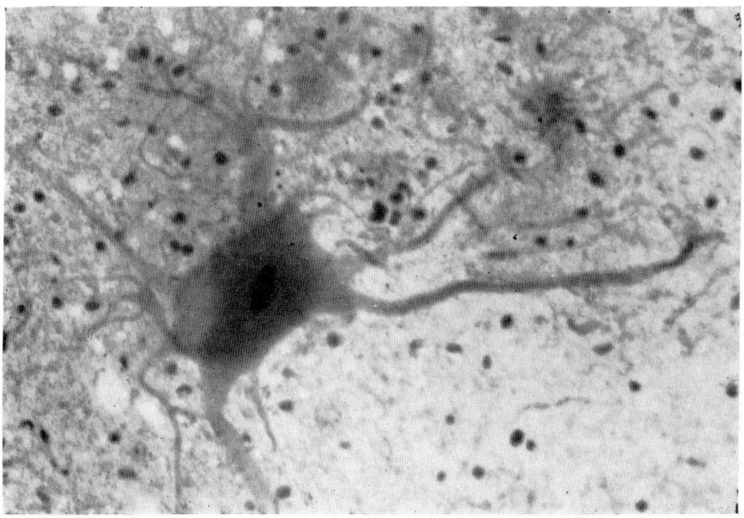

(b)

III Some types of neuron (i)

(a) Purkinje cell of the cerebellum (×480). The small dark spherical objects in this micrograph are granule cells (*see* Chapter 11).

(b) Multipolar motor neuron from the spinal cord (×480). It is not possible in this micrograph to distinguish the axon from the numerous dendrites.

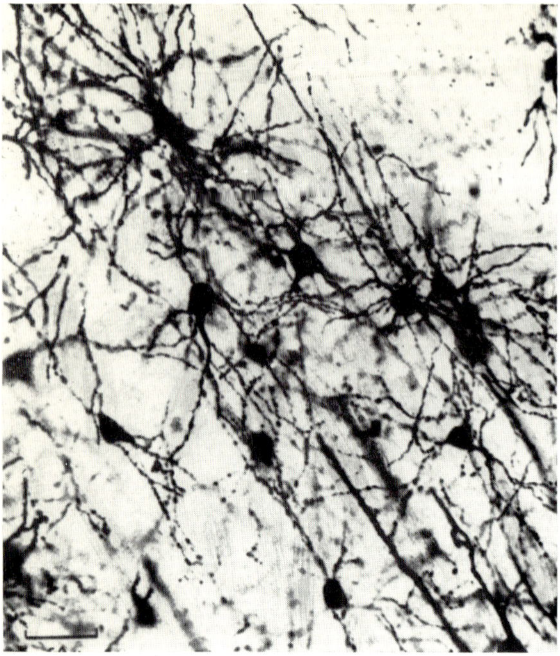

IV Some types of neuron (ii)

(a) Stellate cells in the visual cortex of a cat. The scale marker measures 50μ. (From D. A. Sholl, *The Organisation of th Cerebral Cortex*, Methuen and Co. Ltd (1956).)

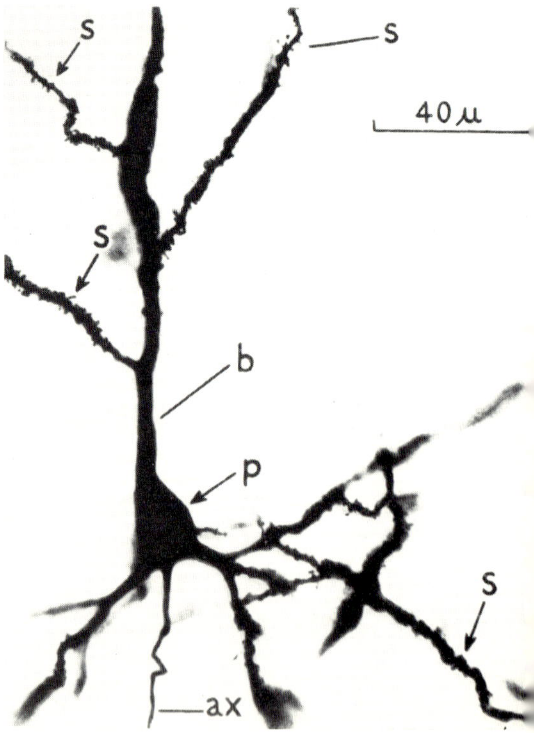


(b) Pyramidal cell of the mammalian cerebral cortex. This plate shows the development of spines (s) on the dendrites. It has been shown that these spines make synaptic contact with the axons of other cells. ax = axon, b = basal region of apical dendrite. (From Whittaker, V. P. and Gray, E. G. (1962), 'The synapse: biology and morphology', *British Medical Bulletin*, **18**, 223–7.)

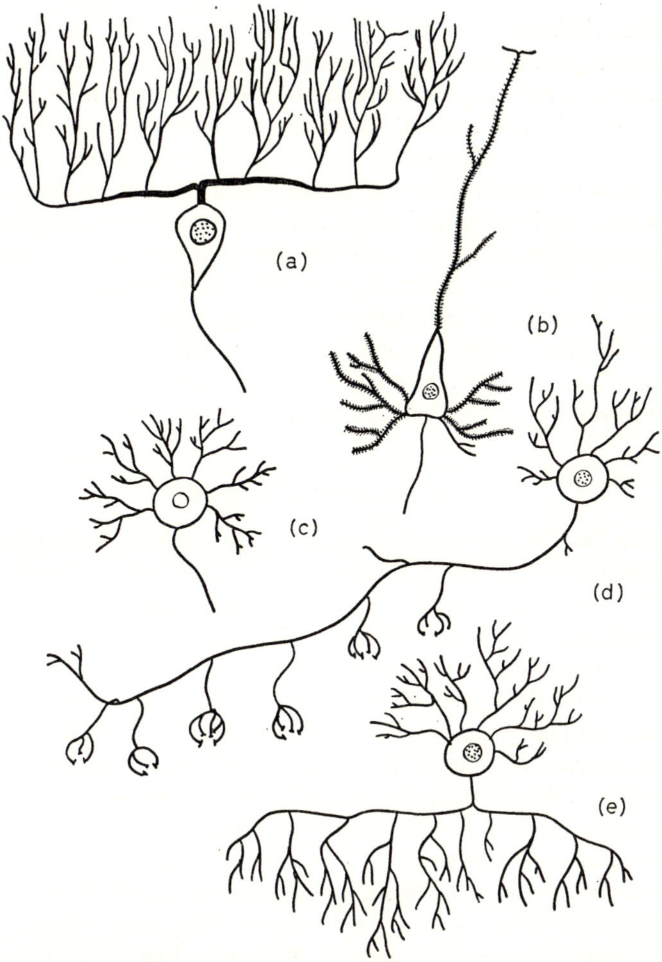


4.2 Some types of interneuron found in vertebrate brains.
(a) Purkinje cell, (b) pyramidal cell, (c) granule cell, (d) basket cell, (e) Golgi cell.

telodendria of interneurons ramify over the dendritic zones of other neurons.

Fig. 4.1 shows that a unified terminology may be applied to widely different types of nerve and neurosensory cell. This generalized terminology is due to Bodian.[1] It ensures that regions of different cells having similar functions are given similar names. Thus the dendritic zone is in all cases responsive to some form of stimulation; the axon hillock is the region where the action potential is initiated; the axon conducts the impulse without decrement; the telodendria, when an impulse arrives, secrete a small quantity of transmitter substance.

Finally the five cells shown in Fig. 4.1 by no means exhaust the known varieties of neuronal morphology. Some neurohistologists have identified nearly a hundred different forms of neuron in the brain. Some of these many forms are shown in Fig. 4.2. In all cases it is possible to apply Bodian's terminology.

### 4.3 The ultrastructure of perikarya

Under the electron microscope the nerve cell body shows all the ultrastructural features of a metabolically highly active cell (Fig. 4.3).

Fig. 4.3 shows that all the usual cellular organelles—lysosomes, endoplasmic reticulum, ribosomes, Golgi apparatus, etc.—are to be found in the perikarya of nerve cells. Optical microscopists had long noticed that the cytoplasm of nerve cell bodies was very granular. These granules were called, after their discoverer, Nissl granules. The electron microscope shows that this Nissl substance in fact consists of large masses of endoplasmic reticulum with attached ribosomes. Now it is well known that a diagnostic feature of the protein-manufacturing cells of metazoa is the presence of a strongly developed, ribosome-studded, endoplasmic reticulum. The presence of Nissl substance is thus good evidence that nerve cells actively manufacture proteins throughout their life. Indeed according to Caspersson[2] the neuron is one of the very few cell types which retains in the adult its embryonic capacity for protein synthesis. This characteristic of nerve cells has, as we shall see in Chapter 15, interesting implications.

Electron microscopy has also thrown light on the nature of the

[1] Bodian, D. (1963), 'The generalised vertebrate neuron', *Science*, *137*, 323.

[2] Caspersson, T. (1947), 'The relations between nucleic acid and protein synthesis', *S.E.B. Symposium*, *1*, 127–151.

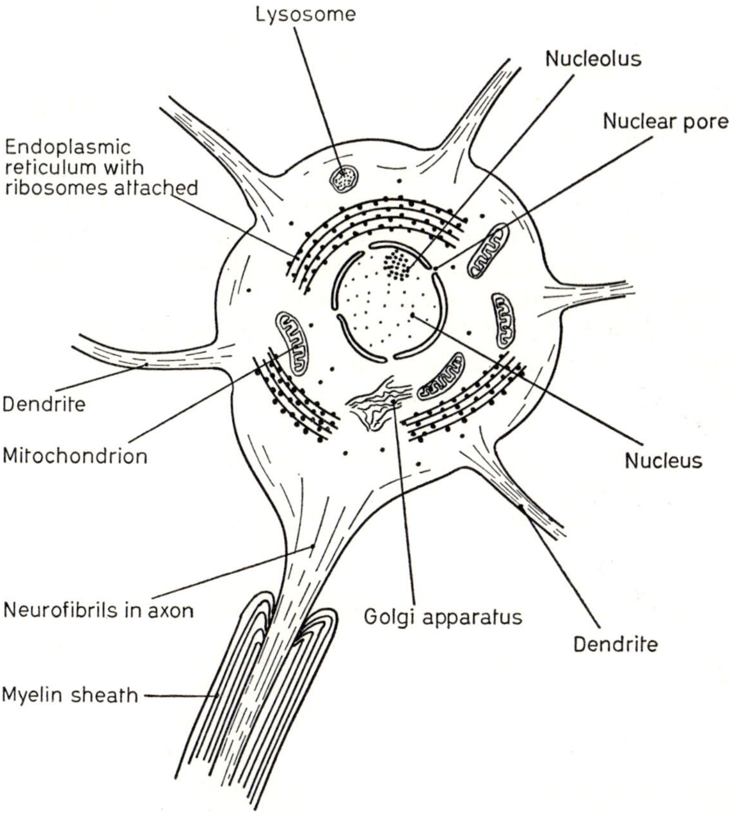


4.3 Ultrastructure of a neuron's perikaryon.

neurofibrils which had also been observed for many years through the optical miscroscope. The staining techniques which had made these fibrils visible to the optical microscopist are nowadays believed to have caused the aggregation of large numbers of submicroscopic filaments and tubules: indeed neurofibrils have never been observed in living neurons. These minute neurofilaments and neurotubules have been revealed by the much greater resolving power of the electron microscope. Neurofilaments are about 100A in diameter and neurotubules about 230A. Both these dimensions are well below the resolving power of the best optical microscopes. It is also nowadays known that tubules similar in dimensions to neurotubules can be observed in the cytoplasms of many other types of cell. The function of these fine proteinaceous threads is at present much debated: some authorities favour a mechanical, strength-giving function; others suggest a contractile activity possibly tied in with cytoplasmic streaming; yet others regard them as minute communication channels connecting the parts of a cell together.[1]

The diagram of a neuron's perikaryon in Fig. 4.3 is a diagram of a very active cell. It is very far from resembling the passive, uniformly reacting components of which electronic computers are built. Indeed, as Bullock points out,[2] neurons are undoubtedly the functional units of the nervous system but they are units in the sociologist's sense rather than in the physicist's sense. Neurons are the units of the nervous system rather as people are the units of society. The reactions of such individualistic units to given stimuli are very difficult to predict.

However, if perikarya are liable to react in manners 'rich and strange', axons are far more dependable. This fact, too, is mirrored, as we shall see in the next section, in their ultrastructure.

## 4.4 The ultrastructure of axons

The axon might be regarded simply as a lengthy tube filled with a viscous fluid—the axoplasm. The walls of the tube are formed of typical lipoprotein unit membranes about 75A thick. The physico-chemical constitution of the axoplasm, which is of paramount importance in the conduction of the nerve impulse, will be set out in Chapter 5. The only ultrastructural features visible in this otherwise homogeneous fluid are neurotubules.

It is frequently found, both in invertebrates and in vertebrates, that the axon is itself wrapped in a lipoprotein sheath. This feature, as we shall see in section 5.9, allows the axon to conduct impulses at a rather more rapid rate than would otherwise be the case. In many instances, especially amongst invertebrates, this fatty sheath is extremely tenuous. In other animals, however, especially amongst vertebrates and certain crustacea, the sheath is very strongly developed. In these latter instances it is called a *myelin sheath.*

The way in which a myelin sheath is formed is interesting. In

[1] There is evidence to show that more neurotubules occur in the dendrites than elsewhere in the nerve cell.

[2] Bullock, T. H. (1959), 'The neuron doctrine and electrophysiology', *Science*, *129*, 997–1002.

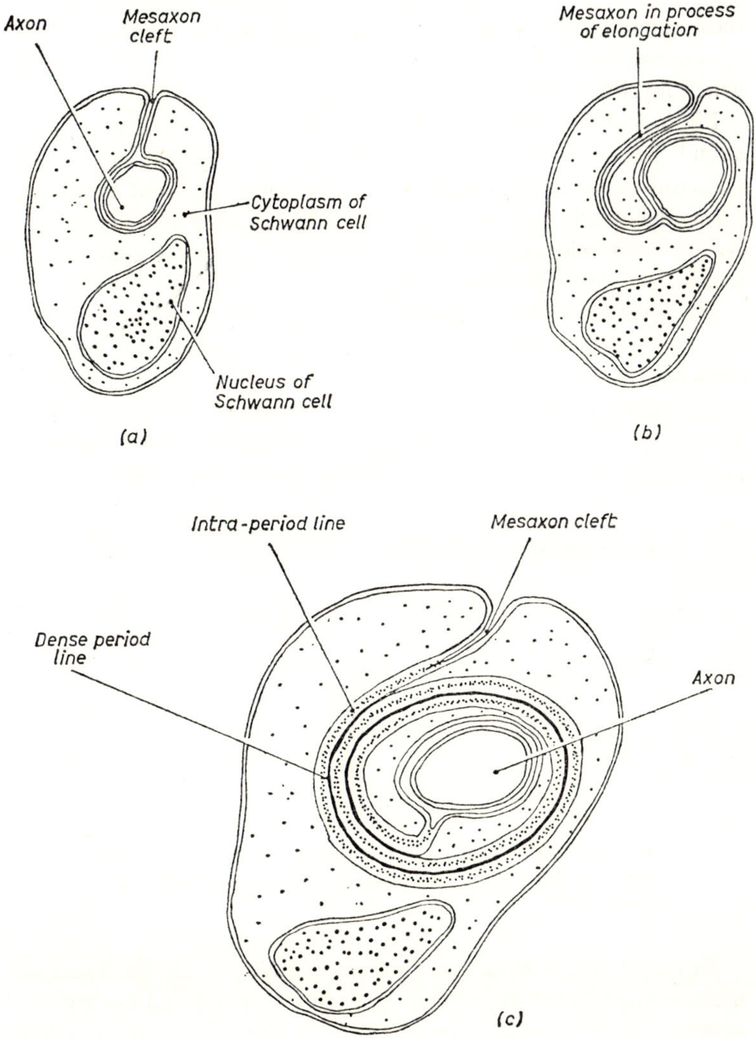


4.4 Myelination. For explanation see text. From *The Architecture of the Body*, Faber and Faber, 1964.

essence it originates by the membrane of a satellite cell wrapping itself round and round an axon. In the case of peripheral nerves these satellite cells are called Schwann cells. In the central nervous system the same job is done by glial cells. Fig. 4.4 shows the way in which myelination occurs around peripheral axons.

Fig. 4.4 shows that the Schwann cell slowly rotates around the axon.[1] The groove leading down to the axon 'gutter'—called the mesaxon cleft—in consequence increases in length and eventually forms the closely packed spiral of membranes shown in Fig. 4.4 (c). An electron micrograph of a vertebrate myelinated axon cut in transverse section is shown in Plate VI(b).

The myelin sheath around the axon of a peripheral nerve is always formed from a number of Schwann cells. It is found that at the junctions between these cells the axon is left bare. These gaps in the otherwise continuous myelin sheath are called nodes of Ranvier (Fig. 4.5). They are, as we shall see in Chapter 5, of considerable importance in speeding the transmission of impulses along nerve fibres.

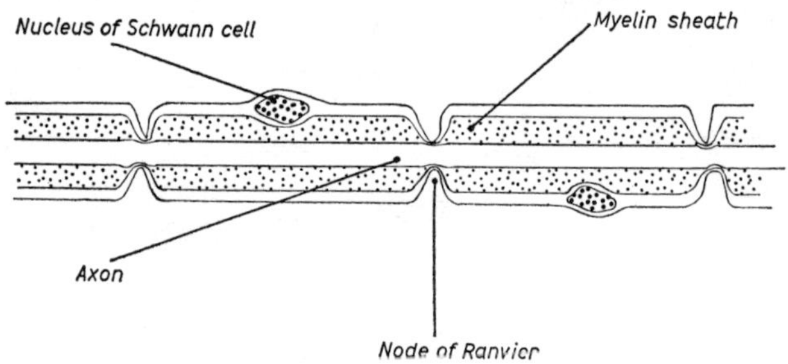


4.5 The myelin sheath is interrupted at intervals by nodes of Ranvier. From *The Architecture of the Body*, Faber and Faber, 1964.

Not all axons, however, are sheathed in layers of myelin. There are many unmyelinated nerve fibres in both vertebrate and invertebrate animals. Nevertheless it is found that even these fibres are associated with satellite Schwann cells. As Fig. 4.6 shows, the mesaxon of the Schwann cell does not become wrapped round the axon to form the tight myelin sheath of a myelinated neuron.

[1] In tissue culture Schwann cells can be shown to complete the circumnavigation of an axon once every 44 hours.

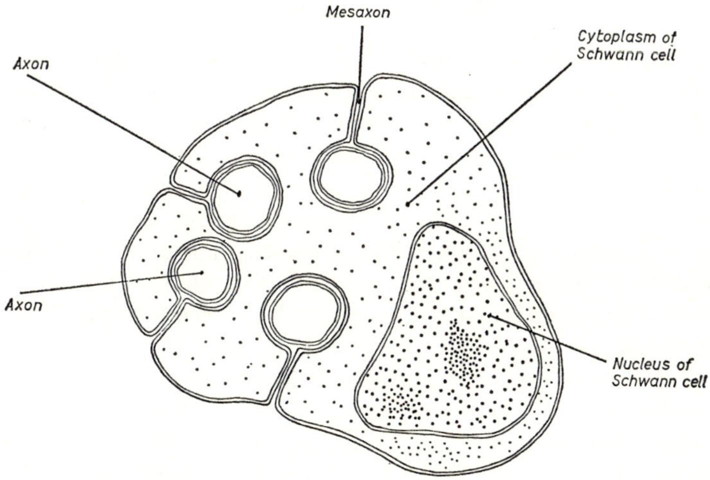


4.6 Transverse section through several unmyelinated axons lying within a single Schwann cell. Compare this with Plate VI(a). From *The Architecture of the Body*, Faber and Faber, 1964.

Returning to the more or less homogeneous axoplasm within the axon, it is very interesting to note that there is good evidence for a flow outwards from the perikaryon to the telodendria.[1] In embryonic chick embryos, for example, it can be shown that granules proceed along the axon at a rate of about 25$\mu$ every 14 seconds. The mechanism(s) producing this movement have been much debated. Many workers favour a peristaltic action: this may be achieved by the Schwann or glial cells, or it may, conceivably, be effected by the abundant neurotubules. Whatever the mechanism the fact that a flow occurs is possibly of considerable physiological significance. We have seen that the perikaryon is a centre of intense biochemical activity. It may well be that the products of this activity are carried in the axoplasmic stream out to the telodendria. Conceivably they influence the structure or the function, perhaps both, of this vital region. We shall return to this concept in Chapter 15 where we discuss that most intriguing of neurological topics: the physical basis of memory. It is logical here, however, to turn next to a consideration of the ultrastructure of this vastly important terminal region.

[1] Weiss, P., Taylor, A. C. and Pillai, P. A. (1962), 'The nerve fibre as a system in continuous flow', *Science*, *136*, 330.

## 4.5 The ultrastructure of synapses

In structure and embryological origin the cells of the central nervous system are more closely related to epithelial than to any other type of cell. It is thus interesting to find that epithelial cells frequently form specialized junctions with each other. Electron microscopists recognize three types of junction: the tight junction, the intermediate junction and the desmosome. All these junctions are believed to confer mechanical strength on epithelial sheets. In spite of this solely mechanical rôle it is suggestive to find that the electron microscope image of a synapse is in many respects rather similar to some of these junctional complexes. It may be that the sites of impulse transmission between neuron and neuron, without which a nervous system is impossible, are evolutionary developments of epithelial junctions.

Neuroanatomists nowadays recognize several different sorts of synapse. The most usual type is shown in Fig. 4.7 and Plate VII(a).

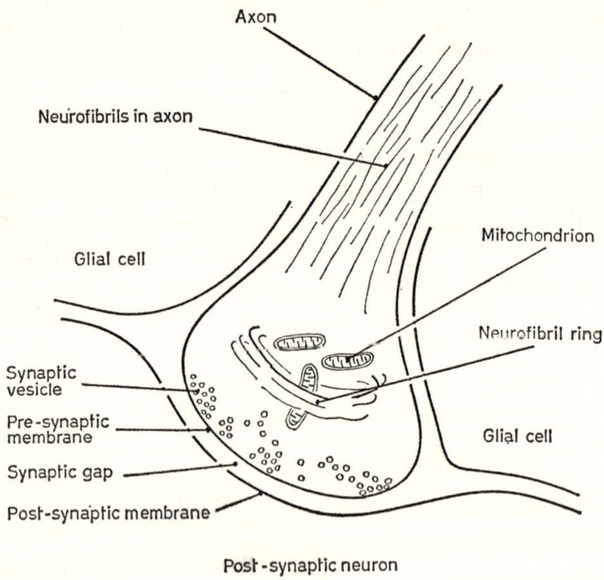


4.7 Schematic diagram of synaptic ultrastructure.

The figure shows that the end of the axon is commonly swollen into a small 'knob' or 'bouton'. The knob is situated in close juxtaposition with a dendron or perikaryon of another neuron. Fig. 4.7 shows that this juxtaposition is very close indeed. The synaptic gap or cleft is believed to be no more than 200A across. This fact is of considerable importance for the physiology of the junction as we shall see in Chapter 6.

Within the synaptic knob are to be found mitochondria and also a large number of small vesicles. The number of mitochondria varies greatly in synaptic knobs derived from synapses in different parts of the brain. Synaptic vesicles are, however, always very plentiful. They are about 500A in diameter and, as we shall see in Chapter 6, are believed to contain small quantities of chemical transmitter substances. In addition to their physiological significance these vesicles are of considerable importance to the neuroanatomist. For, with a few small exceptions, they allow him to determine the 'polarity' of a synapse. Transmission always proceeds from the region containing the vesicles to the adjacent cell and never vice versa.

This recognition of the polarity of the structure seen by the electron microscopist makes it possible to define pre- and post-synaptic membranes. These two membranes are labelled in Fig. 4.7. In some electron micrographs dense material can be observed beneath the post-synaptic membrane. Sometimes fine filaments appear to be attached to this material.

Electron microscopy of fixed and embedded material is not the only means available for the study of the intimate details of synaptic structure. It has proved possible to extract these junctional complexes from the brain and to study them in isolation. This is done by homogenizing portions of the brain and centrifuging the homogenate on a sucrose gradient. Careful adjustment of the conditions allows a reasonably pure suspension of synaptic knobs, often with portions of post-synaptic membrane still adhering, to be obtained. These organized elements are called synaptosomes.

By a further refinement of technique it has proved possible to release the vesicles from suspensions of synaptosomes and to analyse their contents. It can be shown that they are rich in acetyl-choline. This is known to be a transmitter substance (Chapter 6).

We shall see in later chapters of this book that there is good evidence for two types of synapse in the brain: excitatory and inhibitory. Many parts of neurophysiology depend heavily on this distinction. Is it possible to detect any anatomical correlative of this functional difference with the electron microscope? Some investigators have suggested that there is such a difference. These microscopists believe that whereas excitatory synaptic knobs contain rounded vesicles, inhibitory knobs contain rather flattened vesicles. If this distinction can be established it will clearly be of considerable importance for the working out of brain 'wiring diagrams' at the ultrastructural level.

A third type of synapse which is well known in the nervous system of several animals is the electrically conducting junction. The identification of this type of junction in the electron microscope is well established. The 200A synaptic gap of the chemically conducting synapse is lacking. The pre- and post-synaptic membranes abut each other much more closely. Indeed there may be actual physical contact between the two membranes. As Gray and Guillery[1] point out, this type of junction is highly reminiscent of the tight junctions to be observed between epithelial cells.

This leads us on to the next section where we consider another epithelia-like cell which is widely distributed in central nervous systems. These are the neuroglial or glial cells.

### 4.6 Glial cells

In the vertebrate central nervous system glial cells outnumber neurons by about ten to one. In spite of their vast numbers their exact functions have long remained obscure. In recent years, however, it has been suggested that they may play important rôles in the functioning of central nervous systems.

Many different forms of glial cells have been recognized. The most numerous and important are the astroglia, the oligodendroglia and the microglia. Of these the first two, sometimes lumped together as the macroglia, have attracted more interest than the last.

The astroglia, as the name suggests, are cells with several radiating processes. Fig. 4.8 shows that some of these processes may make close contact with brain capillaries whilst others end near nerve cell bodies.

It is tempting to suppose that materials pass from the capillaries to the neurons via the cytoplasm of astroglial cells. This supposition is supported by the finding that there is no intercellular space in the brain[2] and also by the existence of a 'blood-brain barrier'. The existence of this barrier has been known since 1885 when Ehrlich showed

[1] Gray, E. G. and Guillery, R. W. (1966), 'Synaptic morphology in the normal and degenerating nervous system', *Int. Rev. Cytol.*, *19*, 111–173.

[2] de Robertis, E. and Gerschenfield, H. M. (1961), 'Submicroscopic morphology and function of glial cells', *Int. Rev. Neurobiol.*, *3*, 1–61.

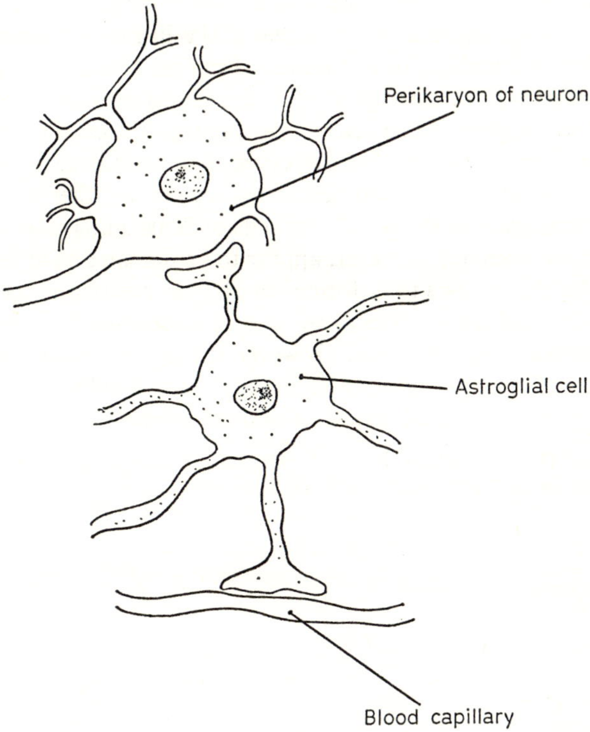


4.8 A possible function for astroglial cells. For explanation see text.

that intravenously injected dyes do not stain brain tissue. In other words, there is no escape of dye molecules into an intercellular space as is found in other parts of the body. It looks as though the cytoplasms of astroglial cells are analogous to the intercellular fluid of other tissues.

It may be, too, that the passage of materials from brain capillaries to neurons via astroglial cells is not the mere passive diffusion which occurs in the intercellular tissue fluid of other organs. Hyden, for example, has suggested[1] that neurons and astroglia may be metabolic symbionts. He proposes that astroglial cells may pass partially metabolized nutrients into nerve cells, having obtained the necessary 'raw materials' from the blood, and thus support in quite an active way

[1] Hyden, H. in *The Cell*, Vol. 4, edited by Brachet and Mirsky, Academic Press, New York and London (1960), Chapter 5: 'The Neuron'.

the functioning of the nervous system. More recently, too, Hyden has put forward evidence to show that glial cells may play some part in storing information, or memories, within the brain.[1]

The other type of macroglial cell—the oligodendroglia—have, as their name suggests, rather fewer processes than the astroglia. One of the most important functions of this type of glial cell is the production of myelin sheaths for central neurons. They are, in other words, the central analogues of the peripheral cells of Schwann. The *process* of myelination does not, however, appear to be the same as at the periphery. Myelin appears to be formed not by any rotation of the oligodendroglial cell around the axon, but in association with the glial cell's endoplasmic reticulum. However it may be formed, the importance of central myelination is very great. Faulty myelination leads to the usually fatal disease of multiple sclerosis.

[1] Hyden, H. and Egyhazi, E. (1963), 'Glial RNA changes during a learning experiment in rats', *P.N.A.S.* (*Wash*), *49*, 618–624.

# CHAPTER FIVE

# The Nerve Impulse

## 5.1 Animal electricity

That the activity on ferves and muscles is accompanied by electrical phenomena has been known for well over a century and a half. It is interesting to note that the early researches into the nature of animal electricity sparked off both the great science of neurophysiology and the equally great science of electromagnetism with all its attendant technology. Yet it is not difficult to appreciate that the experiments of Galvani and Volta on decapitated frogs and their isolated limbs were repugnant to many of the savants living at the end of the eighteenth century. However this early work showed that not only could the muscles and nerves of frogs be stimulated by electrical means, but also that their normal activity was accompanied by electrical phenomena. Indeed du Bois-Reymond, one of the great early nineteenth-century pioneers in this field, believed that he had 'succeeded in realizing in full actuality (albeit under a slightly different aspect) the hundred years' dream of physicists and physiologists, to wit, the identity of the nervous principle with electricity'.[1]

It is, however, only in very recent times that the nature of 'animal electricity' has been finally elucidated. The solution to this age-old problem depended on two developments: the discovery and use of an appropriate biological preparation, and the invention of sophisticated scientific apparatus.

It turns out that the animal body does indeed signal between its parts by electrical means. However the method adopted is altogether different from that employed in the transmission of messages along telephone or telegraph wires. This must, indeed, be so for the 'telegraph wires' of the body are extremely poor conductors of electricity.

[1] Quoted by M. A. B. Brazier in *Handbook of Physiology*, Section 1, Volume 1, American Physiological Society (1959), p. 22.

Hodgkin[1] has calculated that one metre of an average human axon has an electrical resistance equivalent to $10^{10}$ *miles* of 22 gauge copper wire. This distance, as Hodgkin points out, is about ten times that between the Earth and the planet Saturn. This, of course, is the price the animal organism has to pay for being constructed of materials held together by covalent bonds. Only very rarely in materials of this type are electrons free to drift through the atomic lattice. This, on the other hand, is the hallmark of materials based on the metallic bond. In consequence it is only in the latter materials that the overall electron drift which we recognize as an electric current can be induced. It follows that the brain and the nerves function in a radically different manner from the artefacts of the telecommunications engineer. The next sections of this chapter outline the technologically alien mechanisms evolved by living organisms.

### 5.2 Surface recording from nerve and muscle

It was emphasized in the foregoing section that a deep understanding of the physico-chemical nature of the nerve impulse awaited both the discovery of an appropriate biological preparation and the development of sophisticated observational techniques.

Most axons, and in particular mammalian axons, are exceedingly minute. Human axons, for example, range from about 0·1μ to about 20μ in diameter. To isolate such minute fibres from a nerve trunk and determine their electrical characteristics is a task which it would be unwise to undertake lightly. Indeed it is only in the last decade that techniques have been developed which make such an endeavour at all possible. However in 1936 J. Z. Young demonstrated that certain large tubular structures known to occur in the squid and other cephalopods were in fact 'giant' axons. Instead of being only a few micra in diameter these giant fibres averaged 0·5 mm. and in some cases reached as much as 1 mm. across. It is not difficult to see that this anatomical discovery revolutionized the experimental situation.

With the giant axon preparation it became for the first time possible to actually insert electrodes into a nerve fibre. (See Plate VIII.) Before the era of the giant axon the electrical activity of nerves and muscles could only be recorded by externally applied electrodes. The only way in which a record of the electrical potential across a

[1] Hodgkin, A. L. (1958), 'The Croonian Lecture: Ionic movements and electrical activity in giant nerve fibres', *Proc. Roy. Soc. B, 125*, 1–37.

membrane could be obtained was by observing the so-called 'injury potential'. This was done by inserting one electrode into the cut end of a muscle and connecting it, via a suitable recording instrument, to another electrode placed on the uninjured surface of the muscle (Fig. 5.1).

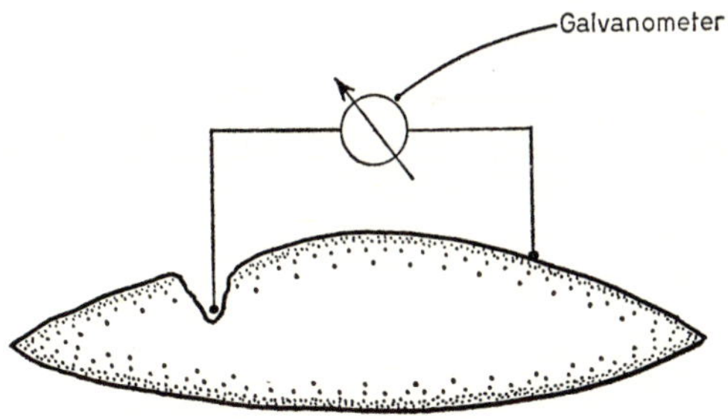


5.1 Detection of the injury potential.

By means of this rather crude technique it is possible to show that current flows (in the conventional sense) from the outside of the membrane into the cut. In other words the external surface of the muscle membrane is at a higher electrical potential than the interior.

Another type of experiment which it is possible to carry whilst still restricted to externally applied electrodes is depicted in Fig. 5.2.

The essence of the experiment schematized in Fig. 5.2 is to place both electrodes on the surface of a nerve or muscle and then to stimulate the tissue. This is shown in Fig. 5.2 (a). Milliseconds later, Fig. 5.2 (b), the galvanometer shows a flow of electricity from electrode *Y* towards electrode *X*. This flow is only very transient and in Fig. 5.2 (c) the galvanometer shows that both electrodes are once more at the same potential. Next we find, Fig. 5.2 (d), that there is a short pulse of current from *X* to *Y* and that this is succeeded, Fig. 5.2 (e), by a permanent quiescence.

This sequence of events can be explained if it is supposed that stimulation of the tissue causes a wave of 'negativity' to spread rapidly down the fibre. This wave is represented in Fig. 5.2 by the cross-hatched rectangle. This wave will first cause *X* to become negative to *Y* and thus induce a flow of current in the observed direction, later it will cause *Y* to become negative to *X* thus inducing a flow of current in the reverse direction.

Full elucidation of the nature of this 'wave of negativity' or *action*

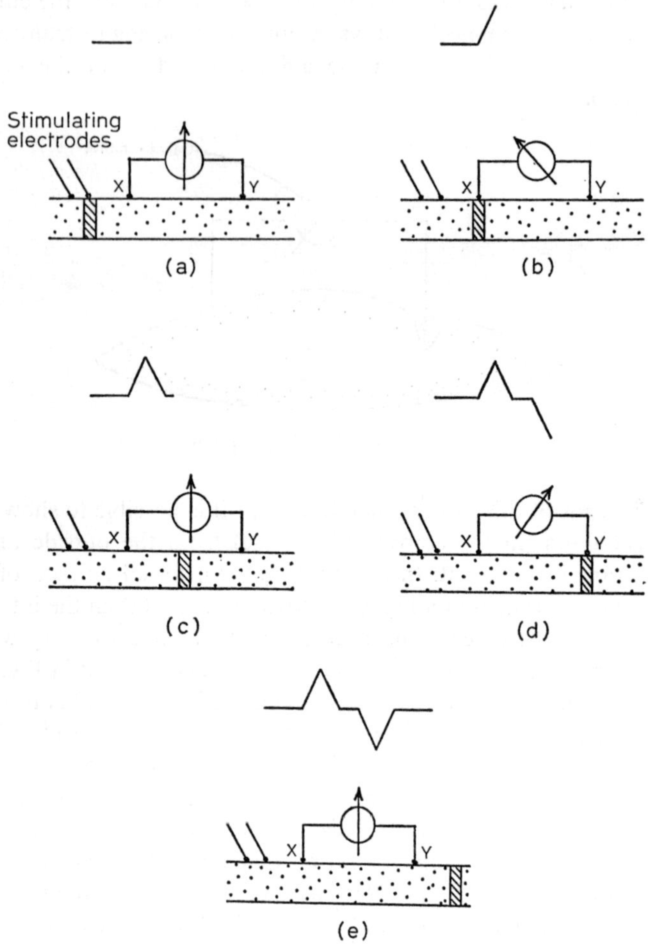


5.2 Surface recording of the action potential. The cross-hatched region represents the action potential. The relevant portion of an oscilloscope trace is drawn above each of the figures. Further explanation in text.

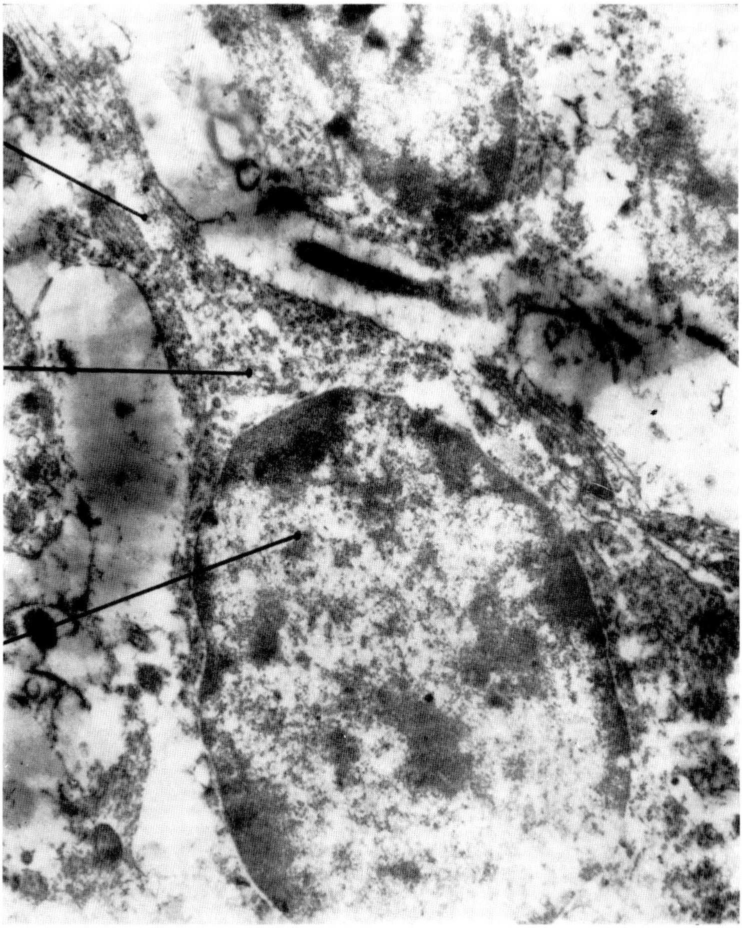


V The fine structure of neurons (i)

Electron micrograph of a granule cell in the cerebellum ($\times$ 8,600). As the plate shows, most of the perikaryon in this type of neuron is taken up by the nucleus. The cytoplasm can, however, be seen to be very granular and to contain mitochondria. The axon running off towards the top left hand corner of the micrograph can be seen to contain a number of neurofibrils.

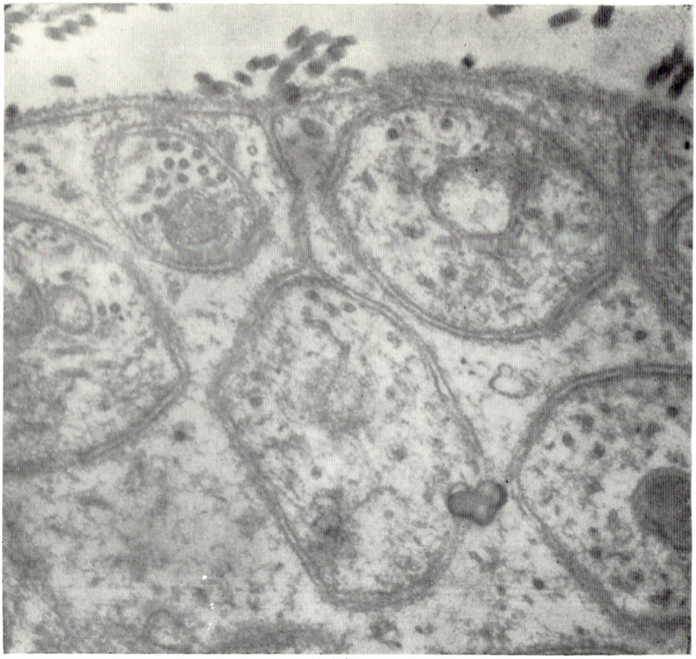

(a)

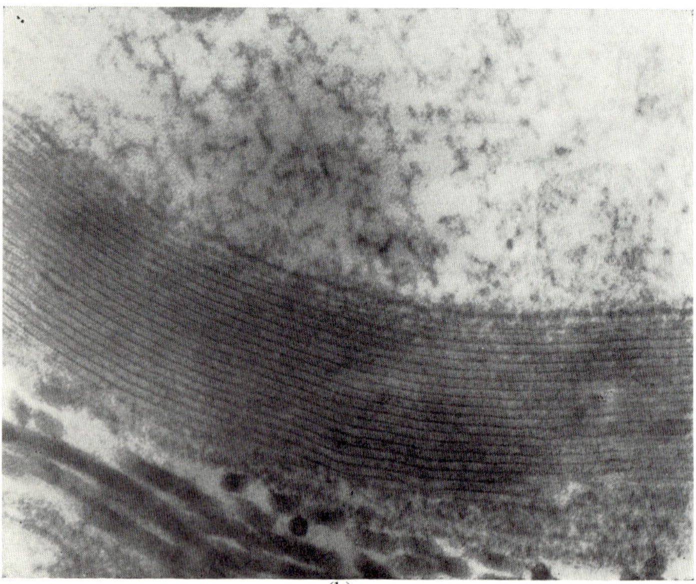

(b)

VI The fine structure of neurons (ii)

(a) Several unmyelinated axons lying in a single Schwann cell (compare with Fig. 4.6). The mesaxons are well-shown and the axoplasm contains numerous neurofibrils and also mitochondria (×43,000).

(b) Portion of the myelin sheath of an axon in the sciatic nerve of a mouse (compare with Fig. 4.4 (c) ). (×68,000).

*potential*, as we may now call it, was only achieved when neurophysiologists turned to the study of cephalopod giant axons. By inserting an electrode into a giant axon it was possible to obtain an unambiguous value for the resting potential (Plate VIII). It could be shown that this procedure does no great harm to the axon as action potentials can be conducted for several hours after the electrode insertion. The value of the resting potential obtained in this way was about 45 mV. By convention the exterior of the axon is taken to be at zero potential, hence the interior of the resting axon is —45 mV.

It was next confirmed that the 'wave of negativity' we have been speaking of, the action potential, was in fact a complete reversal of this polarity. At the peak of the latter potential the interior of the axon is about 40 mV positive to the outside. Thus during the action potential the polarity of the membrane changes from —45 mV to +40 mV, a total change of some 85 mV. This change is very rapid and the membrane returns to its resting state after a few milliseconds. These events are shown in Fig. 5.3.

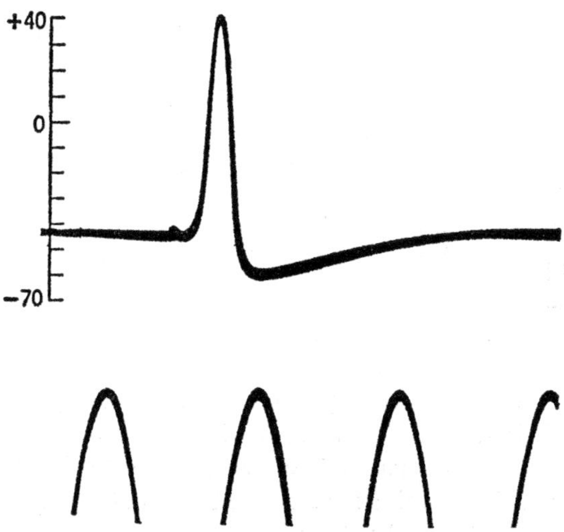


5.3 Action potential recorded from a squid giant axon. Time marker 500 c/s. The vertical scale indicates the potential of the internal electrode (mV), the sea-water outside is taken as having zero potential. In addition to its scientific interest this figure has historic value as it is one of the first pictures of a complete action potential ever to be published. From Hodgkin, A. L. and Huxley, A. F. (1939), 'Action potentials recorded from inside a nerve fibre', *Nature, 144*, 710–711.

Our next questions must be: What are the causes of these electrical phenomena? What, in other words, are the physical bases of resting and action potentials?

### 5.3 The ionic bases of the resting potential

Before we can begin to understand the physical bases of the action potential we must examine the causes of the resting potential. Fortunately we have already laid the foundations for this examination in Chapters 1 and 2. It will be recalled that we were able to show that if and when a membrane is differentially permeable to ions the distribution of even the permeable ions becomes distorted. It also emerged that an asymmetric distribution of permeable ions across a membrane results in a counterbalancing electrical potential. This potential, to a first approximation, is given by the Nernst equation (equation 2.9).

Now it can be shown that the axonal membrane *is* differentially permeable to ions. If the permeability of the squid giant axon membrane to potassium is set (arbitrarily) at unity then its permeability to chloride is 0·45 and to sodium is 0·01. Its permeability to larger ions such as amino-acids and proteins is normally zero. Clearly we have here the necessary and sufficient conditions for the asymmetrical or Gibbs-Donnan equilibrium which we discussed in Chapter 2. But with living membranes in general and axonal membranes in particular there is a complicating factor. It can be shown, as we shall see later, that many of the ions, and in particular sodium and potassium, are actively pumped across the membrane. This accentuates the asymmetry of the ionic distribution and influences still further the equilibrium position of any passively diffusing ion. However it is still possible to fit the internal and external concentrations of one of the passively diffusing ions into the Nernst equation and calculate a value for the membrane potential. We can then compare this calculated value with the value observed. If the two roughly coincide and if, moreover, alteration of the internal or external concentrations alters the membrane potential, we need look no further for the cause of the resting potential. At root it is due to an asymmetrical distribution of electrically charged ions.

One of the great virtues of cephalopod giant axons is that the axoplasm can be squeezed from the axon rather like toothpaste from a toothpaste tube. It is thus not difficult to obtain a sufficient quantity for a detailed chemical analysis. The results of such an analysis are shown in Table 5.1.

TABLE 5.1

Distribution of ions across the freshly isolated squid giant axon (from Hodgkin, A. L., 1958)

| *Substance* | *Axoplasm* | *Blood* | *Sea water* |
|---|---|---|---|
| $H_2O$ | 865 gm/kgm | 870 gm/kgm | 966 gm/kgm |
| $K^+$ | 400 mmoles/kgm | 20 mmoles/kgm | 10 mmoles/kgm |
| $Na^+$ | 50 mmoles/kgm | 440 mmoles/kgm | 460 mmoles/kgm |
| $Cl^-$ | 40 mmoles/kgm | 560 mmoles/kgm | 540 mmoles/kgm |
| $Ca^{2+}$ | 0·4 mmoles/kgm | 10 mmoles/kgm | 10 mmoles/kgm |
| $Mg^{2+}$ | 10 mmoles/kgm | 54 mmoles/kgm | 53 mmoles/kgm |
| isethionate | 270 mmoles/kgm | — | — |
| aspartate | 75 mmoles/kgm | — | — |
| glutamate | 12 mmoles/kgm | — | — |
| succinate<br>fumarate | 17 mmoles/kgm | — | — |

Note that mmole is short for millimole, that is one thousandth part of a mole.

It is clear from the table that the distribution of ions across the axonal membrane is markedly asymmetrical. Of the cations there is far more $K^+$ within than without; vice versa, there is far more $Na^+$ without than within. The major internal anions are organic and consequently large—isethionate $^-$, aspartate $^-$, etc. The major external anion is $Cl^-$. Restricting our attention to the major inorganic ions we can display the ionic situation as follows:

| | Internal | External |
|---|---|---|
| $Na^+$ | 50 mM/l | 460 mM/l |
| $K^+$ | 400 mM/l | 10 mM/l |
| $Cl^-$ | 40 mM/l | 540 mM/l |

5.4 Distribution of the major inorganic ions across the membrane of a squid giant axon. Concentrations are given in millimoles per litre (mM/1). From Hodgkin, A. L. (1957), 'Ionic movements and electrical activity in giant nerve fibres', *Proc. Roy. Soc. B.*, *148*, 1–37.

Now it can be shown that in most nerves and muscles the chloride ion is in free equilibrium across the membrane.[1] Consequently if the concentrations of $Cl^-$ set out in Fig. 5.4 are substituted in the Nernst equation a value for V, the membrane potential, can be calculated.

$$V_{Cl} = \frac{RT}{-F} \ln \frac{[Cl]_o}{[Cl]_i} = -64mV$$

The value of $-64mV$ for $V_{Cl}$ is in fact in very close agreement with the value of the resting potential across the squid axon *in vivo.* The rather lower values mentioned in the previous section of this chapter were obtained from axons dissected out of the squid. It is probable that the dissection damages the very fragile membrane so that ions escape into and out of the fibre.

Next let us substitute $K^+$ into the equation:

$$V_K = \frac{RT}{F} \ln \frac{[K]_o}{[K]_i} = -93mV$$

Clearly $V_K$ is rather higher than the observed value of the resting potential. In other words the distribution of $K^+$ ions across the membrane is rather more asymmetrical than the observed electrical potential suggests. We shall see in section 5.6 that there is good evidence that $K^+$ ions are actively pumped into the axon. This flux is additional to the free movement of $K^+$ across the membrane and accounts for the unexpectedly high concentration of the ion within the axon. It can be shown, however, that the resting potential depends to a large extent on the free diffusion of potassium. If the concentration of $K^+$ in the external medium is increased then the resting potential falls as the Nernst equation predicts.

Finally, what happens if we substitute the observed $Na^+$ concentrations in the Nernst equation? Instead of obtaining a potential in the region of $-60mV$, the equation predicts a potential of about $+56mV$. Clearly there is something very wrong here. It turns out that the axonal membrane is both relatively impermeable to $Na^+$ and that any $Na^+$ which does leak in is quite rapidly extruded again

[1] The squid axon is in fact an exception to this rule. It seems that chloride is actively transported across the membrane. The true situation in the squid axon, as in other excitable cells is, as may be guessed, somewhat more complicated than this outline treatment suggests. The resting potential is due to the team work of a number of different ions. Readers interested in a fuller account of what is rather a technical subject should consult one of the books listed in 'Further Reading'. The method of calculating $V_{Cl}$, $V_K$ and $V_{Na}$ is set out at the end of the book.

by a 'pumping' mechanism. Thus the membrane is certainly not freely permeable to $Na^+$: indeed calculations show that it is some 75 times less permeable to sodium than it is to potassium. It therefore follows, as we stressed in Chapter 2, that the Nernst equation cannot be used.

Thus we may conclude this section by stating that the resting potential across nerve cell membranes is largely due to the asymmetrical distribution of $K^+$ and $Cl^-$ ions. Alteration of $K^+$ concentrations either inside or outside the axon causes a predictable change in the value of the membrane potential. The other major inorganic ion, $Na^+$, plays, however, very little, if any, part in the maintenance of a resting potential.

### 5.4 Electrotonic potentials

Action potentials, as we shall see in the next section, are very specialized features of certain, electrically excitable, membranes. Of far more general occurrence are the so-called electrotonic potentials.

Consider first the experimental arrangement depicted in Fig. 5.5. Two microelectrodes are inserted into a single nerve or muscle fibre. One electrode, *S*, is used to stimulate the fibre, the other, *R*, for recording.

Suppose that a small electrical stimulus is given to the preparation by electrode *S*. Suppose that this stimulus is sufficient to cause a small depolarization of the membrane—some 5 or 10 mV. If the

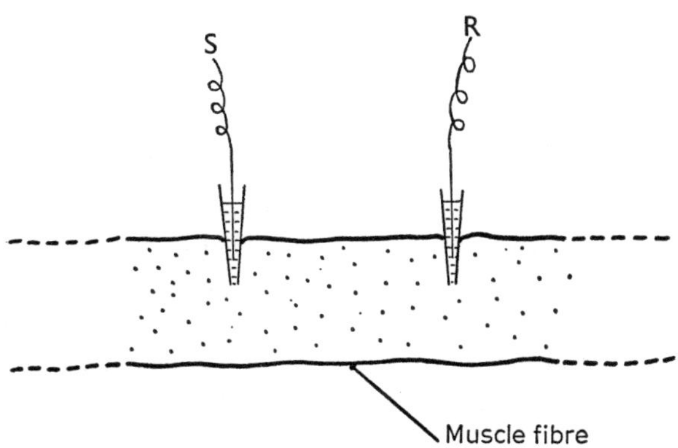


5.5 Experimental arrangement for the detection of electrotonus. S = stimulating electrode, R = recording electrode.

recording electrode, *R*, is only some one or two millimetres distant from this small stimulus it will pick up a minute depolarization. As *R* is moved further away from *S* the size of the recorded depolarization will decrease until it disappears altogether.

There is evidence to show that this rapidly attenuated spread of depolarization from the point of stimulation is caused by the development of small 'local circuits'. The meaning of the latter term is shown in Fig. 5.6. This figure indicates that the region of the membrane immediately beneath the stimulating electrode is, by definition, at a different potential from adjacent parts of the membrane. Our knowledge of elementary physics assures us that in such a situation electric currents will flow. These currents are represented in Fig. 5.6 by broken lines. The figure shows that charge is removed from the outside of the membrane and added to the inside. Thus regions of the membrane neighbouring the stimulated region also become depolarized.

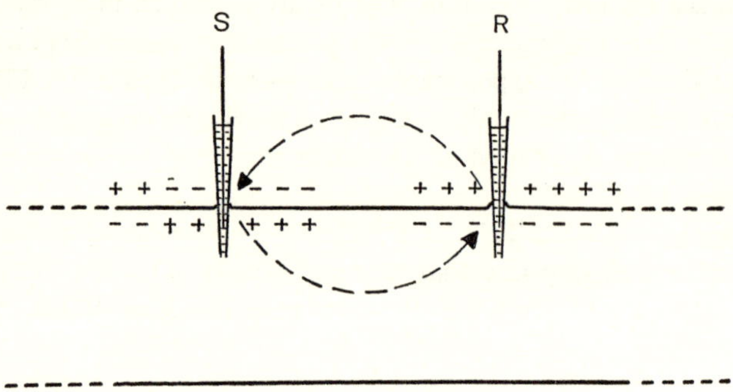


5.6 The physical basis of electrotonic conduction.
**S** = stimulating electrode, **R** = recording electrode.

The depolarization of a membrane by electrotonic 'conduction' immediately disappears when the stimulus is turned off. It is clear that this type of 'conduction' is of little use for rapid signalling over relatively long distances. It is believed, however, that it is of considerable importance in the spread of excitation over the minute distances of dendrites and perikarya (see section 6.3). For long distance communication, on the other hand, a much more efficient mechanism is necessary. This is achieved by one of the most significant advances in animal evolution: the development of electrically excitable membranes and the propagated action potential.

### 5.5 The physical basis of the action potential

It is in the elucidation of the physical basis of the action potential that cephalopod giant axons have played perhaps their most crucial rôle. We shall see in this section that a combination of these axons and some clever electronic circuitry led, in the hands of Hodgkin, Huxley and others, to a complete solution of the nature of the nerve impulse.

One of the most decisive steps on the path towards our modern understanding of the nerve impulse was the realization that it was not merely a depolarization of the nerve membrane but a repolarization. Before this was realized it seemed possible to account for the electrical phenomena of the impulse by postulating a generalized breakdown in membrane permeability. If this were to occur a universal flux of all the inorganic ions—$K^+$, $Na^+$, $Cl^-$, $Ca^{2+}$, etc.—along their electrochemical gradients would result. The consequence of this would be an overall depolarization of the membrane. This is indeed what happens when a cell dies and the integrity of its membrane is lost. But it is not, as we have been at pains to stress, what happens when a nerve impulse is transmitted. The fact that the action potential consists in a radical *repolarization* of the axonal membrane puts this earlier theory out of court.

A hint of what nowadays is believed to occur was dropped in section 5.3. There we noted that the membrane potential predicted when sodium ion concentrations were inserted into the Nernst equation was about +56mV. We also noted that this procedure is invalid for the resting membrane as it is virtually impermeable to this ion. But suppose the membrane should suddenly become selectively permeable to sodium ions. The Nernst equation should then be applicable. The Nernst prediction should be observed. And this, of course, is very much what is observed at the peak of the action potential.

Our working hypothesis, therefore, is that the electrical phenomena observed during the action potential are caused by a sudden, transient, increase in the membrane's permeability to sodium ions. One possible way of determining the truth of this hypothesis would be to alter the quantity of sodium ions in the external solution. This would alter the value of the logarithmic term in the Nernst equation and thus alter the value of the potential predicted. It follows from our hypothesis that the magnitude of the action potential would also be altered. This experiment was tried by Hodgkin and Katz in 1949.[1] The results are shown in Fig. 5.7. They are fully consistent with the hypothesis developed in these last paragraphs.

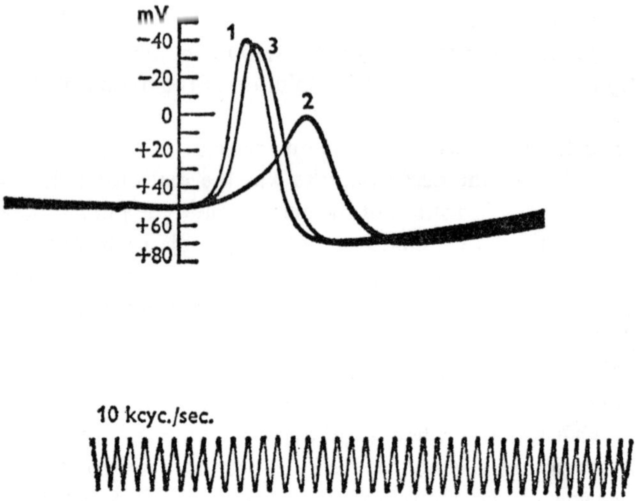


5.7 Effect of altering the external sodium concentration on the action potential. Trace 1 was obtained when the axon was bathed in normal sea water; trace 2 when the axon was bathed in 0·33 sea water/0·67 isotonic dextrose; trace 3, finally, was obtained when the axon was replaced in normal sea water once again. From Hodgkin, A. L. and Katz, B. (1949), 'The effect of sodium ions on the electrical activity of the giant axon of the squid', *J. Physiol.*, *108*, 37–77.

It has been emphasized that the action potential is a transient, explosive, event. It is over and done with in a matter of milliseconds. This multiplies the difficulties of neurophysiological investigation. Consequently it was a very considerable development when in the late nineteen-forties Cole, Marmont and Huxley introduced a technique for slowing down the action potential.

This technique is called the 'voltage clamp technique'. In essence it consists of a clever piece of electronics whereby the voltage across a nerve cell membrane can be 'set' at any desired value and *held at that value*. For example one can select any membrane potential one is interested in, say +30mV, displace the resting potential to this value and then hold the membrane at this desired potential. Whilst the

[1] Hodgkin, A. L. and Katz, B. (1949), 'The effect of sodium ions on the electrical activity of the giant axon of the squid', *J. Physiol.*, *108*, 37–77.

membrane is being held at this potential its physico-chemical characteristics—for example, its permeability—may be examined. It has been pointed out that this technique is comparable to time lapse cinematography. By clamping the membrane at different potentials the various phases of the action potential may be dissected apart from each other and studied at leisure.

Some of the most revealing analyses have been carried out whilst the membrane is clamped at a potential corresponding to a depolarization of about 60mV. When the membrane is clamped at this potential it can be shown that there is an initial inward flux of electric current through the membrane, followed by an increasing and sustained outward flux. This important finding is shown in Fig. 5.8 where an inward current is represented by a downward displacement.

It was quickly established that the initial inward flux of electricity was carried by sodium ions. This could be demonstrated by progressively decreasing the quantity of sodium in the external medium.

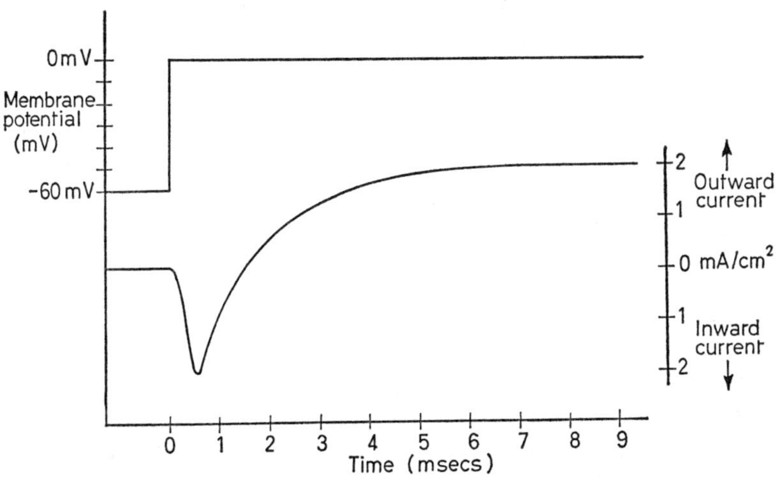


5.8 Use of the voltage clamp technique to examine the flux of electricity across a giant axon membrane. In the upper part of the figure the fact that the membrane has been depolarized from about −60mV to OmV is symbolized. In the lower part of the figure the flow of current across the membrane consequent upon this depolarization is depicted. An upward curve represents an outward current. After Hodgkin, A. L., Huxley, A. F. and Katz, B. (1952), 'Measurement of current voltage relations in the membrane of the giant axon of *Loligo*', *J. Physiol.*, *116*, 424–448.

When this was done the initial inward current was progressively reduced and finally, when external sodium was removed altogether, extinguished. These observations thus confirmed the work of Hodgkin and Katz mentioned above.

Reduction of external sodium concentrations did not, however, affect the externally directed current. It follows that this current must depend on some other mechanism. It was shown by Hodgkin and Huxley, using radioactive tracer techniques, that this outward flux is carried by potassium ions. It is this outwardly directed potassium current which normally restores the membrane to its original resting potential. Indeed the mark is somewhat overshot. Immediately after the action potential has passed on, the membrane possesses a potential corresponding to the full Nernst potassium potential. This, it will be remembered (p. 100), is rather higher than the normal resting potential.

These ion fluxes all happen very rapidly in the normal action potential—a matter of a few milliseconds. Whilst the membrane is recovering its resting potential it is incapable of carrying a second action potential. The few milliseconds required for recharging the membrane constitute the absolute refractory period of the fibre. Furthermore, because the membrane is hyperpolarized immediately after the recharging has ceased it is more difficult to stimulate. The reason for this fact is explained later in this chapter. Thus following the absolute refractory period there follows a relative refractory period of a further few milliseconds. These characteristics clearly restrict the number of impulses a fibre can carry in a given time.

Let us now return to our discussion of the results obtained by using the voltage clamp technique. We have already seen that the inward current responsible for the initiation of the action potential can be eliminated if the nerve fibre is bathed in a sodium-free solution. In Fig. 5.9 the currents across a giant axon's membrane clamped at a depolarization of 56 mV are recorded first in the presence of, and second in the absence of, external sodium. Hence by subtracting the first curve (A) from the second curve (B) the current due to sodium *alone* (C) can be determined. Curve B shows the current carried by potassium alone. It is worth noting in Fig. 5.9 that the sodium and potassium curves are not contemporaneous. The sodium current rises and falls very rapidly. The potassium current lags some 500 microseconds behind the sodium current and is then sustained as long as the membrane remains depolarized.

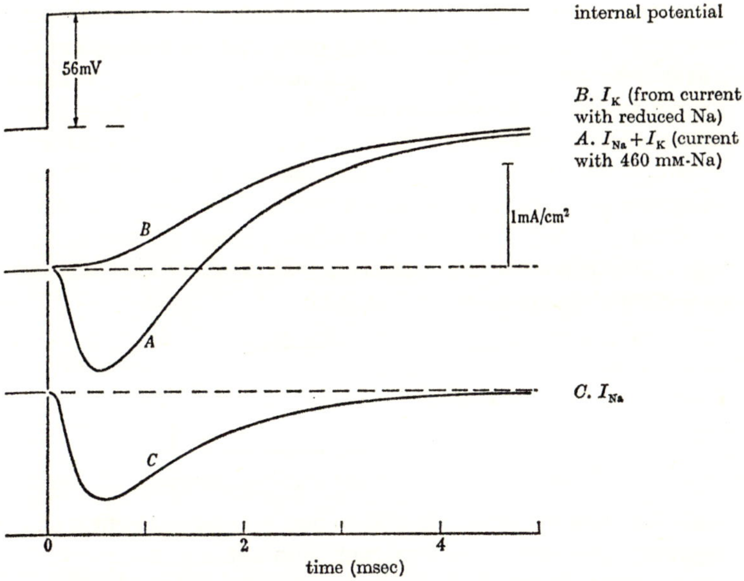


5.9 Analysis of the membrane current into components carried by Na+ and by K+ alone. At the top of the figure the membrane is shown to be clamped at a depolarization of 56 mV. Curve A shows the flux of current across the membrane when held at this depolarization. Curve B shows the flux at the same depolarization when the medium outside the giant fibre has been depleted of sodium. The current represented by this curve must thus of necessity be that carried by K+ alone. It follows that 'subtraction' of curve B from curve A yields a curve representing the current carried by Na+ alone. This curve, labelled C, is shown at the bottom of the figure. Outward current, as in the previous figures, is represented by an upward curve. From Hodgkin, A. L. and Huxley, A. F. (1952), 'Currents carried by sodium and potassium ions through the membrane of the giant axon of *Loligo*', *J. Physiol.*, *116*, 449–472.

We mentioned earlier in this chapter that the axonal membrane is permeable to potassium ions. Hence it follows from the considerations of Chapters 1 and 2 that these ions will diffuse out of the axon if the membrane is de- or re-polarized. This movement of potassium ions down their electrochemical gradient will continue until the membrane achieves the potassium potential, $V_K$. When this potential is attained the overall movement of ions out of the axon ceases. If, however, the axon is clamped at a depolarization of 56mV, as in Fig. 5.9, the flux will continue indefinitely. *In vivo* the pump mentioned on p. 113 causes potassium and sodium ions to move into and out of the axon against their electrochemical gradients and hence restores the membrane to its normal resting potential.

It is clear from the above paragraph that *in vivo* the potassium current automatically switches itself off. To use engineering jargon there is *negative feed-back*. The opposite is the case with the sodium current. Here the relation between membrane permeability and membrane potential is the other way about. The more the membrane is depolarized the more it is permeable to sodium ions. In other words there is *positive feed-back*. This vital characteristic of excitable membranes is schematized in Fig. 5.10.

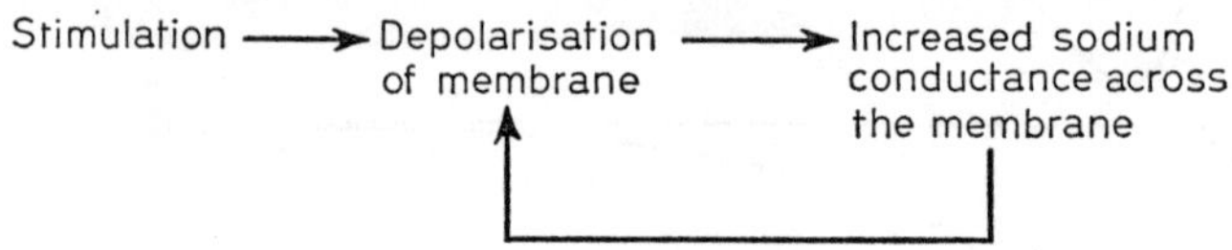


5.10 Positive feed-back in excitable membranes.

The fact that the sodium flux has a positive feed-back effect on the membrane potential has important implications. So far in this chapter we have seen how an ingress of sodium ions causes a depolarization of the membrane. Now we see that the process feeds on itself. Depolarization of the membrane, in turn, causes increased sodium permeability.

If the depolarization is only slight the sodium permeability will not be very greatly increased. An outflow of potassium along its electrochemical gradient will quickly re-establish the resting potential. If, however, the depolarization is rather greater a critical point may be reached. At this point the influx of sodium ions may just counterbalance the restorative potassium current. At a depolarization a fraction greater than this critical, or threshold, value the increased sodium permeability overbalances the membrane's restorative powers. The inward flux of sodium now depolarizes the membrane still further and this, in turn, opens the sodium 'gates' yet wider. The depolarization flares up into a full-scale repolarization or action potential. The critical or threshold value in most muscle and nerve membranes is some 20mV below the resting potential.

Fig. 5.11 shows the sodium and potassium currents underlying an average action potential. In this figure the broken line represents the total voltage change across the membrane. The sodium and potassium currents are represented by the curves labelled $g_{Na}$, and $g_K$ respectively. The fact that the membrane is slightly hyperpolarized immediately after an action potential has passed is also clear from the figure. We are now in a position to understand why this hyperpolarization is responsible for a relative refractory period. Clearly it requires a greater depolarization to reach the threshold of an action potential than if we were starting from a membrane at its normal resting potential level.

Finally, to conclude this section, it is worth noting that the action potential, in spite of its explosive character, depends, in fact, on the movement of a comparatively small number of ions. Hodgkin and Huxley have calculated that about $4 \times 10^{-12}$ moles of sodium and potassium traverse a square centimetre of neuronal membrane during

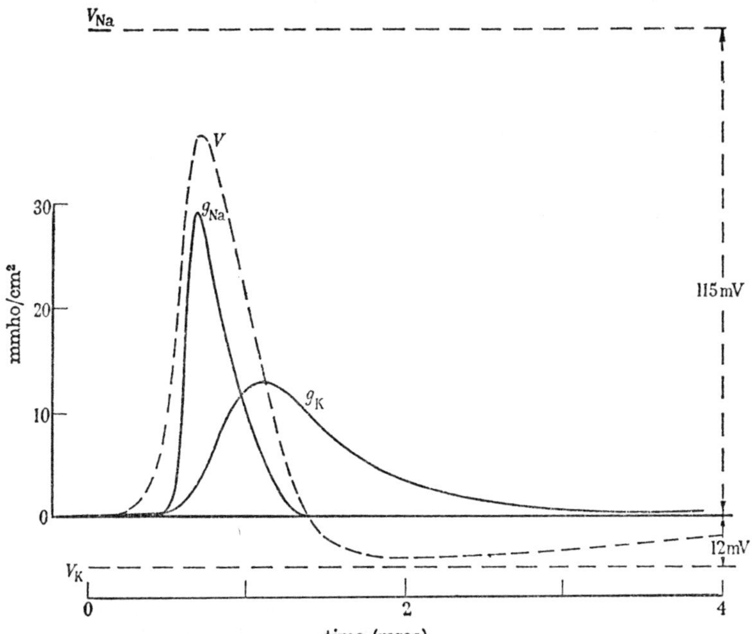


5.11 Theoretical prediction of the ionic currents responsible for a typical action potential. The left-hand ordinate shows the conductance of the membrane for Na + and K+ ions; the right-hand ordinate shows the voltage across the membrane. The curve labelled $g_{Na}$ represents the conductance of the membrane for sodium during the action potential, the curve labelled $g_K$ represents the membrane's conductance for potassium during the same period. The broken line shows the total voltage change across the membrane as the action potential proceeds. From Hodgkin, A. L. and Huxley, A. F. (1952), 'A quantitative description of membrane current and its application to conduction and excitation of nerve', *J. Physiol.*, *117*, 500–544.

a single action potential. $4 \times 10^{-12}$ moles is equivalent to about $2 \times 10^{12}$ ions: an almost negligible quantity when compared with the total numbers of ions in the vicinity. Katz[1] points out that a loss of $2 \times 10^{12}$ potassium ions through a square centimetre of squid axonal membrane represents a loss of only about a millionth part of the potassium present in that segment of giant axon.

### 5.6 Ionic pumps and restoration of the *status quo ante*

One axon in its life carries many million impulses. In the analogous case of heart muscle Overton pointed out as long ago as 1902 that, in humans, about two and a half billion contractions occur during the allotted span and yet the muscle contains as much potassium and as little sodium at the end as it did at the beginning. It looks as though there must be some mechanism for extruding the sodium which has flowed in during the rising phase of the action potential and for recapturing the potassium which escapes during the falling phase. Only in this way can the *status quo ante* be achieved.

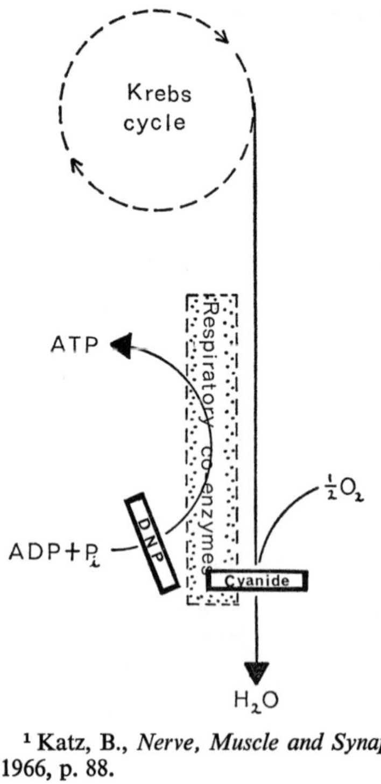


5.12 Points of action of some metabolic inhibitors used in neurophysiology. The major energy resource in the cell is the Krebs cycle. From intermediates in this cycle hydrogen atoms are detached, pass over respiratory coenzymes and finally combine with oxygen to form water. During their passage over the respiratory coenzymes some of their energy is harnessed for the synthesis of ATP from ADP and $P_i$ (shorthand for $H_3PO_4$). The figure shows how DNP and cyanide interfere with these processes. For further explanation see text.

[1] Katz, B., *Nerve, Muscle and Synapse*, McGraw-Hill Book Co., New York, 1966, p. 88.

There is nowadays much convincing evidence to show that such a mechanism does indeed exist. Several conceptually quite simple experiments indicate that a metabolically driven pump extrudes sodium and recaptures potassium. The most impressive of these experiments are based on the creative use of metabolic inhibitors. The points of action of some of the inhibitors used are shown in Fig. 5.12.

It will be observed in Fig. 5.12 that cyanide ($CN^-$), by blocking the terminal oxidase enzyme of the respiratory chain, effectively inhibits the whole of oxidative metabolism. DNP (dinitrophenol), on the other hand, uncouples the connections between oxidative metabolism and the phosphorylation of ADP to form ATP. It will be recalled from elementary biochemistry that ATP (adenosine triphosphate) is the form in which readily available energy is stored in living cells.

Now let us see how these two inhibitors have been used in the analysis of ion movements during the period when an axon is recovering from the transmission of an action potential. First it can be shown that in the presence of DNP the extrusion of radioactively labelled sodium ($^{24}Na$) is very nearly eliminated. The results of such an experiment are shown in Fig. 5.13.

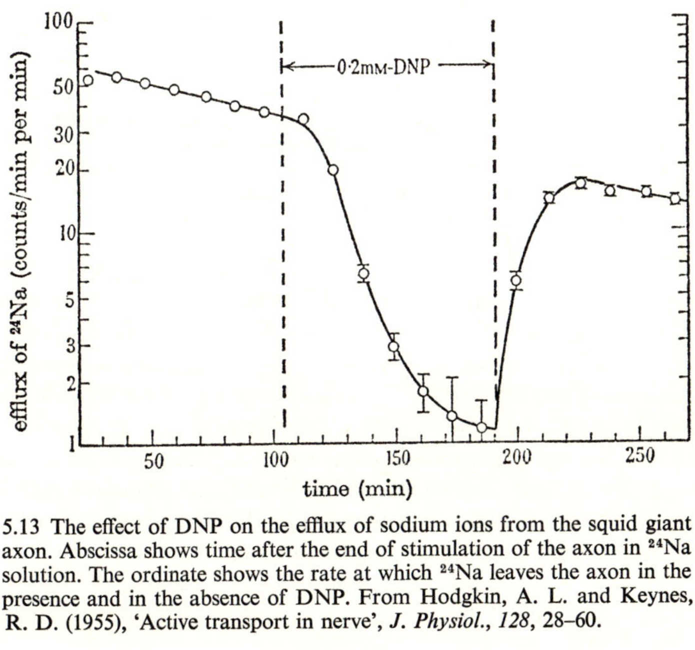


5.13 The effect of DNP on the efflux of sodium ions from the squid giant axon. Abscissa shows time after the end of stimulation of the axon in $^{24}Na$ solution. The ordinate shows the rate at which $^{24}Na$ leaves the axon in the presence and in the absence of DNP. From Hodgkin, A. L. and Keynes, R. D. (1955), 'Active transport in nerve', *J. Physiol.*, *128*, 28–60.

That the drop in $Na^+$ extrusion shown in Fig. 5.13 is due to the lack of ATP can be confirmed by a second experiment in which the axon is poisoned with cyanide. When this is done, as Fig. 5.14 shows, the expulsion of $Na^+$ from the axoplasm is once again drastically reduced; if, however, ATP is injected into the poisoned axon it starts afresh.

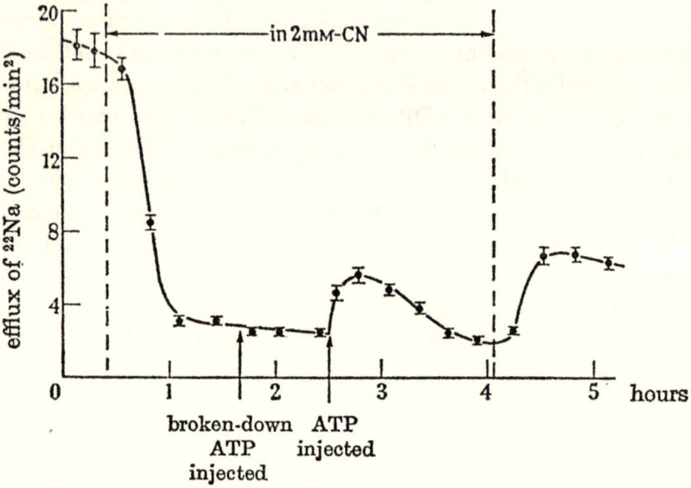


5.14 Effect of ATP on the rate at which labelled sodium leaves a squid axon which has been poisoned with cyanide. The figure shows that only undenatured ATP is effective in increasing the rate of sodium efflux. For further explanation see text. From Caldwell, P. C. and Keynes, R. D. (1957), 'The utilisation of phosphate bond energy for sodium extrusion from giant axons', *J. Physiol.*, *137*, 12P.

It can be shown that the quantity of $Na^+$ extruded is roughly proportional to the quantity of ATP injected. Careful experiments show that approximately 0·7 $Na^+$ ions are expelled for each molecule of ATP injected.

There is thus convincing evidence to show that sodium ions are *actively* extruded from an axon's interior after the passage of an impulse. This active extrusion depends on the energy stored in ATP molecules and this, in turn, normally depends on oxidative metabolism. It is clear that this flux is radically different from the passive, thermodynamic, fluxes discussed in Chapters 1 and 2 and in section 5.5. Next let us see if there is any evidence to show that the inflow of $K^+$ ions after an action potential is also due to an active mechanism.

It turns out that inhibitors which prevent the extrusion of sodium also reduce the ingress of potassium. Even more strikingly it can be shown that if potassium ions are removed from the external solution the pumping of sodium ions out of the interior is almost brought to a halt. The construction normally put on these experiments is to say that the expulsion of sodium ions is coupled to the capture of potassium ions. In other words the two ions are exchanged, sodium moving outwards as potassium moves inwards. This concept is illustrated in Fig. 5.15. In addition to this active pumping of potassium ions inwards there is also evidence to show that a passive flux of these ions also occurs down their electrochemical gradient.

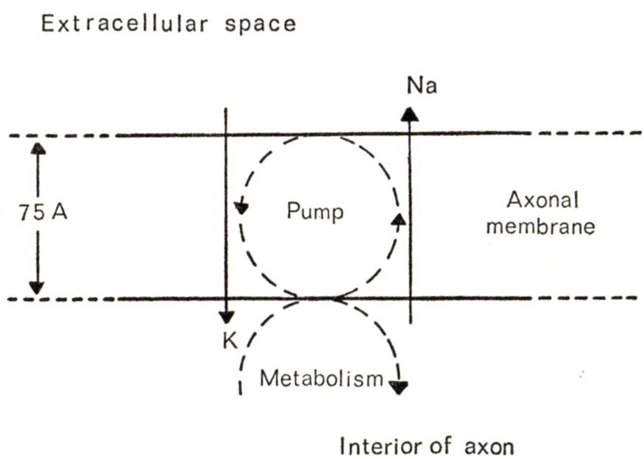


5.15 Diagram to show the nature of the putative pump in the axonal membrane.

Although there have been many suggestions as to the nature of the 'pump' shown in Fig. 5.15 there is, as yet, no certain knowledge. It remains one of the oustanding areas of biophysical research.

## 5.7 A summary and an analogy

Before going any further let us sum up our account of the physical basis of the nerve impulse. We have seen that it consists of two separable phases. First there is the sudden self-exciting increase in permeability to sodium, followed quickly by a movement of potassium in the opposite direction. These explosive ion movements first completely repolarize the membrane and then bring it back to its original polarity. After these sudden instabilities, normally all over and done with in a few milliseconds, comes the slower[1] more sustained work of the sodium-potassium pump which eventually restores the initial ionic concentrations.

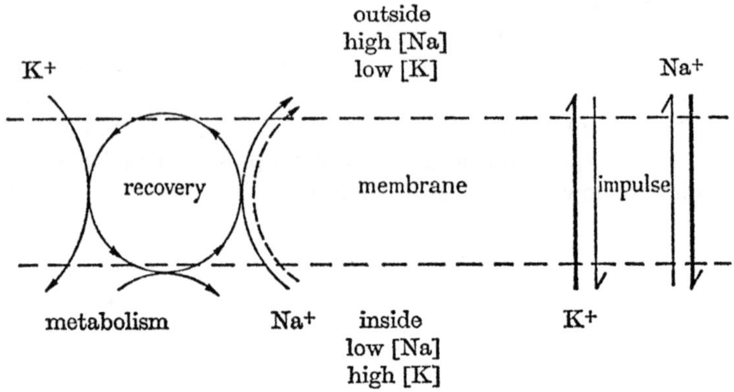


5.16 Summary of the movements of the major ions through the axonal membrane during and after an action potential. The 'downhill' movements which occur during an action potential are shown on the right; the 'uphill' movements, requiring metabolic energy, which take place during recovery are shown on the left. The broken line represents the component of the sodium efflux which is not abolished by removing external potassium ions. From Hodgkin, A. L. and Keynes, R. D. (1955), 'Active transport in nerve', *J. Physiol.*, *128*, 28–60.

It is not difficult to demonstrate that the two phases are quite independent of each other. For example an axon is capable of conducting many thousands of impulses whilst its ion pump is inactivated by DNP or cyanide. Vice versa, changes in the external concentration of divalent ions like $Ca^{2+}$ which have very marked effects on a neuron's excitability have no effect at all on the pumping mechanism.

We may thus regard the membranes of excitable cells, and amongst these are numbered neurons, some muscles and sensory cells, as being in a peculiar state of tension. This inherent instability is due to the asymmetrical distribution of sodium ions across the membrane and to the existence of sodium 'gates' which open when the membrane potential falls. An asymmetrical distribution of sodium

[1] The metabolic pump has a maximum throughput of about 50 p.moles/cm$^2$ sec $^{-1}$ compared with a flux of about 10,000 p.moles/cm$^2$ sec $^{-1}$ which occurs during an action potential. (1 p.mole = 1 x $10^{-12}$ moles.)

ions is a feature of most if not all cell membranes. It is the development of electrically actuated sodium gates which makes the excitable membrane. On this development hangs the evolution of nervous systems and brains.

The axonal membrane has been compared to a gunpowder trail. The chemical energy stored in the gunpowder is analogous to the electrochemical energy stored in the ionic asymmetry across the membrane. A lowering of the membrane potential is analogous to putting a match to the trail. Unlike the trail, however, the axonal membrane is endowed, as we have seen, with a regenerative mechanism. It is as though a few milliseconds after the passage of a flame along the gunpowder track the burnt-out powder is removed and replaced by a fresh unburnt trail.

We have, however, in this analogy strayed on to a topic we have not yet discussed. A topic fundamental, moreover, to the working of a nervous system. This topic is, of course, the means whereby an action potential propagates itself along a nerve fibre.

### 5.8 Propagation of the action potential

The mechanism responsible for the transmission of a nerve impulse is, in fact, implicit in the physico-chemical nature of the nerve impulse as described above. It is a straightforward consequence of the fact that sodium permeability is a function of membrane polarity.

We saw in section 5.4 that a slight depolarization of any region of a cell membrane creates the condition for a local electric circuit. Clearly this circuit is much more strongly developed when a repolarization rather than a mere depolarization of the membrane occurs. Electric currents (carried by ions) will flow in the directions indicated in Fig. 5.17.

It is clear that the local circuits depicted in Fig. 5.17 will remove charge from, and thus depolarize, the axonal membrane in regions adjacent to the active (shaded) area. It is easy to see the consequence of this. In section 5.6 we saw that at a certain critical level of depolarization—some 20mV below the resting potential—the linked increase in sodium permeability becomes self-regenerative. The depolarization flares up into the full-scale repolarization of an action potential. Thus we see that the local circuits set up by an action potential in one section of an axonal membrane automatically excite an action potential in neighbouring regions of the same membrane.

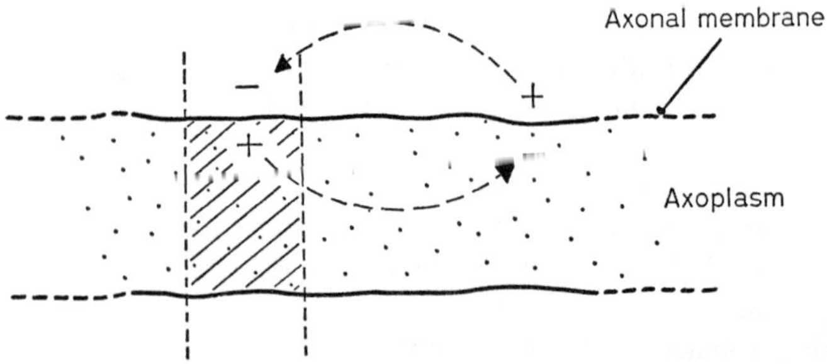


5.17 Propagation of the action potential. The cross-hatched region represents the repolarized segment of the nerve cell membrane, in other words the segment carrying the action potential. The figure shows that a local circuit is set up between this active region and the resting membrane immediately adjacent. For further explanation see text.

This physical mechanism accounts very satisfactorily for the long known fact that an action potential travels in both directions from the point of stimulation. In this respect the axonal membrane may, once again, be compared to a gunpowder trail. And, to continue the analogy, each action potential, once it has started, travels, like the gunpowder flame, in only one direction. Behind each gunpowder flame lies a trail of burnt-out powder. Behind each action potential lies a region of refractory, inexcitable, membrane. The refractory state is, it will be remembered, only transient. Its existence is, however, quite sufficient to ensure that there are no 'strike-backs' once the impulse has got under way.

### 5.9 Rates of impulse propagation

It is clear from Fig. 5.17 that the sizes of the local circuits underlying impulse propagation have an important influence on transmission velocity. Now the magnitudes of these circuits are governed by two physical parameters. First the size of the circuit is inversely proportional to the quantity of electric charge held in the membrane. The less charge there is the easier it will be to discharge it, to depolarize it, to the required threshold. The quantity of charge held is proportional to the membrane capacity. The second physical parameter determining the size of the circuit is the electrical resistance of the internal and external media. The smaller these resistances are the greater will be the dimensions of the local circuits. Now it can be shown that, in general, where '*r*' is the radius of a nerve fibre the resistance of the internal medium varies in proportion to $1/r^2$, whilst the capacity of the membrane varies in proportion to *r*. Hence as the diameter of an axon increases the internal resistance falls off much more rapidly than the capacity of the membrane increases. In consequence a given local circuit is able to depolarize regions of the axon further and further away from the active region. In other words the greater the diameter of the fibre, other things being equal, the greater the velocity of propagation. This, of course, is the reason for the development of giant fibres among so many phyla of invertebrates.

A giant fibre some 0·5 mm. in diameter has, however, many disadvantages. These go far towards counterbalancing the important advantage of rapid impulse propagation. A tube half a millimetre or so in diameter is ungainly; the amount of information it can transmit in a given time is severely limited. Indeed in most invertebrates giant fibres are used merely to signal emergency flight and avoidance reactions. Clearly the earthworm feeling the sudden shock of beak or spade need signal only one command to its body musculature!

In many cases, however, a nerve trunk some 0·5 mm. in diameter is required to signal a complex of information to the brain. The optic nerve of a rat, for example, has approximately this diameter and yet is required to transmit a plethora of information relating to the visual scene to the rat's cortex. To do this the optic nerve is composed of several hundred thousand axons running in parallel. It follows that the diameter of each of these axons must be small. But just as in the case of the earthworm, velocity of conduction is still of considerable survival value. It would usually be too late if an appreciable time lag occurred between the retina picking up the patterned image of terrier or tom-cat and the arrival of this vital information in the visual cortex.

Nature has found an ingenious way out of this dilemma. In the vertebrates and in some of the invertebrates a means of increasing the velocity of impulse transmission whilst at the same time keeping the girth of nerve fibres small has been evolved. This means depends on myelination. We discussed the nature of myelination in Chapter 4. It will be recalled that the myelin sheath around an axon is interrupted at intervals by gaps—the nodes of Ranvier. Now the fatty layers of the myelin sheath form a good electrical insulation around an axon. Only at the nodes is the excitable membrane exposed. In consequence the action potential can only propagate itself by depolarizing adjacent nodes. This type of impulse propagation is called 'saltatory': the action potential 'sparks' from node to node. Clearly this greatly speeds the transmission.

Now although myelination greatly increases the rate of impulse propagation the diameter of a fibre still has an important effect. Hence the most rapidly conducting nerve fibres in the animal kingdom are the largest mammalian myelinated fibres. These have transmission rates of up to 120 metres/second and diameters of over 20 μ. The smallest mammalian fibres, on the other hand, are only a fraction of a micron in diameter and transmit impulses at only about 0·5 metres/second.

Most parts of the mammalian nervous system consist of a mixture of fibres varying in diameter from the smallest to the largest. There is evidence to show that the smallest fibres belong to the phylogenetically oldest parts of the nervous system and that the larger fibres have been superimposed at later stages in evolutionary history. If the diameters of the nerve fibres in a mammalian nerve trunk are tabulated they are found to fall into a number of overlapping groups. Three main groups are recognized: A (subdivided into α, β, γ and δ), B, and C. The most important characteristics of these different types of fibre are set out in Table 5.2.

TABLE 5.2

Some characteristics of mammalian nerve fibres

| | A | B | C |
|---|---|---|---|
| Fibre diameter (μ) | 1–22 | 3 | 0·3–1·3 |
| Conduction speed (metres/second) | 5–120 | 3–15 | 0·6–2·3 |
| Absolute refractory period (msecs) | 0·4–1·0 | 1·2 | 2·0 |

(After Schadé and Ford, *Basic Neurology*, Elsevier, 1966)

The different velocities at which fibres conduct impulses is clearly a complicating factor in both the sensory and motor communication channels of the nervous system. This complication is compounded by the different lengths of the nerve fibres innervating different parts of the body. Consider, for example, the complex musculature which controls the rapid progress of human speech. Some ten to fifteen thousand neuromuscular events are believed to occur during each minute of normal human discourse.[1] And continuous speech may be sustained for many hours, even, for example in some U.S. filibusters, for over a day's length. Now if we examine the nerves controlling the muscles responsible for speech we find that they vary not only in length but also in the average diameters of their constituent fibres. The recurrent laryngeal nerve to the muscles of the larynx is, for example, about 32 cms. in length and the mean calibre of its fibres is about 5·4 μ. In contrast the trigeminal nerve to the jaw musculature is only about 10 cms. long and consists of fibres having a mean diameter of some 9·5 μ. Clearly the brain is presented with a considerable timing problem in co-ordinating the hundred or so different speech muscles many times a second by such disparate communication channels. The wonder is that we are not all of us stutterers and stammerers! Similar remarks could be made about the sensory nerves carrying information in to the brain from the periphery. It seems likely that, in both cases, temporal patterns considerably different from the patterns observed at the periphery occur in the brain: perhaps these as yet unknown patterns enable the brain to achieve some of its legendary feats of sensory discrimination and muscular control.

[1] Lenneberg, E. H.: *Biological Foundations of Language*, John Wiley and Sons, Inc., New York, 1967, p. 107.

# CHAPTER SIX

# The Synapse

## 6.1 The physiological significance of synapses

In Chapter 4 we saw that the functional 'contacts' between two neurons are called synapses. The term was coined by Sherrington in 1897 from a Greek root meaning 'I clasp'. The clasping, however, as we saw is in most cases virtual rather than actual. In the vast majority of cases there is no continuity between neurons, only contiguity. A small gap, the synaptic gap, or cleft, remains between one neuron and the next.

This gap is of very great significance. We shall see in this chapter that the nerve message is transmitted from one neuron to another by means of a chemical mediator. Only in a few synapses has direct electrical transmission been demonstrated.

Chemical mediation has important biological consequences. We have seen that the action potential is very much a yes/no, all-or-nothing, phenomenon. The threshold is either reached or it is not reached. If it is reached or surpassed an action potential is initiated. If it is not reached the axon remains quiescent. This reminds us of the binary code of a digital computer. The toothed wheel turns or does not turn, the electric current flows or does not flow. There are no intermediate states.

Yet one of the most noticeable features of living brains is their extreme flexibility, their adaptiveness. Buriden's ass starving between two equally tempting heaps of food is a logician's not a mammalogist's creature. The question thus has been: how does a system built of inflexible on/off units give a flexible, adaptive response? Doubtless by complexifying the interconnections and multiplying the units such an output could, in principle, be obtained from a digital computer. However in living brains a very important contributory factor is the flexibility chemical mediation confers on the synaptic junction.

### 6.2 A technique for the study of synaptic function

Although much work had been done on the analogous mechanisms operating at the neuromuscular junction, a precise understanding of synaptic action in the CNS awaited the development, in the early nineteen-fifties, of microelectrode techniques. This technique, developed by Eccles and his colleagues in Australasia,[1] consists in pushing a very fine glass capillary (tip diameter 0·5 μ), filled with an electrically conducting KCl solution, actually into the perikaryon of a neuron within the CNS. It is believed that the cell membrane automatically seals itself around the microelectrode (Fig. 6.1) thus preventing the flow of any short-circuit current out of the cell. Indeed so resilient is the cell that many have been known to behave normally for several hours after being impaled.

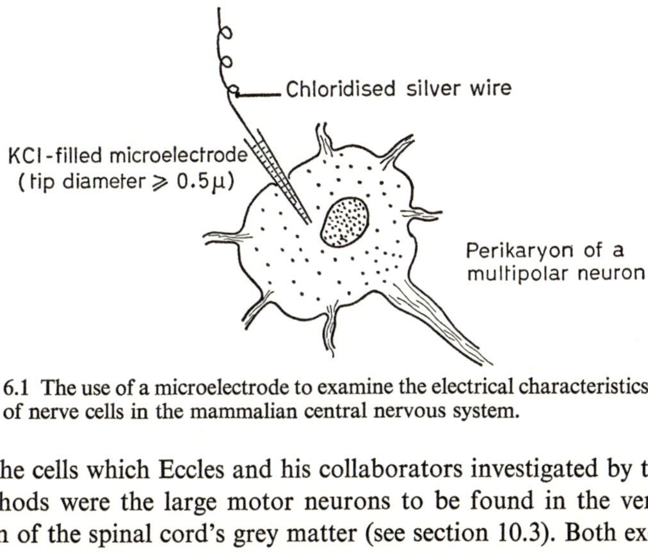


6.1 The use of a microelectrode to examine the electrical characteristics of nerve cells in the mammalian central nervous system.

The cells which Eccles and his collaborators investigated by these methods were the large motor neurons to be found in the ventral horn of the spinal cord's grey matter (see section 10.3). Both excitatory and inhibitory synapses were identified and investigated. More recently several other types of neuron have been investigated *in situ* within the central nervous system. These cells include, as we shall see in Chapter 14, neurons of the cerebral cortex. In this chapter, however, we shall outline first the results of work on spinal excitatory and inhibitory synapses, and conclude by reviewing what is known of chemical transmitter substances and their psychotomimetic analogues.

[1] See Eccles, J. C. (1964), 'Ionic mechanisms and post-synaptic inhibition', *Science*, *145*, 1140–1147.

### 6.3 The excitatory synapse

Let us begin by considering the excitatory synapse. And first let us look at the anatomical system used by Eccles and his co-workers. In section 9.7 the complex system developed by vertebrates to control muscular movement will be described in some detail. We shall find that in each skeletal muscle are embedded sense organs responsive to stretch. On stimulation impulses travel up axons springing from these stretch receptors to the spinal cord. In the cord these fibres terminate on the perikarya of motor neurons which innervate that particular muscle. These neuronal pathways are shown in Fig. 6.2.

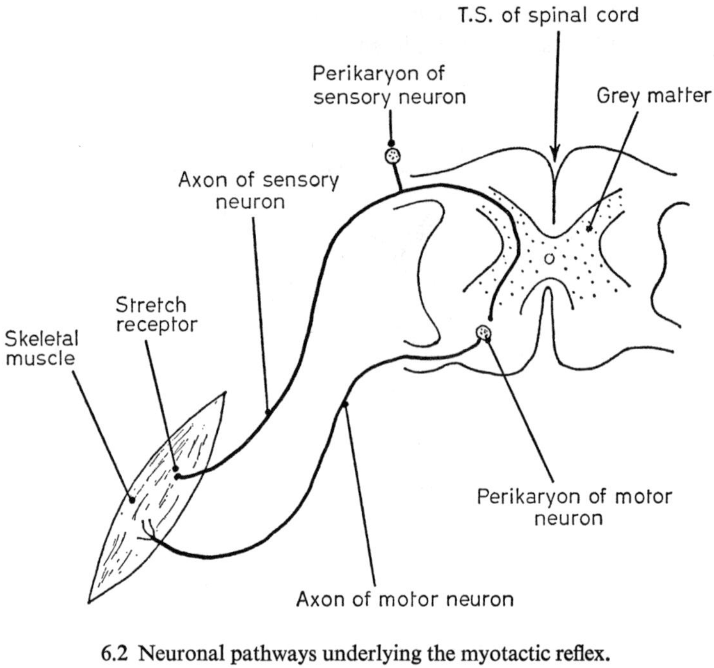


6.2 Neuronal pathways underlying the myotactic reflex.

The outcome of the circulation of impulses in the neuronal circuit of Fig. 6.2 is that the muscle attempts to contract when it is stretched. In other words the 'monosynaptic' circuit is responsible for what is called the 'myotactic' reflex. It is clear that this system provides an excellent preparation for studying the mechanisms of the excitatory synapse.

In essence the technique developed consists in impaling the perikaryon of the motor neuron on a microelectrode and then stimulating the sensory fibre. Any change in the electrical polarity of the perikaryal membrane may then be detected and measured.

From our account of the initiation of the nerve impulse in Chapter 5 it is clear that such a change in potential would be expected. Our expectations, moreover, are not disappointed. It is found that the membrane is indeed depolarized. This depolarization is referred to as an excitatory post-synaptic potential or, more shortly, as an EPSP.

The EPSP differs in one very important respect from the action potentials we discussed in Chapter 5. It is not an all-or-nothing event. It is essentially a graded response. And this characteristic is, as we shall see, of very great importance in the working of the central nervous system.

Frequently it is found that more than one sensory fibre synapses with a single motor neuron. It can then be shown that the EPSP varies in magnitude in direct proportion to the number of sensory fibres activated. In other words EPSPs show the property of spatial summation. This finding is schematized in Fig. 6.3.

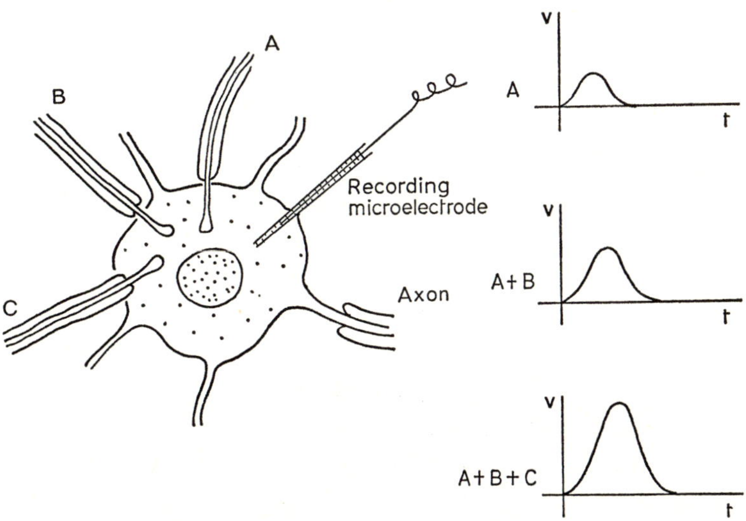


6.3 Spatial summation of EPSPs. The figure shows three fibres—A, B and C—synapsing with a single motor neuron. The graphs in the lower part of the figure show the process of spatial summation when impulses arrive in one, two or three of the fibres simultaneously.

This property of spatial summation is, of course, an aspect of the graded character of EPSPs. It stands in strong contrast to the all-or-none characteristic of the action potential. It will be remembered that increasing the value of the stimulus above a certain threshold does not lead to an increase in the size of the resulting action potential.

Not only do EPSPs summate spatially, they also summate temporally. In other words if two impulses arrive at the termination of a sensory fibre in rapid succession the ensuing EPSP is greater than that developed in response to either impulse on its own. We shall find that these properties of temporal and spatial summation are of considerable importance in the working of central nervous systems and brains.

We have emphasized that the EPSP is very different from an action potential. We know, however, that the end result of (successful) synaptic transmission is an action spike in the post-synaptic neuron. It follows that an EPSP must in certain circumstances lead to an action potential. It is not difficult, following the discussion in Chapter 5, to guess what these conditions are. Quite simply the initiation of a spike in the motor neuron depends on the EPSP reaching or exceeding a certain threshold. Now it appears that an action potential is not normally developed on the perikaryal membrane itself. The site of spike initiation seems to be the axon hillock at the beginning of the axon (see section 4.2). Clearly the depolarization of the perikaryal membrane which we have been calling the EPSP must act as one pole of the type of local circuit we discussed in section 5.4. When this local circuit removes sufficient charge from the axon hillock the axonal membrane in that region 'explodes' into the repolarization of the action potential (Fig. 6.4).

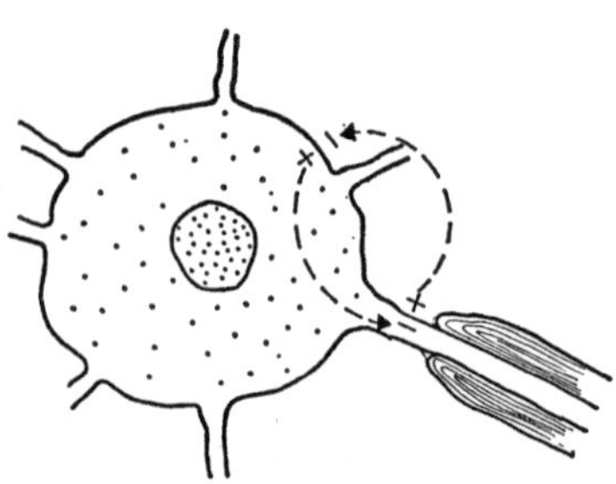

6.4 Local circuits are responsible for generating an action potential at the axon hillock.

Thus far in our account of the EPSP we have shown that the arrival of an impulse at a synaptic junction causes a depolarization of the post-synaptic membrane. The question of the molecular and ionic mechanisms responsible for this depolarization has not yet been broached. Before however taking up this rather fascinating topic it is important to describe the other type of synapse commonly found in the central nervous system. This is the inhibitory synapse.

### 6.4 The inhibitory synapse

Ever since the phenomenon of inhibition in the central nervous system was discovered by the Russian worker Sechenov in the nineteenth century it has attracted the attention and interest of physiologists. It will be mentioned frequently in the subsequent pages of this book. Some of its importance in the working of the central nervous system may be gathered from the following simple example.

In the previous section of this chapter the nerve pathways underlying the myotactic reflex were described (Fig. 6.2). Now it is found that skeletal muscles are invariably arranged in antagonistic groups. In other words if a muscle is positioned to flex a joint, another muscle is positioned to extend it. A well-known example of this antagonism is to be found in the grouping of muscles activating the elbow joint. The biceps muscle in front of the humerus flexes this joint; the triceps muscle behind extends it. It follows from this anatomical disposition that it would be futile and, in fact, probably disastrous if both muscles contracted and relaxed simultaneously. In a properly organized system we would expect to find that the contraction of the 'agonist' muscle was accompanied by the inhibition of the 'antagonist'. And this is indeed what is found.

Let us look, first, at the 'wiring diagram' on which this mutual inhibition depends. This is shown in outline in Fig. 6.5. It will be appreciated that a similar pathway exists to inhibit the agonist muscle when the antagonist contracts.

Fig. 6.5 shows that a short inhibitory neuron runs through the grey matter from the sensory to the motor neuron controlling the antagonist muscle. This fibre prevents the antagonist neuron firing at the same time as the agonist neuron.

Now how is this prevention, this inhibition, achieved? It was for researches designed to elucidate the physico-chemical mechanisms responsible for this type of inhibition that Eccles was awarded the

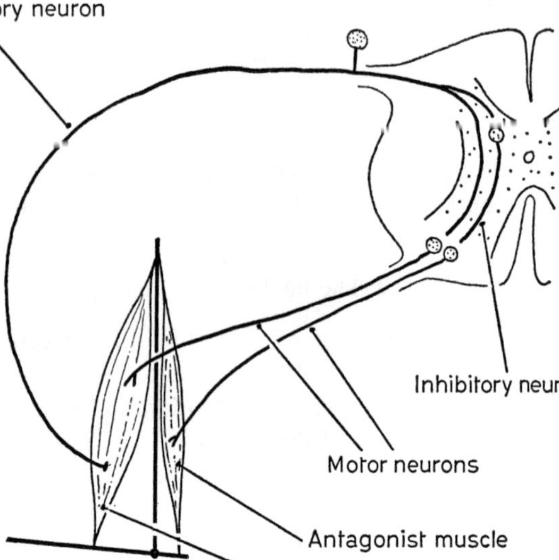


6.5 Highly simplified 'wiring diagram' for the innervation of pairs of antagonistic muscles. The true situation is in fact far more complicated including an important negative feed-back loop from the motor neuron axons back on to their perikarya. This loop has been omitted in the interests of simplicity.

Nobel prize in 1964.[1] Eccles' technique, as we have seen, was to introduce microelectrodes into the relevant motor neuron and to record the electrical changes consequent upon synaptic transmission. He was able to show that activation of an inhibitory synapse produced, instead of a depolarization, a slight hyperpolarization of the post-synaptic membrane. Instead of the resting potential being reduced from, say, —70mV to, say, —55mV, it was increased to —75mV or even —80mV.

It is easy to see that such a hyperpolarization of the membrane potential would make the post-synaptic cell less stimulable than usual. This type of potential is, in consequence, called an inhibitory post-synaptic potential, or IPSP. It can be shown that IPSPs share many of the general properties of EPSPs. For instance IPSPs, like EPSPs, are graded, not all-or-nothing, responses; furthermore IPSPs, like EPSPs, show both temporal and spatial summation.

[1] Eccles' Nobel oration is reprinted in *Science*, *145*, 1140–1147 (1964).

Perhaps most important of all, EPSPs and IPSPs interact. In other words a number of EPSPs and IPSPs on a single post-synaptic membrane will summate algebraically. Thus, taking the resting potential of a typical post-synaptic membrane as —70mV, we may imagine that two IPSPs of —5mV each occur contemporaneously with three EPSPs of +3mV. The algebraic sum —(70 − 3 − 3 − 3 + 5 + 5) gives the resultant potential on the membrane: —71mV. These relations are schematized in Fig. 6.6.

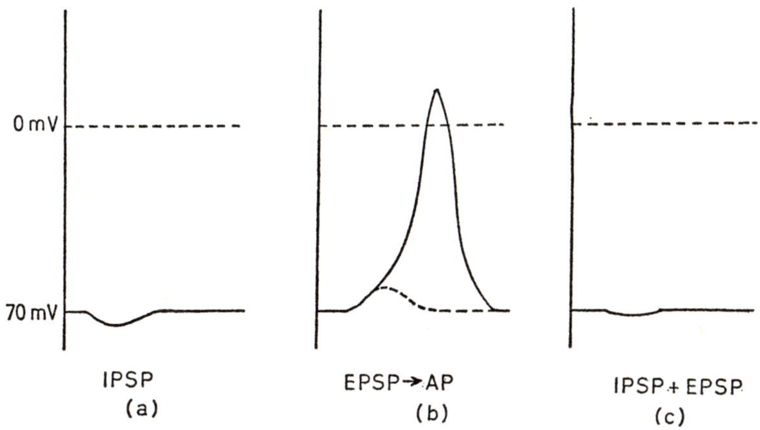


6.6 Interactions between IPSPs and EPSPs. The figure shows an IPSP on its own at (a), an EPSP leading to an action potential (AP) at (b) and, at (c), the result of an interaction between an IPSP and an EPSP initiated on the neuronal membrane simultaneously.

It is clear that the possibilities for interaction between EPSPs and IPSPs are legion. That the multiplicity of these possible permutations and combinations is extraordinarily rich follows from the fact that the dendritic zones of some neurons may make synaptic contact with over sixty thousand synaptic knobs. This almost overwhelming complexity ensures that the brain will not quickly yield its secrets to the neurophysiologist. Today we stand only at the threshold and it is for this reason that the present volume bears its somewhat tentative title.

## 6.5 Axo-axonic synapses

A further complication is introduced by the recognition in the electron microscope that a synapse may be provided with synaptic vesicles on both sides of the synaptic gap. It has been suggested that these electron microscopical observations are of 'axo-axonic' synapses. It is proposed, in short, that the termination of one axon synapses with the termination of another (Fig. 6.7). It is easy to see the physiological consequences of this organization. One axon may, in this way, bias the action of the other. This is particularly the case if the axons are of different type; one inhibitory and the other excitatory.

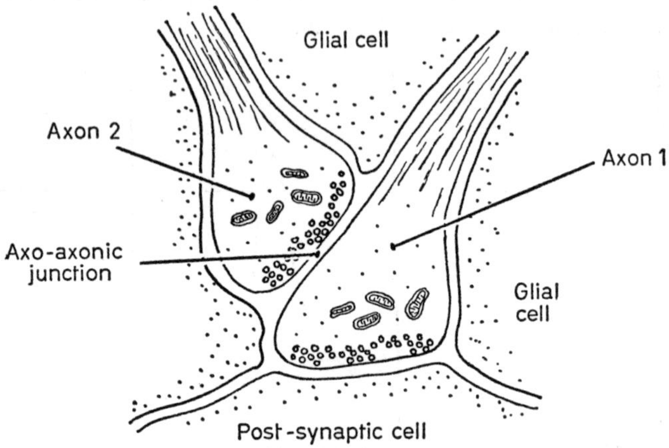


6.7 Ultrastructure of an axo-axonic synapse.

(a) This electron microcraph is of the two types of synaptic contact made with one of the giant axons of the electric catfish *Malapterus electricus*. One synaptic knob ($A_1$) makes both electrical and chemical junctions with the giant axon. The chemical synapse (indicated by an arrow) is characterized by a definite gap between the pre- and post-synaptic membranes. This gap is missing in the electrical synapse; this is also shown at higher magnification in the inset. The second synaptic knob ($A_2$) makes a chemical synapse with the giant cell. Large numbers of synaptic vesicles can be seen in both synaptic knobs. ($\times$20,000, inset $\times$61,000). (From Bennett, M. V. L., Nakajima, Y. and Pappas, G. D. (1967), 'Physiology and ultrastructure of electrotonic junctions. III. Giant electromotor neurons of *Malapterus electricus*', *J. Neurophysiol.*, *30*, 209–300.)

(b) Electron micrograph of a spine synapse on the dendrite of a pyramidal cell of the cerebral cortex (see Plate IV). den = dendrite, m = mitochondrion, mt = thickened region of synaptic membrane. s = spine, sa = spine apparatus (an ultrastructural feature often found in dendritic spines), sv = synaptic vesicles. (From Whittaker, V. P. and Gray, E. G. (1962), 'The synapse: biology and morphology', *British Medical Bulletin*, *18*, 223–227.)

(c) Electron micrograph of a reptilian neuromuscular junction. The diameter of this motor nerve ending is about 2·5$\mu$ (scale marker 1$\mu$). In the centre of the nerve ending is a mass of mitochondria; surrounding the mitochondria are numerous synaptic vesicles. (From Robertson, J. D. (1956), 'The ultrastructure of a reptilian myoneural junction', *J. Biophys. Biochem. Cytol.*, *2*, 381–393. Reprinted by permission of the Rockefeller University Press.)

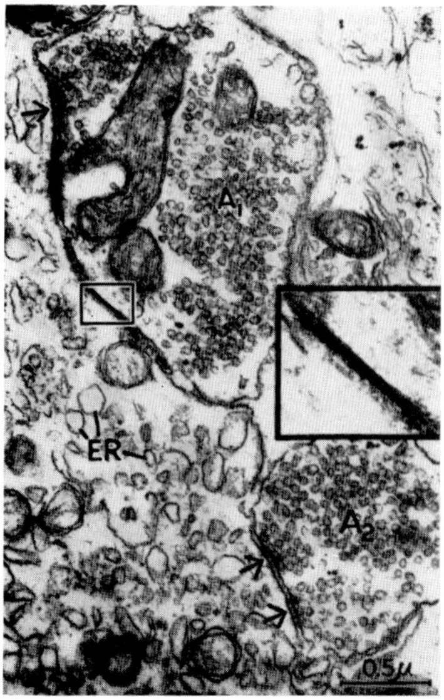


(a)

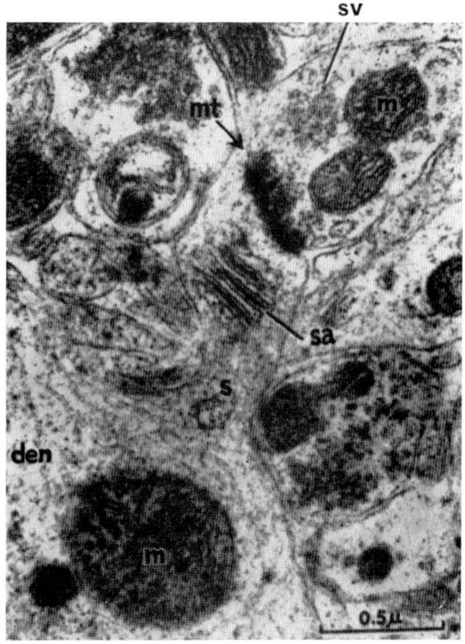


(b)

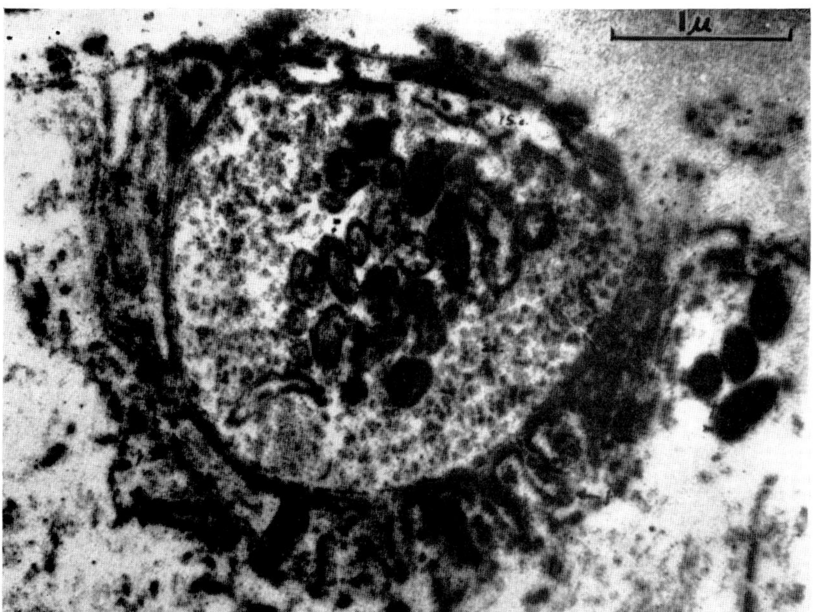


(c)

VII Ultrastructure of synapses (*See opposite*)

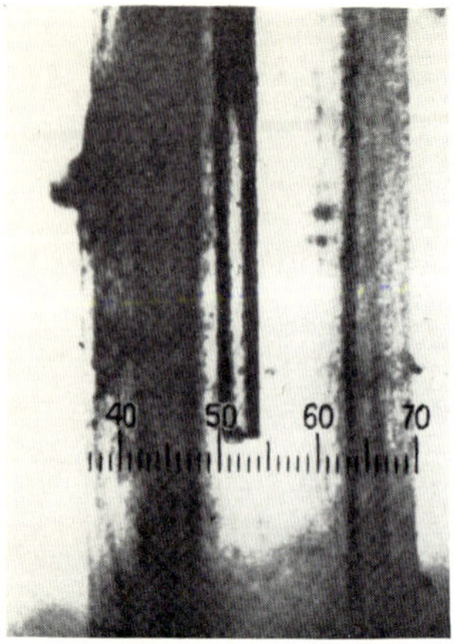


(a)

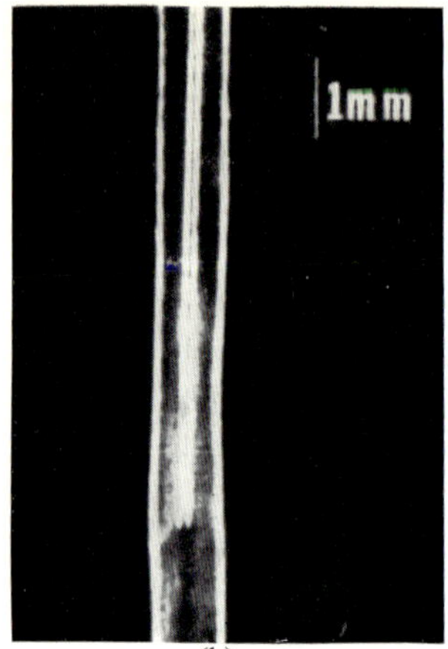


(b)

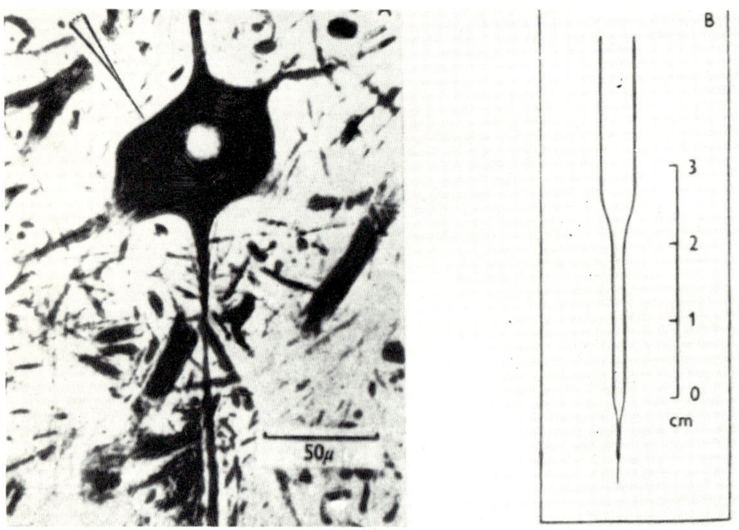


(c)

VIII Techniques for recording electrical phenomena in nerve cells

(a) and (b) Giant axons of the squid *Loligo forbesi* into which have been inserted glass microelectrodes. In (a) one division of the scale equals 33 microns. The giant axon shows as a translucent cylinder in the centre of the plate. The wall of the axon in (b) is largely composed of connective tissue, the unit membrane permeability barrier is invisible at this magnification. (From Hodgkin, A.L. (1964), 'The ionic basis of nervous conduction', *Science*, *145*, 1148–1153. Copyright 1964 by the American Association for the Advancement of Science.)

(c) Superimposed on this micrograph of a cat spinal motor neuron is a tracing of a microelectrode tip at the same magnification.
(From Brock, L. G., Coombs, J. S. and Eccles, J. C. (1952), 'Intracellular neuronal potentials', *J. Physiol.*, *117*, 431–460.)

This physiological outcome is believed to be responsible for some of the otherwise paradoxical effects physiologists and pharmacologists sometimes observe at synaptic junctions. The biasing action of one axon on another may also be of considerable significance in the adaptive changes responsible for learning. It is not difficult to see that the nerve pathways underlying a behavioural activity may be either facilitated or inhibited by junctions of this type.

## 6.6 The ionic bases of EPSPs and IPSPs

Let us next pursue the problems of synaptic transmission to their roots in biophysics and molecular biology. Let us see what has been discovered about the causes of EPSPs and IPSPs.

In Chapter 5 we saw that the resting potential across a nerve cell membrane is due to an asymmetrical distribution of ions. We saw, moreover, that sub-threshold depolarizations and the action potential itself were both caused by an alteration of this asymmetric *status quo*. Accordingly it will come as no surprise to learn that analogous mechanisms lie behind EPSPs and IPSPs.

First let us recall the anatomical structure of the synapse (section 4.5). It will be remembered that at least some of the vesicles observable in the synaptic knob are believed to contain acetyl-choline. Now it is well established that the terminations of motor neurons on muscles also contain acetyl-choline vesicles. The structure of a typical neuromuscular junction is shown in Fig. 6.8. The intricately folded region of the muscle fibre's membrane immediately beneath the nerve ending is called the motor end plate. These junctions are much more accessible than central synapses and hence more convenient to investigate. Accordingly much of the early work on synaptic transmission was carried out on these structures. Indeed these junctions are well qualified to be regarded as honorary synapses.

It can be shown that when an impulse reaches the nerve ending acetyl-choline cascades across on to the underlying muscle membrane which is, in consequence, depolarized. This depolarization is called an end-plate potential (EPP). In most vertebrate muscles the EPP initiates an action potential on the muscle membrane (sarcolemma) which, in turn, triggers the contractile machinery within. Neurophysiologists see the EPP as a close analogue of the EPSP. Hence they believe that the arrival of an impulse at the synaptic knob results in a shower of transmitter substance across the synaptic

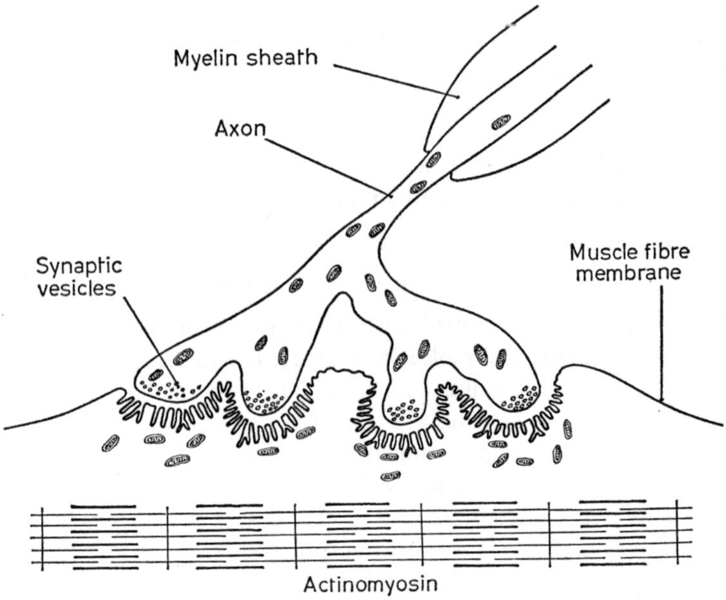


6.8 Ultrastructure of a myoneural junction. After Coens, C. (1967), 'Structure and organisation of the myoneural junction', *Int. Rev. of Cytol.*, *22*, 239–267.

gap. If the transmitter substance is acetyl-choline an EPSP results.

So far, so good. Arrival of an impulse at the pre-synaptic membrane in some way causes the synaptic vesicles, or some of them, to release their contained chemical. This rapidly diffuses across the 200A synaptic gap and depolarizes the post-synaptic membrane. But how is the depolarization, the EPSP, brought about? What is the mechanism?

Here we are very rapidly approaching the frontiers of present-day knowledge. No one can yet answer this question. No one can yet say what the precise mechanism is. It is known, however, that it is an ionic mechanism. It seems that the EPSP is caused by a total breakdown of the post-synaptic membrane's permeability barrier. Instead of being virtually impermeable to sodium ions the membrane suddenly becomes very leaky. Sodium ions, and with them potassium ions, chloride ions and all the other small inorganic ions in the vicinity can suddenly proceed along their electrochemical gradients. In consequence the potential difference across the membrane decreases towards zero.

In parenthesis here it is important to notice the difference between this mechanism and that underlying the action potential. The latter phenomenon, it will be remembered, is due to a sudden *selective* increase in permeability to a single ion—sodium. Hence a repolarization rather than a depolarization ensues.

How the post-synaptic membrane's impermeability is destroyed by acetyl-choline, or other excitatory transmitter substance, is as yet unknown. It is speculated that the excitatory transmitter in some way 'unplugs' pores in the post-synaptic membrane. Through these pores the various inorganic ions can then flux (Fig. 6.9).

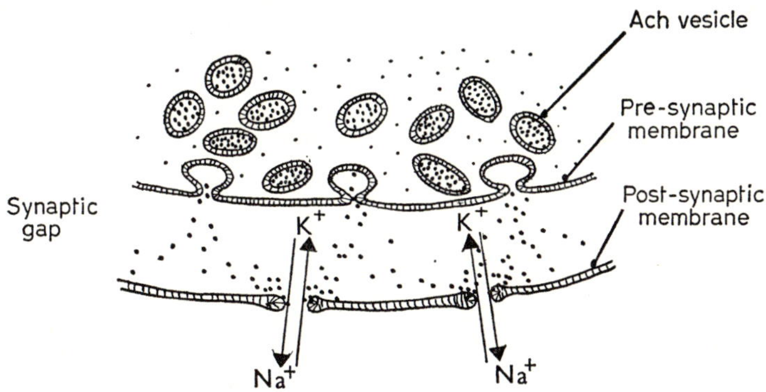


6.9 Biophysics of the EPSP. For explanation see text.

The action of acetyl-choline is very brief. An enzyme is present in the synaptic gap—cholinesterase—which very quickly cleaves acetylcholine into two parts. More will be said of this in the next section of this chapter.

Next let us look at the IPSP. Is there any evidence that an ionic mechanism is responsible for this synaptic potential also? The answer is yes. The IPSP is believed to be due to a very interesting case of selective permeability change. Instead of an increase in sodium permeability, as in the case of the action potential, the hyperpolarization of the IPSP is thought to be caused by a sudden increase in permeability to potassium and chloride ions.

It will be recalled from Chapter 5 that potassium is actively pumped *into* resting nerve cells against its electrochemical gradient. If the membrane were inactive with respect to potassium so that the concentrations inside and outside the neuron could be fitted into the Nernst equation a potential of about —93mV would be predicted

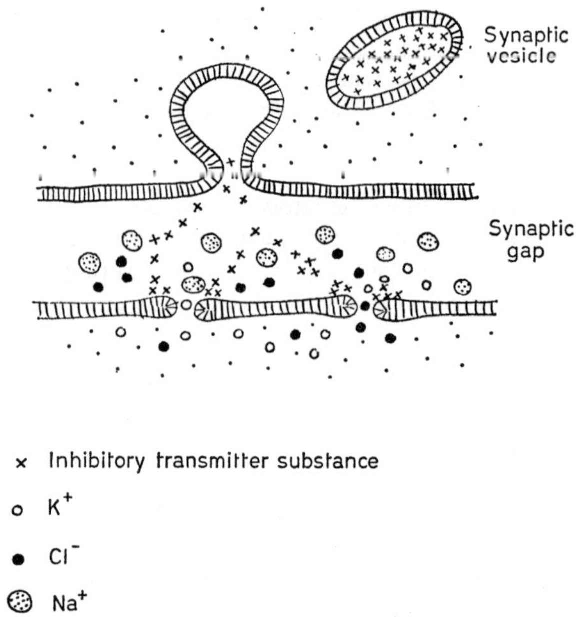


6.10 Biophysics of the IPSP. For explanation see text.

(see section 5.3). This is suggestive as it is towards this value that the membrane potential moves during the hyperpolarization of an IPSP. It is clear that if pores specific to potassium were to open in the post-synaptic membrane a hyperpolarization would ensue.

Now it is very interesting to note (Table 2.1) that the hydrated radius of the potassium ion is considerably less than that of the sodium ion. The chloride ion, which is very plentiful in the extra-cellular environment, is smaller still. J. C. Eccles and his colleagues provide evidence[1] to show that an IPSP is caused by the opening of pores in the post-synaptic membrane which are large enough for potassium and chloride, but too small for sodium. It looks as though the discrimination may be based merely on the relative magnitudes of the ions.

Fig. 6.10 shows, diagrammatically, that whilst potassium and chloride ions are able to move along their electrochemical gradients through the hypothetical pores, sodium, in its hydrated state, is prevented by its bulk. The fact that chloride ions move inwards at

[1] Eccles, J. C. (1964), loc. cit., p. 1145.

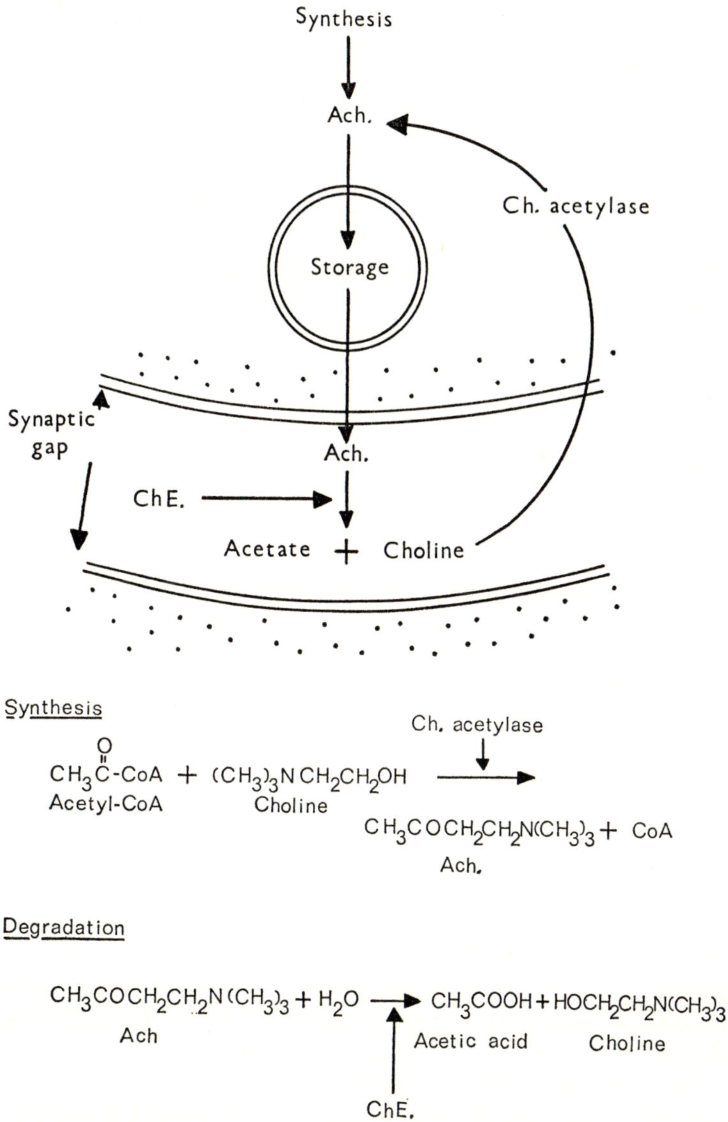


6.11 Biochemistry of a cholinergic synapse. Ach = acetyl choline, Ch. acetylase = choline acetylase, ChE = cholinesterase, CoA = Coenzyme A. For further explanation see text.

the same time as potassium ions move outwards probably accounts for the observation that the IPSP never reaches the potassium potential of about −93mV and, in fact, seldom exceeds −80mV.

Fig. 6.10 indicates that these narrow pores develop in response to an inhibitory transmitter. This transmitter is assumed to be stored in synaptic vesicles in a fashion analogous to acetyl-choline. This idea, however, remains an assumption as, so far, no inhibitory transmitter has been unquestionably identified in vertebrate central nervous systems. Indeed it is not impossible that the difference between inhibitory and excitatory synapses lies not so much in the transmitter involved as in the nature of the post-synaptic membrane (see section 9.3). Different post-synaptic membranes may be designed to react in different ways to the same transmitter substance.

Although there is no indubitable candidate for the rôle of inhibitory transmitter a large number of active chemicals have, nevertheless, been detected in the central nervous system. In addition to acetyl-choline these include nor-adrenalin (=nor-epinephrin), gamma-amino-butyric acid (=GABA), 5-hydroxytryptamine (=5-HT, or serotonin) and a number of acidic amino-acids—glutamic acid, aspartic acid, cysteic acid, etc. With the exception of acetyl-choline and nor-adrenalin none of these molecules has yet passed all the stringent tests required for full admission into the class of transmitter substances.[1] Much however is known of the pharmacology of acetyl-choline and nor-adrenalin and this will be outlined in the next section.

### 6.7 Pharmacology of acetyl-choline and nor-adrenalin

First let us consider the pharmacology of the best established central transmitter: acetyl-choline. We have already noticed that there is good evidence that this substance is stored in the synaptic vesicles of synaptic knobs. Let us now briefly look at its molecular life-history.

Fig. 6.11 schematizes this life-history. The major portion of the acetyl-choline in synaptic knobs is stored in the vesicles, but smaller quantities exist in the surrounding cytoplasm. When the acetyl-choline is liberated into the synaptic cleft it is very rapidly broken down to acetic acid and choline by the enzyme cholinesterase. Its

[1] Eccles, J. C., *The Physiology of Synapses*, Springer-Verlag, 1963, p. 190.

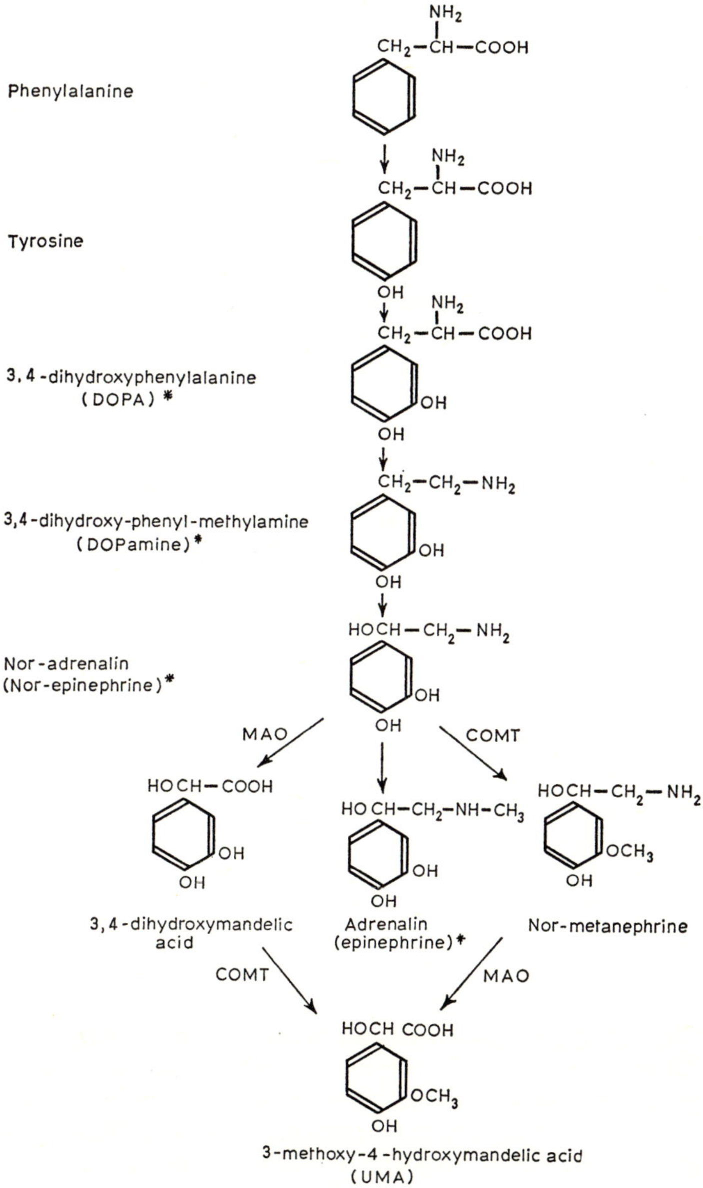


6.12 Biochemistry of nor-adrenalin and its relatives. Molecules with an asterisk against their name possess synaptic activity. COMT = catechol-o-mythyl transferase, MAO = monoamine oxidase.

effect on the post-synaptic membrane is thus very transient. It is not difficult to see that this is very important in the working of a nervous system.

The choline is reabsorbed into the synaptic knob and used over again for the synthesis of acetyl-choline. This resynthesis is catalysed by the enzyme choline-acetylase.

The molecular life-history of nor-adrenalin has also been well worked out. First let us look at the synthesis of this neurohumour. Fig. 6.12 shows that it is formed from the amino-acid phenylalanine. The figure also shows that it is related to quite a number of other neurally active molecules. These molecules are marked with asterisks.

Fig. 6.12 shows that all the neurally active molecules share a common ring structure:

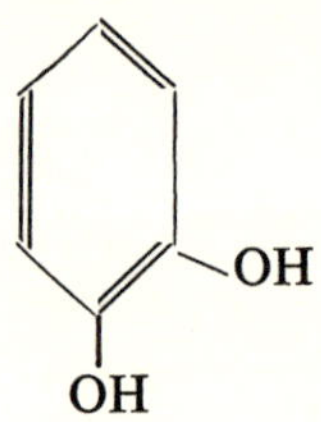


This ring is the substance catechol. Hence it is common to refer to the adrenalin-like molecules as catechol-amines. All the steps shown in Fig. 6.12 are catalysed by enzymes. Elimination or inhibition of any one of these enzymes prevents the synthesis of nor-adrenalin.

In the presynaptic terminals of neurons nor-adrenalin, like acetyl-choline, is believed, in the main, to be stored in vesicles. When an impulse arrives at the termination this nor-adrenalin is released into the synaptic gap. Here it is quickly acted upon by an enzyme—catechol-o-methyl transferase (COMT). COMT methylates nor-adrenalin and in so doing eliminates its synaptic activity. COMT thus plays a part at the adrenergic synapse which is precisely analogous to the part played by cholinesterase at the cholinergic synapse.

COMT is not the only enzyme to which nor-adrenalin may be exposed. Associated particularly with the mitochondria of the synaptic knob is another enzyme—monoamine oxidase (MAO). MAO oxidatively deaminates any free nor-adrenalin in the knob. The products of this oxidation again have no synaptic activity. We thus see that there is at least one very good reason for the sequestration of nor-adrenalin into synaptic vesicles.

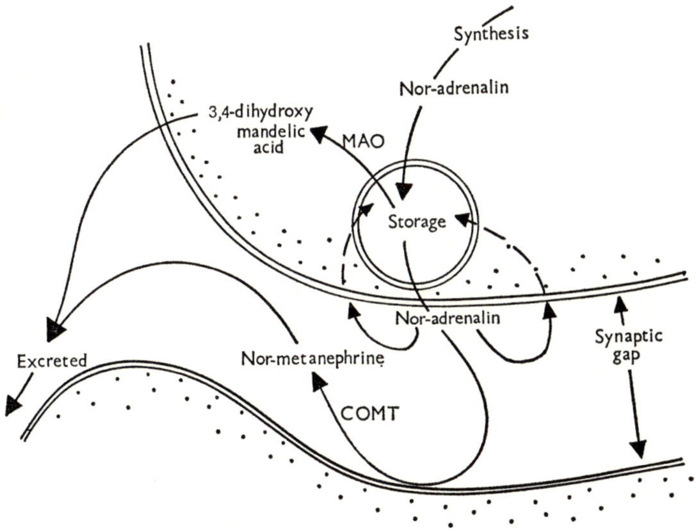


6.13 Biochemistry of an adrenergic synapse.
COMT = catechol-o-methyl transferase, MAO = monoamine oxidase. Further explanation in text.

Fig. 6.13 summarizes the pharmacology of an adrenergic synapse. Note that the arrows indicate that in addition to being destroyed by MAO and COMT some nor-adrenalin is transported back from the synaptic cleft into the vesicles.

These rather intricate transmitter life-histories have, of course, an interest in their own right; in the context of this book, however, they are of considerable significance as they allow the beginnings of an insight into the mechanisms of action of certain hallucinogenic drugs.

## 6.8 Aspects of neuropsychopharmacology

Hallucinogenic, or psychotomimetic, agents have attracted human attention since the beginnings of recorded history. This interest has shown no signs of slackening in more recent years. Let us first of all consider the substance whose effects Aldous Huxley described so graphically in *The Doors of Perception* and *Heaven and Hell*—mescalin.

Mescalin can be extracted from the peyote cactus of central America. The pre-Columban Indians chewing the dried plant were rewarded by hallucinations of a rich and varied nature. When, in later years, the chemical nature of mescalin was worked out a rather remarkable finding emerged. It turns out that the structural formula of mescalin is closely similar to that of nor-adrenalin. This relationship is shown in Fig. 6.14.

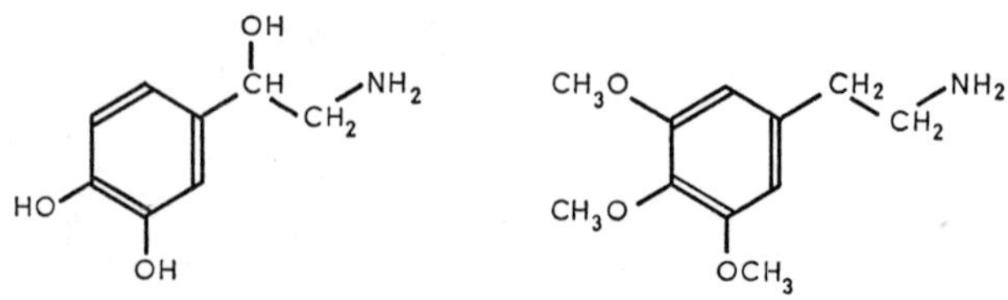


Nor-adrenalin Mescalin

6.14 Structural formulae of nor-adrenalin and mescalin.

It is not difficult to *speculate* that mescalin foxes one or both of the enzymes responsible for the breakdown of nor-adrenalin. The enzyme, mistaking the drug for its normal substrate, finds itself unable to catabolize it. The drug in consequence remains *in situ* blocking the enzyme's active site. Analogous cases of this so-called competitive inhibition are well known in other areas of biochemistry.

If this does indeed happen, and it must be emphasized that the idea is at present no more than a speculation, then nor-adrenalin might well begin to accumulate in the synaptic gap. This, in turn, might lead to increased rates of neuronal firing. The abnormal excitability might well be experienced as some form of vivid hallucination.

Another molecule which, as we saw earlier, is believed to have a transmitter function is 5-HT, or serotonin. This substance can be shown to have the same type of physiological effect as adrenalin although it is rather less powerful. The structural formula of serotonin is shown in Fig. 6.15.

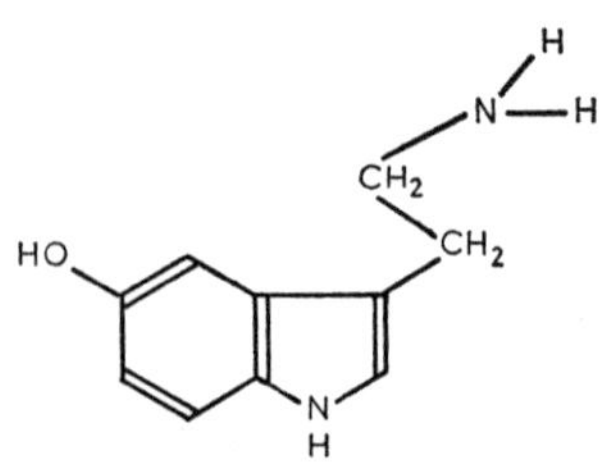


Serotonin

6.15 Structural formula of serotonin.

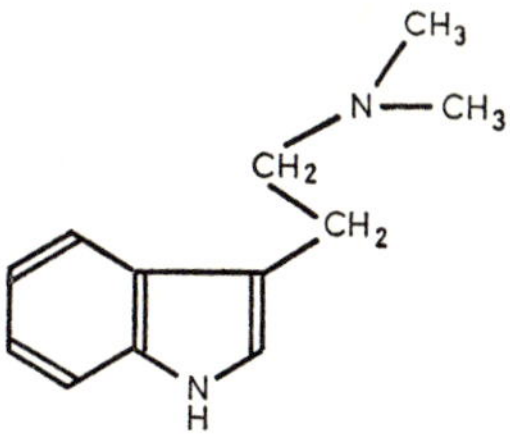

Bufotenine

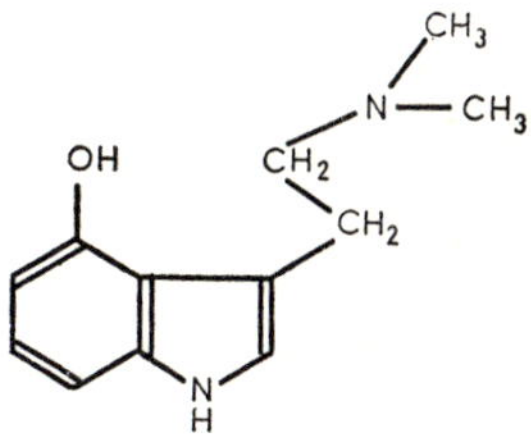

Psilocin

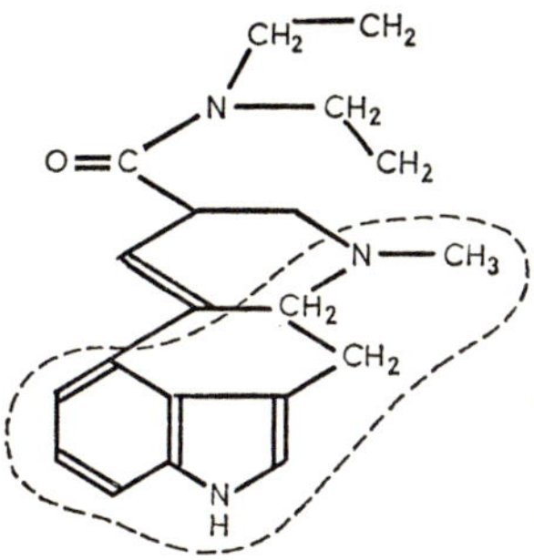

Lysergic acid diethylamide (LSD)

6.16 Structural formulae of some hallucinogenic compounds. The broken line surrounds that part of the LSD molecule which bears a stereochemical resemblance to serotonin. After Ediuson, S. (1967), 'The biochemistry of behaviour', *Science Journal*, *3*, 5, 113–117.

It is fascinating to find that certain structural features of this molecule appear in several psychoactive drugs. Many of these hallucinogens may be extracted from fungi.[1] They include bufotenine, psilocin and lysergic acid diethylamide (LSD). Fig. 6.16 shows the structural formulae of these drugs; comparison with Fig. 6.15 brings out their stereochemical similarity to serotonin.

Once again we may *speculate* that these drugs exert their psychical effects by competing with the enzymes and membranes which are normally involved in the metabolism and activity of serotonin. Of these psychotomimetic analogues of serotonin LSD is the most powerful. Pharmacologists have synthesized many variations on the

[1] Indeed Robert Graves suggests (*The Greek Myths, 1,* Penguin Books Ltd.) that nectar and ambrosia, the ancient 'foods of the gods', were in fact concoctions of edible fungi. Ingestion of the raw mushroom *Ananita muscaria* induces, he says, 'hallucinations, senseless rioting, prophetic sight, erotic energy and remarkable muscular strength', all characteristics, as Graves points out, of the reported exploits of the Maenads and Centaurs.

structural themes shown in Fig. 6.16 and examined their effects on behaviour. Several theories have been advanced to account for these effects and analogies have been drawn with such naturally occurring psychotic states as schizophrenia. The subject matter of neuropsychopharmacology, combining as it does the sciences of biochemistry, neurology and psychiatry, is at present the focus of intense research activity. However, to date, no well substantiated explanation of the action of hallucinogenic drugs exists.[1]

[1] Cohen, S. (1967), 'Psychotomimetic agents', *Ann. Rev. Pharmacol.*, *7*, 301-318.

# CHAPTER SEVEN

# The Sensory Input

'There is no conception in man's mind which hath not at first, totally or by parts, been begotten upon the organs of sense'.

THOMAS HOBBES, 1651.

## 7.1 Sense organs and brains

The concept of mind as *tabula rasa* in fact antedates Hobbes by millennia. Heraclitus in the fifth century B.C. held the same view. Knowledge, he writes, enters 'through the door of the senses'. The concept was also the accepted view of the Stoic philosophers of antiquity and the scholastic tag 'nihil est in intellectu quod non prius in sensu' gained wide currency in medieval times. However, the contrary idea—that knowledge is, to some extent at least, inborn—has also long had powerful advocates. The empiricist view of mind seems always to have been distasteful, as J. S. Mill noted,[1] to those enjoying or accepting hereditary privilege or authoritarian advantage.

It seems clear, however, that whatever inbuilt organization the brain may have a consideration of the sensory input remains an essential prerequisite for any understanding of how it works. Also it has been clear to zoologists since at least the time of Aristotle that sensation is very deeply interfused into the life and evolution of animals. Almost by definition an animal is sensitive: it reacts to environmental stimuli.

We have seen in the earlier chapters of this book that the world is full of a restless energy: it is full, in Whitehead's phrase, of a constant and unending 'stream of happenings'. It is the animal's part to respond to these happenings in an appropriate manner: a manner, in short, which ensures the prolongation of its individual life so that its progeny may perpetuate that of the species.

[1] Mill, J. S. (1873), *Autobiography*, Longmans Green, London, pp. 225–227.

We shall see in Chapter 10 that the brains of animals develop in very close association with the major sense organs. It is a large part of the brain's function to interpret the signals arriving from the sense organs, to sift their significance and biological relevance, and then to compute an appropriate response.

An animal without sense organs is therefore hardly an animal at all. All the dominant members of the kingdom have developed detectors responsive to all the main forms of environmental energy. In many cases these detectors have achieved a remarkable sensitivity and have developed into elaborate and intricate structures.

### 7.2 'Specific nerve energies' and the classification of sensory cells

It is likely that all cells are to some extent responsive to stimuli impinging on them from the environment. The idea that they should be so is closely bound in with our concept of what constitutes a living organism. The cells which act as receptors in the sense organs of higher animals have, however, developed this characteristic to a very high degree. For example, there is good evidence that the photoreceptor cells populating the human retina respond to a single photon of light. It is very interesting to note that the sensitive parts of vertebrate photoreceptor cells, and of a multitude of other receptor cells developed in the animal kingdom, are developed from modified cilia.[1] In a sense, therefore, it seems that from the first sensation and action have been united.

We noticed in section 4.2 that not all the cellular detectors developed by the animal kingdom are, strictly speaking, sensory cells. Indeed the majority of sense receptors in the animal kingdom are neurosensory cells. Even at the level of the mammals only the eye, ear and tongue develop true sensory cells.

However, whether we are examining a sensory or a neurosensory cell one important characteristic remains unaltered. This is that, within limits, each receptor cell responds to only one type of environmental energy flux.[2] An olfactory receptor is sensitive to certain chemical molecules, but not to photic or mechanical stimuli; vice

[1] Vinnikof, J. A. (1965), 'Principles of the structural, chemical and functional organisation of sensory receptors', *Cold Spring Harbor Symposium, 30*, 293–300.

[2] Sensory receptors may be stimulated by stimuli other than those for which they are designed if the former are intense. We have all 'seen stars' after the receipt of a blow on the eyes.

versa, photoreceptor cells are responsive to electromagnetic radiation of certain wavelengths but not to chemical substances in solution.

This devotion of receptor cells to one specific type of energy, to one specific sense modality, is clearly vital to the efficient working of the brain. Consider, for example, the neurophysiological correlatives of admiring the night sky. Jessica may well have been adjured by Lorenzo to note

> '. . . how the floor of heaven
> Is thick inlaid with patines of bright gold'

but the starlight falling on her retinae is transduced into something far more prosaic: patterns of action potentials ascending her optic nerve fibres. Similarly if she could have heard the harmony implicit in 'each smallest orb' this, too, would, on reaching her cochlea, have been transduced into action spikes.

The point, of course, is that one action potential is very much like another. Impulses in the auditory nerve are very similar to those in the optic nerve. Indeed it has been suggested that by re-routing the optic and auditory nerves we should hear lightning as thunder, and see thunder as lightning! Only by a system of 'labelled' lines can the brain distinguish different sense modalities. We shall return to this point in Chapter 11 where we look at some of the fascinating 're-wiring' experiments carried out by Sperry and others.

Clearly, then, the restriction of a sensory cell's sensitivity to just one form of environmental energy is of considerable importance to the physiology of the brain. This restriction also allows us to classify receptors into various different classes.

One type of classificatory division groups receptor cells into exteroreceptors and enteroreceptors. The former monitor changes in the 'external' environment, whereas the latter respond to changes in the 'internal' environment. Another type of classification groups sense organs according to the type of energy flux to which they are sensitive. Thus we can recognize chemoreceptors, mechanoreceptors, photoreceptors, thermoreceptors,etc.

Now whereas distinctions between sense modalities depend, as we have seen, on a system of 'labelled lines', differences in the intensity of a given stimulus are signalled by modulating the frequency of the sensory impulses. In very general terms, the more intense the stimulus the higher is the frequency with which impulses ascend the sensory nerve.

In fact the precise relationship between sensory stimulus and impulse frequency is quite complicated. First we have to take into account the phenomenon of sensory adaptation. It is found, as we shall see more fully later in this chapter, that the frequency of impulses in a sensory nerve exposed to a constant stimulus falls off with time. Second, it can be shown that the increase in sensory magnitude due to an increase in stimulus intensity is related to the intensity of the original stimulus. The sound of a coin dropping on the pavement beside an active pneumatic drill will hardly be heard. The sound of a similar coin dropping on the pavement in the still reaches of the night might well be heard at some distance. This phenomenon was put on a quantitative basis by Weber in the nineteenth century. Weber's law is expressed by equation 7.1 where $I$ is the intensity of the initial stimulus, $\Delta I$ is the smallest discriminable increment in intensity and $k$ is a constant:

$$\Delta I/I = k \qquad \ldots\ldots (7.1)$$

It is nowadays recognized that Weber's law is only correct to a first approximation. The true situation is rather more complicated. However Weber's formulation brings out the essence of the matter and the development of information theory over the last two or three decades has provided an explanation for his law. For we can now see that sensory nerves are, in the terms of information theory, 'noisy' channels. The brain has to decide whether any variation in the frequency of incoming signals is due to random, spontaneous fluctuations or due to a genuine alteration in the stimulus. The more intense the initial stimulus the greater will be the 'spread' of impulse frequencies reaching the brain. Thus the more intense the initial stimulus, i.e. the louder the road drill, the greater the increment must be before the brain recognizes it as significant.

### 7.3 The biophysics of sensory transduction

Let us now look at the business of sensory transduction a little more closely. This is, as usual, much easier said than done. Sensory and neurosensory cells are, on the whole, rather small and often rather inaccessible. In consequence a deep analysis of how environmental energy is transduced into patterns of action potentials in sensory neurons has been accomplished in only a small number of cases.

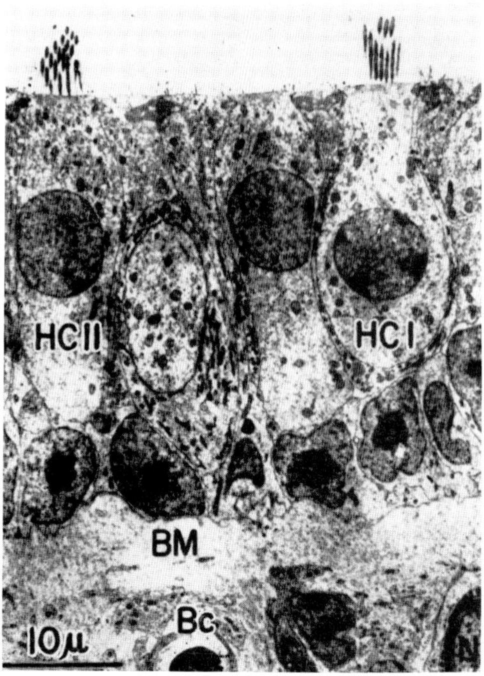


IX Some sensory cells (i)

(a) Hair cells in the crista ampullaris of the semicircular canal of a guinea-pig's ear. Two types of hair cell (HCI and HCII) are shown surrounded by supporting cells. BM = basement membrane, Bc = blood capillary. (From Wersall, J. and Flock, A. (1965) 'Functional anatomy of the labyrinth' in *Contributions to Sensory Physiology*, Vol. 1, Academic Press, 1965.)

(b) Cells of the olfactory epithelium of rabbit (× 10,000). The dendrites (D) of the neurosensory cells end in a number of modified cilia (broken in this electron micrograph). These cilia are the chemosensitive elements of the neurosensory cells. Sandwiched between the neurosensory cells are supporting cells containing numerous vesicles and distorted mitochondria. OR = olfactory rod (From de Lorenzo, A. J. (1957), 'Electron microscopic observations on the olfactory mucosa and olfactory nerve', *J. Biophys. Biochem. Cytol., 3,* 839–850. Reprinted by permission of the Rockefeller University Press.)

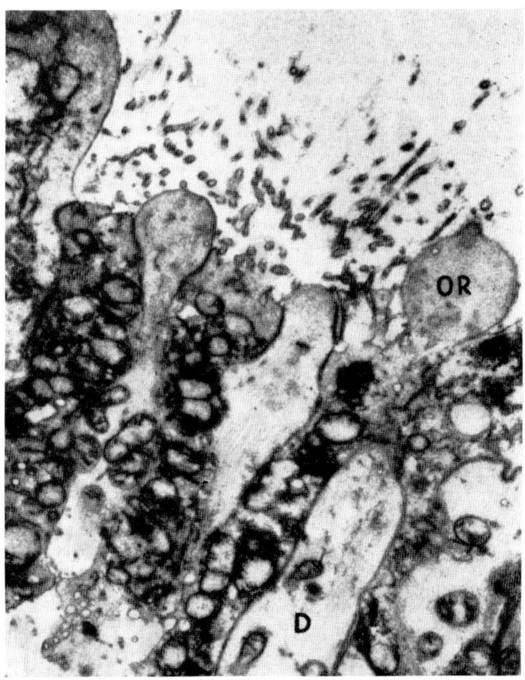

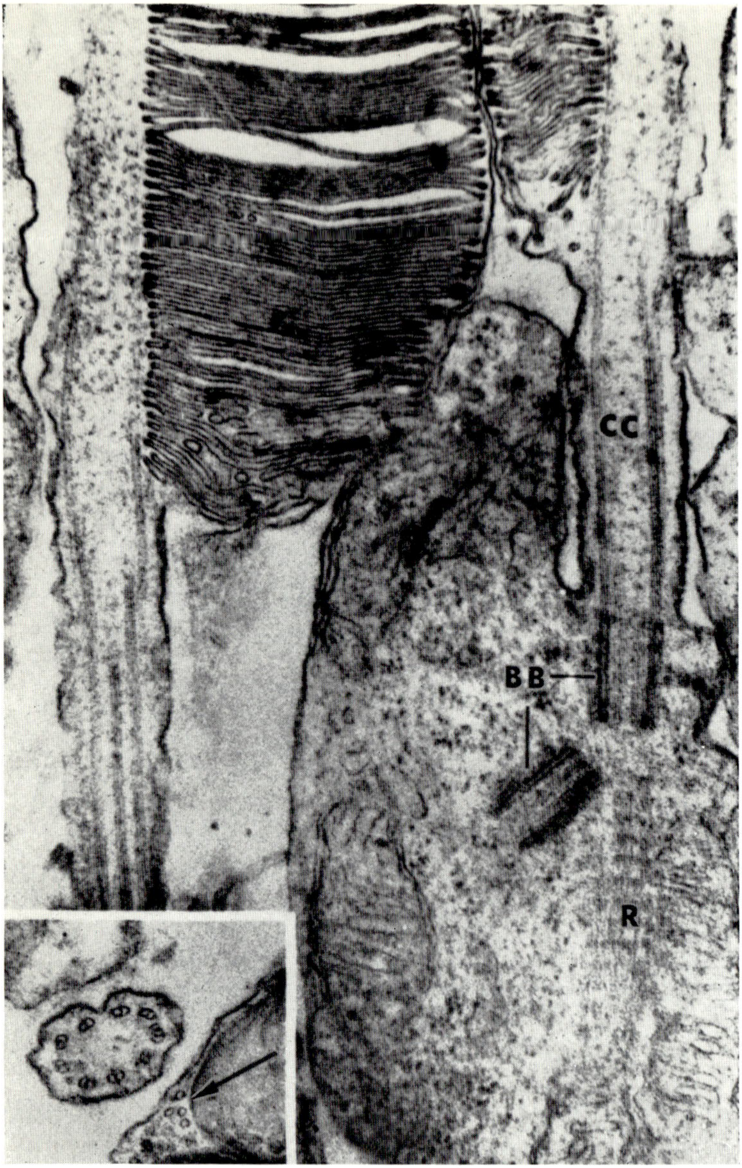


X Some sensory cells (ii)

Electron micrograph (× 48,000) of the junction between inner and outer segments of a vertebrate retinal rod cell (compare Fig. 7.9). The rod discs are well-shown in the upper left-hand part of the plate. Inset is a transverse section through a connecting cilium and portion of an outer segment. BB = basal bodies; CC = connecting cillium; R = rootlet fibre.

(From Dowling, J. E. (1967), 'The organisation of vertebrate visual receptors', Figure 4 in *Molecular Organisation and Biological Function,* edited by John M. Allen. Copyright © 1967 by John M. Allen. Reprinted by permission of Harper and Row, Publishers, Inc.)

Chief among these have been certain mechanoreceptors and the *Limulus* photoreceptor. There seems no reason, however, to suppose that the biophysical mechanisms shown to obtain in these cells should not also obtain in the majority of sensory and neurosensory cells.

First let us look at the fascinating work carried out on the stretch receptors of certain decapod crustacea. In the abdomena of many of these animals are to be found large extensor and flexor muscles. Anyone who has observed how a crayfish, a prawn or a lobster eludes its would-be captor by darting backwards with strong contractions of its abdominal segments, will understand the significance of these muscles.

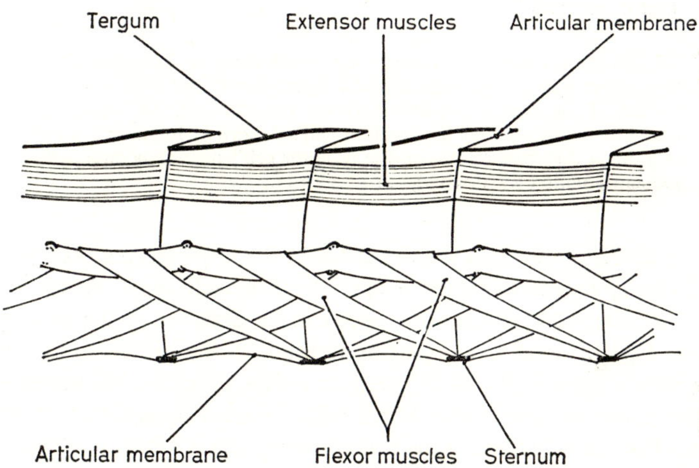


7.1 Abdominal muscles of the crayfish. The rather complicated system of muscles is drawn from the side. Contraction of the extensor muscles straightens the abdomen; contraction of the flexor muscles causes the abdomen to bend beneath the cephalothorax thus shooting the animal backwards out of danger. After Parker, T. J. and Haswell, W. A. (1949), *A Text-Book of Zoology, Vol. 1*, Fig. 369, Macmillan and Co. Ltd., London.

For accurate handling of this important musculature the crustacean nervous system requires precise information on the state of contraction of each muscle. This information is largely provided by stretch receptor cells situated in the extensor muscles. These cells are comparatively large and easily accessible.

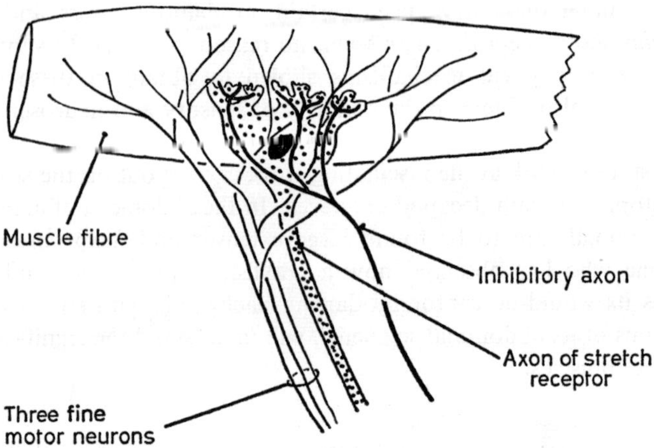


7.2 Schematic diagram of a crustacean stretch receptor. Branches of the thin motor nerve fibres shown in the figure ramify not only over the surface of the muscle but also over the receptor cell. An inhibitory fibre also branches over the receptor cell's dendrites. Impulses travelling down this fibre repolarize the receptor cell's membrane and consequently inhibit the discharge of sensory impulses.

Figure 7.2 shows that the dendrites of the large mechanoreceptor cell ramify extensively over a specialized muscle fibre. When this fibre is put under tension impulses can be detected in the sensory axon. Fig. 7.2. also shows that in addition to the neurosensory cell the muscle fibre is also innervated by motor fibres. In life impulses arriving down these motor fibres will initiate a contraction in the specialized muscle fibre. If the rest of the muscle in which this fibre is embedded is not also contracting to the same degree the specialized fibre will find itself under tension. This fact, as we saw, is signalled to the central nervous system. We shall find in Chapter 9 that an analogous mechanism controls the contraction of our own muscles.

Because this mechanoreceptor is large and accessible several important physico-chemical parameters can be examined. It is possible, for example, to subject the extensor muscle to varying degrees of stretch and to record the frequency of nerve impulses in the axon. It is also possible to introduce a microelectrode into the receptor cell and record any change of potential across its membrane. The results of such experiments throw much light on the physiology and biophysics of receptor cells.

First it can be shown that the impulse frequency in the sensory axon is roughly proportional to the degree of tension applied to the muscle. Second, if the tension on the fibre is maintained at a constant value it is found that the frequency of impulses in the sensory axon falls off with time. This, as we saw earlier in this chapter, is called sensory adaptation, and is characteristic of all sensory systems. These two features of a sense receptor are shown in Fig. 7.3.

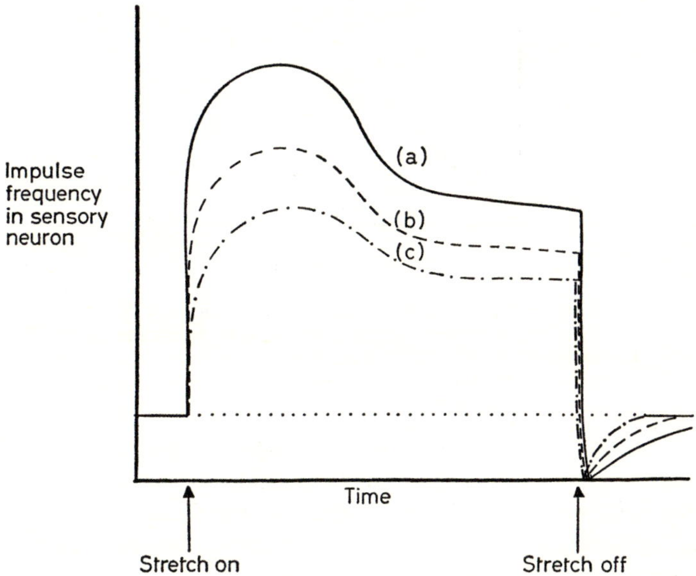


7.3 Impulse frequency in a sensory neuron. The figure shows the impulse frequency in a fibre from the frog's skin when the latter is subjected to three different degrees of tension: (a), (b) and (c). For further explanation see text. After Loewenstein, W. R. (1956), 'Excitation and changes in adaptation by stretch of mechanoreceptors', *J. Physiol.*, *133*, 588–602.

Next let us look at the results of microelectrode recording from the mechanoreceptor. It is very interesting to find that when stretching forces are applied the membrane of the receptor cell is depolarized. The more the fibre is stretched the greater is the depolarization. This electrical change across the sense cell's membrane is called a generator potential. Fig. 7.4 shows how the generator potential varies with the applied tension.

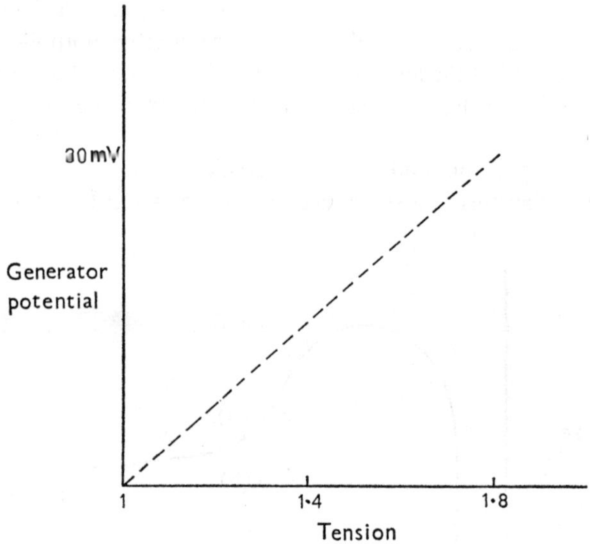


7.4 A straight line relation obtains between tension and depolarization of the crustacean stretch receptor cell membrane. After Loewenstein, W. R. (1965), 'Facets of a transducer process', in *Cold Spring Harbor Symposium on Quantitative Biology*, *XXX*, Cold Spring Harbor, L.I., New York.

Clearly we have here a situation analogous to the EPSPs we discussed when describing synaptic transmission in Chapter 6. It is not difficult to see in the light of our discussion in Chapter 5 that when the depolarization reaches or exceeds a certain threshold an action potential is initiated in the sensory axon.

A similar understanding of the molecular basis of receptor activity has emerged from the study of the Pacinian corpuscle. Pacinian corpuscles are pressure receptors located in mammalian mesenteries. They are very sensitive, being stimulated by displacements of as little as 0·5μ applied over 0·1 msecs. Their histological structure is interesting. Fig. 7.5 shows that they somewhat resemble a minute onion—the sensitive nerve ending is covered by concentric layers of connective tissue.

It has been shown that the sensitive element in this receptor is the unmyelinated axon tip right in the centre of the 'onion'. Slight deformation of the 'onion' causes a depolarization of the axon tip, causes, in other words, a generator potential. Again, as in the case of the crustacean stretch receptor, the generator potential is proportional to the strength of the stimulus. The local circuit (see Chapter 5) which results may, if it is of sufficient intensity, depolarize the axonal membrane at the first node of Ranvier. If this depolarization brings the membrane below its threshold an action spike is initiated which propagates itself in the usual way along the sensory axon to the central nervous system.

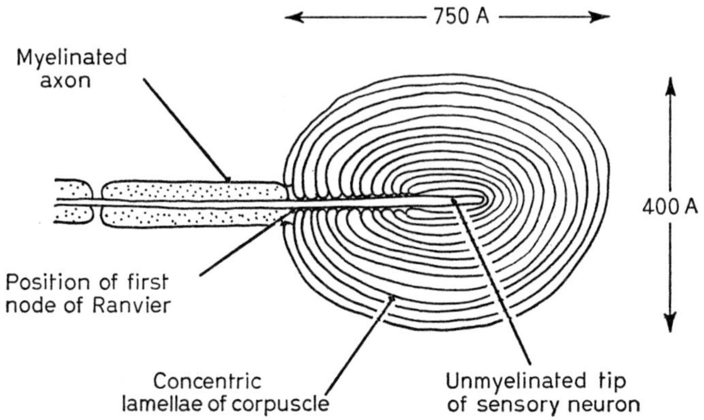


7.5 Sectional view of a Pacinian corpuscle.

The two receptors so far discussed have both been neurosensory cells. However in many important cases sensory rather than neurosensory cells are deployed to detect the environmental energy flux. Let us first examine an example of a mechanoreceptive sensory cell.

In many groups of animals, including the vertebrates, mechanoreceptive cells called hair cells are developed. In many fish, for example, a system of grooves—the lateral line system—develops in the epidermis of the skin. Within this system groups of hair cells are to be found. These cells (Fig. 7.6) respond to pressure changes, particularly low frequency vibrations, in the surrounding water.

There is evidence[1] that the hairs springing from these receptor cells are modified cilia. Whatever their origin it can be shown that if they are distorted the cell is stimulated. The cell's response consists in a depolarization of the boundary membrane. Because it is not a neurosensory cell this depolarization cannot lead *directly* to an action potential and hence, instead of being called a generator potential, it is termed a *receptor* potential.

Fig. 7.6 shows that the dendron of a sensory neuron ends in close

[1] Vinnikof, J. A. (1965), *loc. cit.*

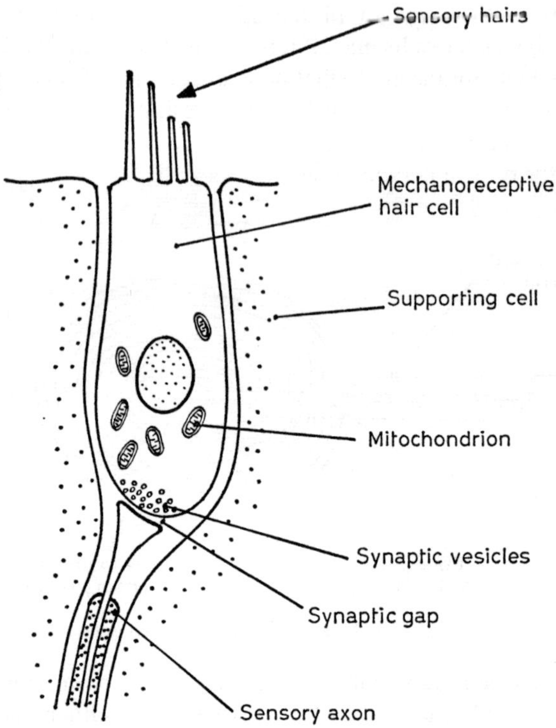


7.6 Ultrastructure of a mechanoreceptive hair cell.

proximity to the sensory cell. It is believed that when the sensory cell is stimulated it releases a chemical transmitter across the synaptic gap on to the underlying dendron. The sequence of events following stimulation of the receptor cell may thus be schematized in the following way:

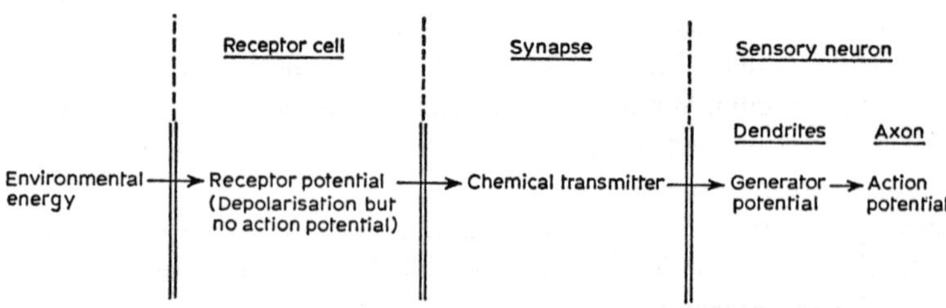


7.7 Summary of events leading to the transduction of environmental energy into the energy of action potentials in sensory nerve fibres. Simplified from Davis, H. (1961), 'Some principles of sensory receptor action', *Physiol. Rev.*, *41*, 391–416.

It is interesting to find that hair cells very similar to those developed in the lateral line canals of fish are to be found in all orders of vertebrate animals. However, instead of providing a general epidermal sensitivity to vibration the hair cells of higher vertebrates are confined to the chambers of the inner ear. Here they play vastly important rôles in detecting acceleration of the head in any of the three dimensions of space, in ascertaining the orientation of the head with respect to gravity and last, but very far from least, in responding to the atmospheric pressure waves which we experience as sound. Some account of this last function will be given in later chapters of this book.

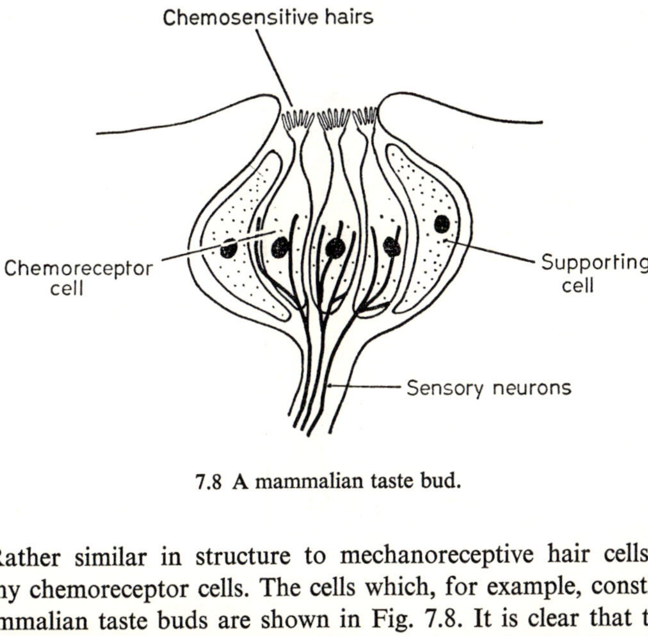


7.8 A mammalian taste bud.

Rather similar in structure to mechanoreceptive hair cells are many chemoreceptor cells. The cells which, for example, constitute mammalian taste buds are shown in Fig. 7.8. It is clear that these cells, like the mechanoreceptors discussed above, develop long hair-like projections. It is believed that these are modified cilia once more and it can be shown that they are the chemosensitive parts of the cell. Despite much research and many theories a physico-chemical basis for the excitation of chemoreceptors has, however, yet to be established.

Yet another type of sensory cell whose sensitive region is developed from a cilium is the photosensitive rod and cone cell of vertebrate retinae. The cilium of this type of sensory cell becomes, however, very extensively modified and in the adult retina is nearly unrecognizable. It seems that the membrane of the cilium grows enormously and invaginates to form a series of lamellae or discs. These discs (Fig. 7.9) have been likened to a stack of pennies. The visual pigments (rhodopsin or iodopsin) are believed to be built into these discs and are thus exposed in a very advantageous manner to incoming electromagnetic radiation. Interaction of a photon of appropriate wavelength with the visual pigment leads to a photochemical reaction which, in turn, results in a receptor potential in the rod or cone. A chemical transmitter then excites the bipolar neuron synapsing with the base of the photoreceptor cell. The ensuing events are considered in some detail in Chapters 8 and 14.

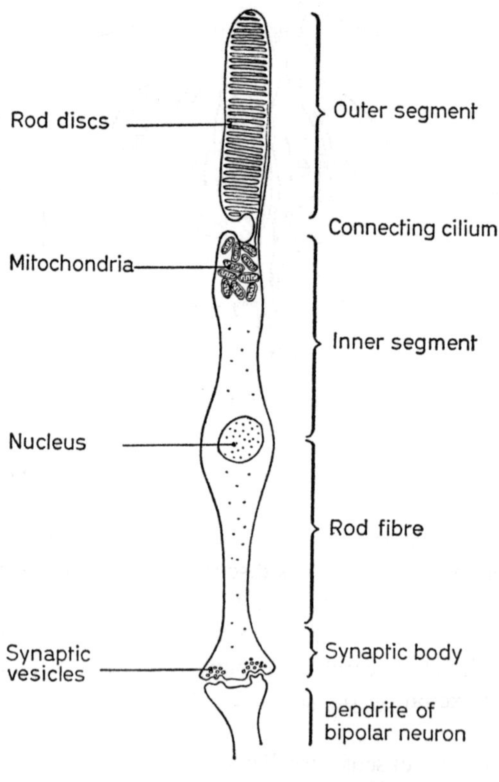


7.9 The rod cell of vertebrate retinae.

Vertebrate photoreceptor cells are, however, very minute and rather inaccessible. In consequence it is difficult to determine their biophysical and physiological properties. Much more amenable to such investigations are the photoreceptor cells to be found in the carapace of *Limulus* the King or Horseshoe crab. These photoreceptor cells are parts of the animal's primitive compound eyes. More will be said of the anatomy and physiology of these eyes in Chapter 8. Here we may note that each compound eye consists of a

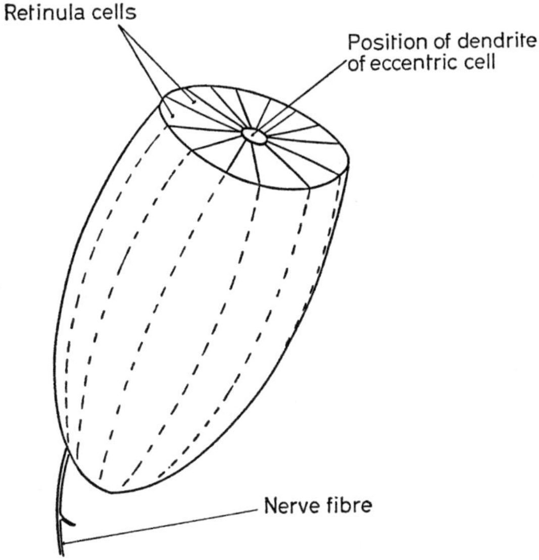


7.10 Schematic diagram to show the arrangement of retinula cells in the ommatidium of *Limulus.*

number of small groups of photoreceptor cells. The photoreceptor cells are called retinula cells. Fig. 7.10 shows that a dozen or so retinula cells form the walls of a cylinder surrounding the dendrite of a so-called eccentric cell. This group of cells constitutes the functional unit of the compound eye and is called an ommatidium.

The eccentric cell whose dendrite forms the centre of the ommatidium is in fact a sensory neuron. Its axon transmits impulses towards the central nervous system.

Fig. 7.11 shows a *Limulus* ommatidium cut in longitudinal section. It can be seen that where each retinula cell abuts the central dendrite its membrane is developed into a large number of minute finger-like

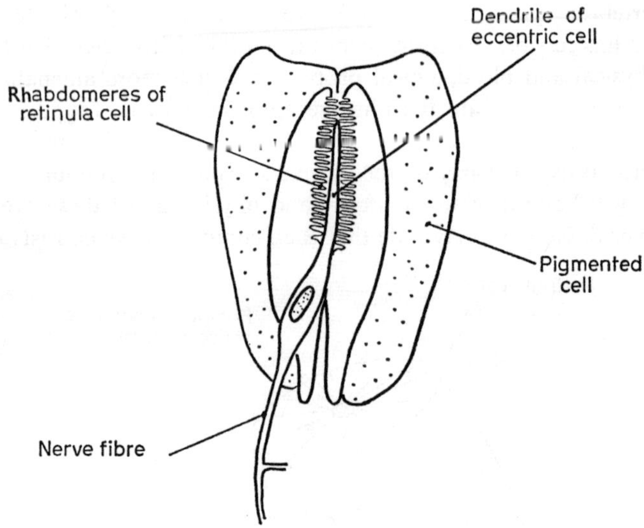


7.11 Longitudinal section of *Limulus* ommatidium. After Davis, H. (1961), *loc. cit.*

processes. These processes are called rhabdomeres. The rhabdomeres of all twelve retinula cells form a region of the ommatidium called the rhabdom. Incident light is focused on to the rhabdom.

There is evidence that a visual pigment similar to rhodopsin is concentrated in the rhabdom. As in the case of vertebrate rod or cone cells an electromagnetic photon of the appropriate wavelength causes a photochemical change in this pigment. This, in turn, leads to a depression in the membrane potential of the retinula cells. Because the eye of *Limulus* is very simple, possessing large and easily accessible retinula cells, this receptor potential can be recorded by microelectrode techniques. Its physico-chemical characteristics are found to be precisely similar to those of the generator potentials we discussed earlier in this section.

Next it can be shown that the development of a receptor potential in the retinula cells leads to a depolarization in the adjacent dendrite. In other words it can be shown to cause a generator potential in the eccentric cell which, if it is of sufficient magnitude, initiates an action potential in the axon. Thus in the compound eye of *Limulus* the sequence of events schematized in Fig. 7.7 can be followed in detail by the physiologist's microelectrode.

# CHAPTER EIGHT

# Systems of Receptor Cells

## 8.1 Information processing in sense organs

In Chapter 7 we saw how the organism is provided with an extensive array of detectors for monitoring the situation obtaining both within and without the body. We saw, moreover, that the various forms of environmental energy were transduced into a single common code: frequency modulated action potentials. By distinguishing between activated and quiet sensory fibres the brain keeps itself informed of which form of environmental energy is interacting with which part of the body.

This account of sensory reception is, however, badly oversimplified. It covers the very simplest of pain and touch receptors where an approximately one-to-one translation of the environmental stress is communicated to the brain. For all the more sophisticated receptors, however, the situation is very considerably more complicated. The senses of hearing and sight, for example, are mediated by complicated sense organs where large teams of sensory cells work together. In the case of the eye, moreover, considerable manipulation and reorganization of the raw 'sense data' occurs actually within the sense organ before any signals are made to the brain. In general, as we shall see, the information communicated to the brain is preselected for its biological relevance. Unimportant and trivial features are weeded out. The brain, like the headquarters of an industrial or political organization, is shielded from insignificant and petty detail. Its decision is required only on matters of importance.

Before, however, examining the physiology of the retina let us look briefly at the rather simpler case of the mammalian ear. This organ is the *ne plus ultra* of mechanoreceptors. Its cells are believed to be responsive to displacements of as little as $10^{-10}$ cms.

## 8.2 The mammalian ear

In Chapter 7 we discussed the biophysical characteristics of some mechanoreceptors. In particular we considered the characteristics of 'hair cells'. It will be remembered that distortion of the hair leads to a receptor potential which, in turn, causes a generator potential and then an action potential in the subjacent sensory nerve fibre.

Now it has long been known that the mammalian sense of hearing depends on arrays of mechanoreceptive hair cells. These cells develop within the cochlea of the inner ear. This organ is normally coiled rather like a minute snail's shell (Fig. 8.1 (a) ). In essence, however, the cochlea is a long tube divided into three canals by a couple of membranes (Fig. 8.1 (b) ).

Fig. 8.1 (c) shows that the hair cells are situated on the basilar membrane. A flap of gelatinous material—the tectorial membrane—rests on the mechanoreceptive hairs. When the vibration which is the physical basis of sound reaches the inner ear the basilar membrane is caused to oscillate. In comparison the tectorial membrane remains fairly stationary. It follows that the sensitive hairs of the hair cells are alternately stretched and compressed. This stress is enough to stimulate them and thus to set up impulses in the fibres of the cochlear nerve which ramify about their bases.

The mammalian ear can, however, do much more than merely detect the presence or absence, the strength or weakness, of a sound. It is also able to discriminate accurately between different pitches or,

---

8.1 The mammalian cochlea. In (a) the relation of the cochlea to the rest of the ear is shown. In (b) the coiled cochlea is straightened out so that the relative positions of the various membranes and cavities can be more easily seen. Lastly, in (c), the cochlea is cut in transverse section so that the organ of Corti, consisting of the tectorial membrane and the hair cells springing from the basilar membrane, can be shown. Atmospheric vibrations channelled down the external auditory meatus to the tympanic membrane (ear drum) are transmitted across the middle ear chamber by the three auditory ossicles: the malleus, incus and stapes. Vibration of the stapes causes the membrane covering the oval window to vibrate and this, in turn, causes pressure changes in the fluid (perilymph) filling the scala vestibuli. These oscillations of pressure are transmitted through the vestibular membrane to the fluid (endolymph) filling the scala media. This leads to oscillations of the basilar membrane and the variation in pressure is thus transmitted to the perilymph of the scala tympani and finally results in movement of the membrane covering the round window. The latter membrane thus moves in a direction opposite to that of the membrane covering the oval window. In this way the hair cells on the basilar membrane, whose ends are attached to the comparatively stationary tectorial membrane, are subjected to an oscillating stimulus as is explained further in the text.

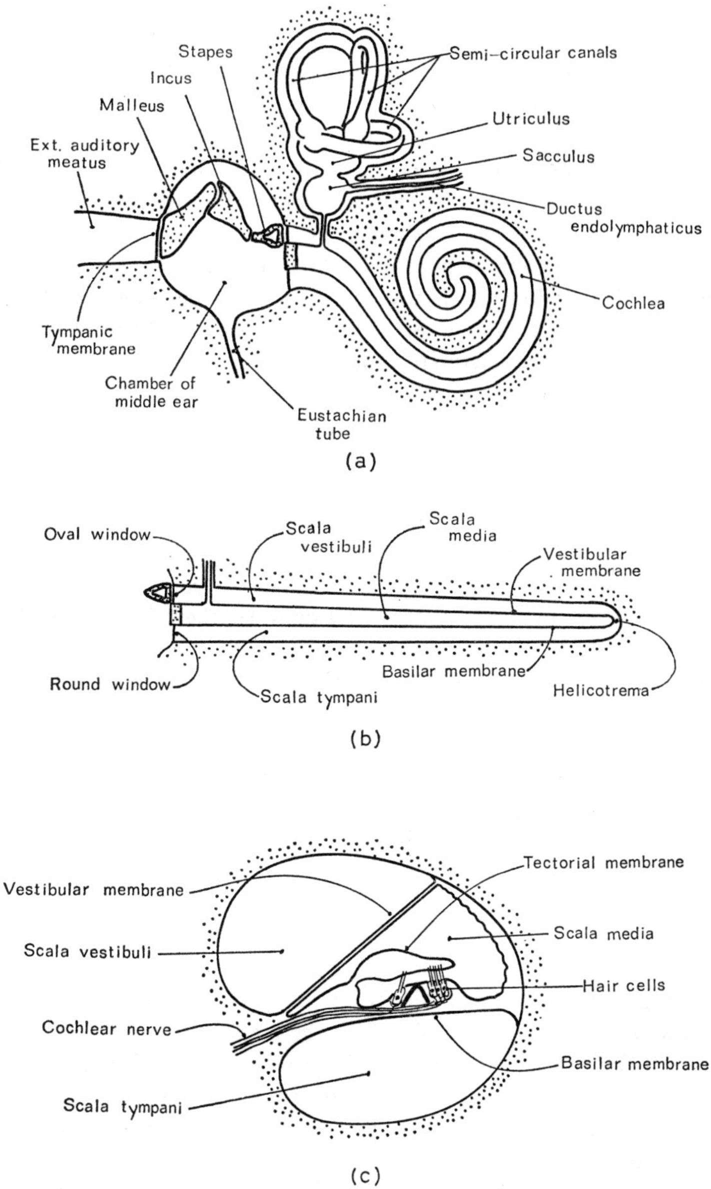
Stapes
Incus
Malleus
Ext. auditory meatus
Semi-circular canals
Utriculus
Sacculus
Ductus endolymphaticus
Cochlea
Tympanic membrane
Chamber of middle ear
Eustachian tube
(a)
Oval window
Scala vestibuli
Scala media
Vestibular membrane
Round window
Scala tympani
Basilar membrane
Helicotrema
(b)
Vestibular membrane
Scala vestibuli
Cochlear nerve
Scala tympani
Tectorial membrane
Scala media
Hair cells
Basilar membrane
(c)

*Fig. 8.1*

to use physical terms, frequencies. The precise way in which it draws these important distinctions is not yet fully understood. However although the detailed physiology remains obscure the general type of mechanism adopted is fairly well established. Indeed it was in essence worked out by Helmholtz as far back as the mid-nineteenth century. It depends on the fact that the position at which maximal oscillation of the basilar membrane occurs varies with the incoming sound frequency. It can be shown, for example, that high frequency sounds cause maximal vibration toward the base of the basilar membrane, whereas low frequency sounds lead to maximal oscillation near the helicotrema (Fig. 8.1 (b) ). It follows that different groups of hair cells will be maximally stimulated by different frequencies of sound. By attending to which auditory nerve fibres are firing and which are quiescent the brain is able to discriminate between notes varying in pitch.

Frequency discrimination has been developed to a very high degree in both mammals and birds. Humans can distinguish between tones of 1000 c/s and 1003 c/s. Clearly this ability is of considerable importance to the many higher vertebrates which use sound as a means of communication. We shall consider the topic of auditory perception further in Chapter 14 where we shall see that the information transmitted by the cochlea is 'sharpened up' by the auditory centres in the brain.

When we turn to the next of the important sensory organs—the eye—we find that much of the sharpening and sifting of sensory information occurs not in the brain but in the sense organ itself. Perhaps this is not altogether surprising as the vertebrate retina is derived from a part of the brain.

### 8.3 Some invertebrate retinae

The vertebrate retina, as we shall see in Chapter 10, is derived from an outgrowth of the forebrain. It is a portion of the brain pushed out to the periphery and specialized for the handling of visual information. It follows that its structure is very intricate. Before beginning an examination of this highly complex tissue it will be wise to look at some of the far simpler retinae developed by invertebrates.

One of the very simplest of invertebrate retinae is developed by the nudibranch mollusc *Hermissenda*. This retina consists of only five photoreceptor cells (Fig. 8.2). In comparison a vertebrate retina may consist of several tens of millions of photoreceptors. Yet in

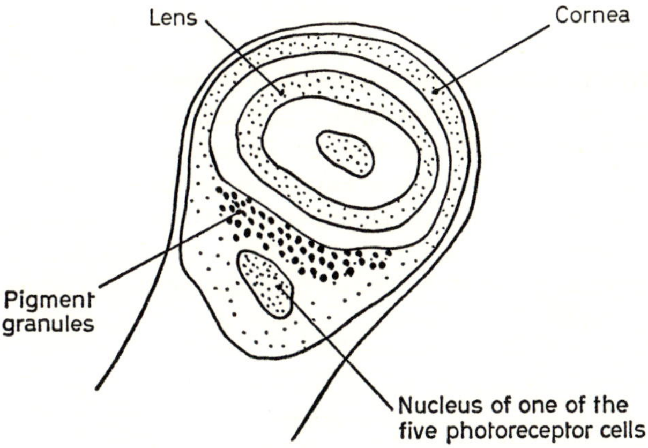


8.2 Section through an eye of the nudibranch mollusc *Hermissenda*. After Barth, J. (1964), 'Intracellular recording from photoreceptor neurons in the eyes of a nudibranch mollusc *Hermissenda crassicornis*', *Comp. Biochem. and Physiol.*, *11*, 311–315.

spite of this vast simplification the retinae of *Hermissenda's* eyes display some of the basic features of more complex retinae.

It can be shown that *Hermissenda*'s retinae are true retinae, not just groups of independent photoreceptors. In other words it can be shown that the five photoreceptors are tied together so that they work as a physiological unit. This interdependence is achieved by a system of inhibitory contacts. If, for example, one of the five photoreceptors is illuminated its activity tends to inhibit the activity of the other four. This phenomenon of mutual inhibition is shown in Fig. 8.3. We shall find that it is of very general occurrence in sense organs of all kinds.

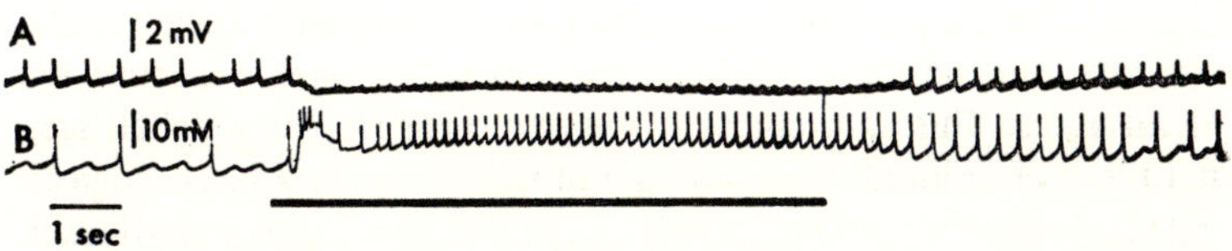


8.3 Lateral inhibition in the primitive retina of *Hermissenda*. Recordings are made simultaneously from two of the mollusc's photoreceptor cells: A and B. Cell B fires faster when illuminated and in so doing inhibits cell A. Horizontal bar at bottom of figure indicates duration of illumination. From Dennis, M. J. (1967), 'Interactions between the five receptor cells of a simple eye', in *Invertebrate nervous systems*, edited by C. A. G. Wiersma, University of Chicago Press, Chicago and London.

The sense organ in which mutual inhibition has been most exhaustively studied is the compound eye of *Limulus*. We noticed in Chapter 7 that this eye is composed of a number of fairly widely separated units called ommatidia. This in fact is the great virtue of the compound eye of *Limulus*—the ommatidia can be examined individually. The compound eyes of more advanced forms[1] such as insects and crustacea possess large numbers of ommatidia in very close juxtaposition with one another. It would be very difficult to conduct electrophysiological experiments on individual ommatidia in these eyes.

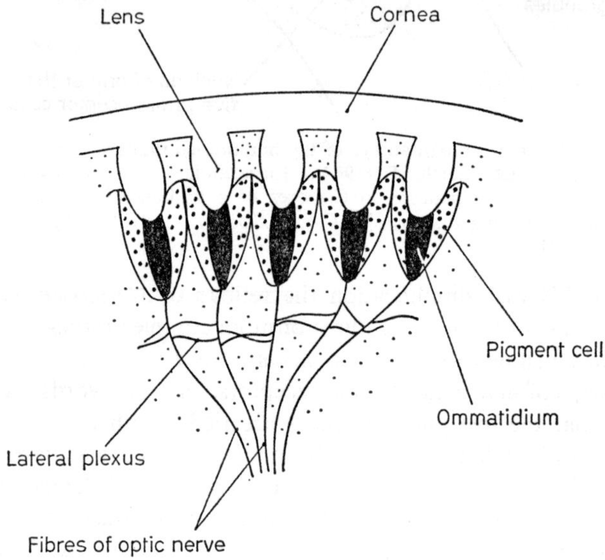


8.4 Part of the compound eye of *Limulus*.

Fig. 8.4 shows a section through one of the compound eyes of *Limulus*. The figure shows that although the ommatidia are widely separated the neurons leaving their bases are interconnected by lateral fibres. This anatomical arrangement ensures, as we shall see, that the several hundred ommatidia of the eye act as a physiological unit: that they form, in fact, a retina. The action of each ommatidium is to some extent affected by the condition, whether active or inactive, of all its neighbours.

[1] Although commonly called the King or Horseshoe crab, *Limulus*, in point of fact, is not zoologically speaking a crab at all. It is more nearly related to the spiders and is in consequence classified with them in the class Arachnida. *Limulus* is a largish marine form not uncommon on the eastern seaboard of the U.S.A.

As in the case of *Hermissenda* it is found that activation of one photoreceptor unit (ommatidium) tends to inhibit the activity of its near neighbours. Consider, for instance, the situation schematized in Fig. 8.5.

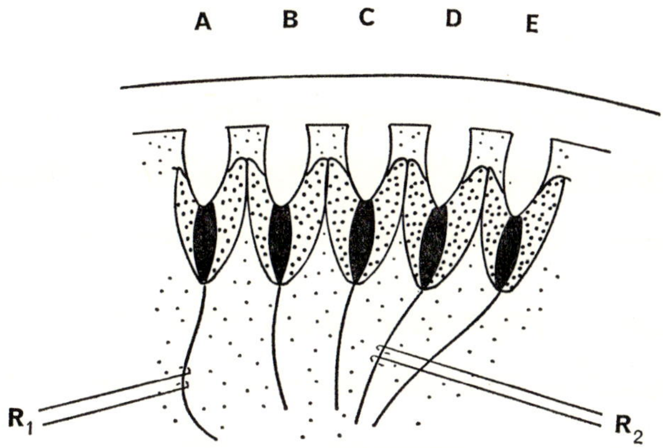


8.5 Experimental arrangement for recording lateral inhibition in the eye of *Limulus*.

In Fig. 8.5 it is supposed that impulses in the nerve fibres leading away from ommatidia A and D are detected by electrodes attached to recorders $R_1$ and $R_2$. The results of a similar experiment carried out by Hartline and Ratliff are shown in Fig. 8.6. It is clear that when two neighbouring ommatidia are simultaneously illuminated the activity of each is reduced.

There can only be one explanation for such a finding. When both ommatidia are activated they must mutually inhibit each other. This mutual inhibition is, moreover, mediated via the lateral fibre plexus. Transection of this plexus abolishes the inhibition.

Various characteristics of this type of inhibition have been discovered by Hartline and his colleagues at the Rockefeller Institute. It can be shown, for instance, that the inhibition rapidly falls off with distance. Ommatidia more than four or five millimetres distant from each other show little or no mutual inhibition. Similarly it can be shown that the degree of inhibition is proportional to the intensity of the light falling on the inhibitor ommatidium. Finally the inhibitory action is additive: the dampening influence on any given ommatidium is greater the greater the number of its near neighbours illuminated.

Now what is the biological significance, if any, of this neurosensory mechanism? The answer to this question is straightforward:

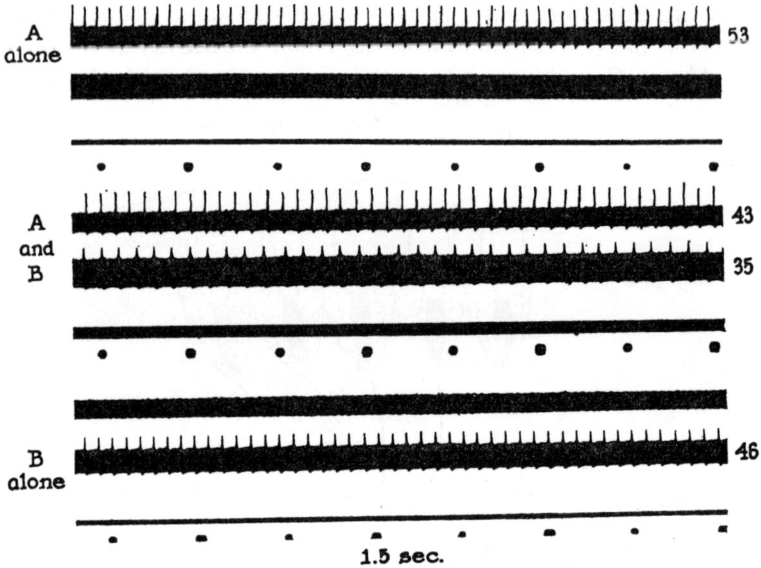


8.6 Discharges from *Limulus* ommatidia under different conditions of illumination. In the top record one ommatidium was illuminated by itself at an intensity which elicited 53 impulses in 1·5 seconds. In the bottom record an adjacent ommatidium was illuminated at a similar intensity which elicited 46 impulses in 1·5 seconds along its nerve fibre. In the middle record both ommatidia were illuminated at the same intensity as before; it can be seen that the discharge from both is markedly reduced. For explanation see text. From Hartline, H. K. and Ratliff, F. (1957), 'Inhibitory interaction in *Limulus* eye', *J. Gen. Physiol.*, *40*, 357–376.

the mechanism serves to enhance contrast. Edges are sharpened up, movement is made more obvious. Let us see how these important advantages flow from the phenomenon of mutual inhibition.

Imagine that an edge is focused on to this primitive retina. In other words a region of abruptly varying colour or intensity is projected on to the retina. Let us consider what happens amongst our array of ommatidia. Mutual inhibition ensures that the ommatidia under the brightly illuminated part of the image strongly inhibit those under the dimmer part. The back reaction from the dimly lit ommatidia to the brightly lit units is, however, much feebler. Thus whilst the brightly lit ommatidia signal strongly to the brain those half in the shadow are completely inhibited. This results in the continuously varying field of illumination being considerably crispened up. The mechanism is shown diagrammatically in Fig. 8.7.

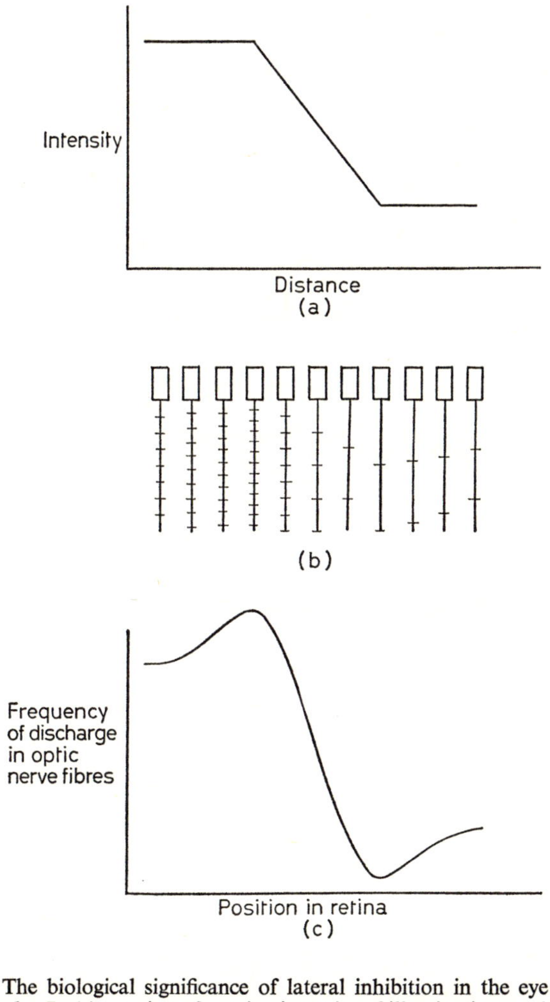


8.7 The biological significance of lateral inhibition in the eye of *Limulus*. In (a) a region of varying intensity of illumination, such as might occur at the transition from a dark to a light area, is graphed. In (b) the response to this variation in the nerve fibres leaving one of the King crab's compound eyes is shown. In (c) the impulse frequency symbolized in (b) is graphed against position in the retina. When graph (c) is compared with graph (a) it is clear that the variation in light intensity falling on the retina is greatly emphasized and crispened up. This is one of the most important consequences of lateral inhibition.

This crispening of edges and contours is of first-rate importance to the organism. Attneave[1] and others have shown that information is concentrated along contours, and particularly at those points where the contour changes direction. A striking illustration of this proposition is shown in Fig. 8.8, taken from Attneave's paper. The figure shows a drawing of a sleeping cat made by abstracting 38 points of maximum curvature and connecting them with straight lines.

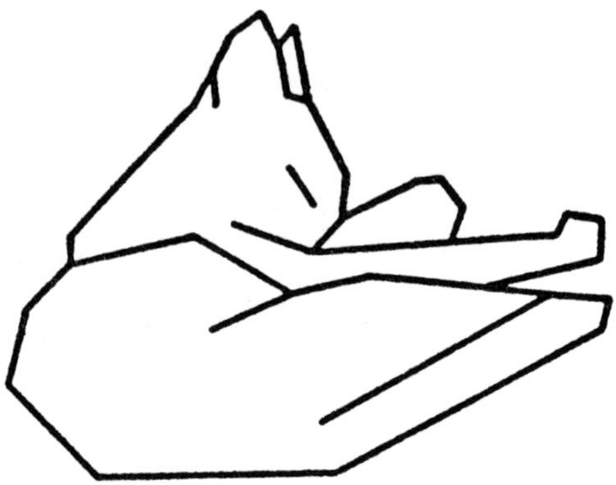

8.8 Drawing made by abstracting 38 points of maximum curvature from the contours of a sleeping cat and connecting these points appropriately with a straight edge. From Attneave, F. (1954), 'Informational aspects of visual perception', *Psychol. Rev, 61,* 182–193. Copyright (1954) by the American Psychological Association, and reproduced with permission.

If a similar number of points of minimum curvature were to be joined by straight lines we should be hard put to it to recognize any animal at all!

Clearly the mutual inhibition which we have seen at work in the eyes of *Hermissenda* and *Limulus* helps to filter out the biologically relevant information from the flux of electromagnetic energy to which the animal is exposed. Mutual inhibition, as we have mentioned before, does not seem to be restricted to retinae. There is evidence to show that it is also at work in auditory and tactile perception. However there is some controversy in both these latter instances as to whether this sharpening up of the raw 'sense data' takes place peripherally at the sense organ, or centrally in the brain.

[1] Attneave, F. (1954), 'Some informational aspects of visual perception', *Psychol. Rev., 61,* 183–193.

## 8.4 The structure of vertebrate retinae

After this brief account of 'information processing' in the primitive eye of a 'living fossil' let us turn to the immensely more complex case of the vertebrate, and in particular, the mammalian retina. In man, for reasons touched on in Chapter 10, vision has become the dominant sense. Almost 40% of all the sensory fibres entering the human central nervous system are concerned with this sense. Yet in spite of this the number of fibres in the optic nerve is, as Table 8.1 shows, very considerably less than the number of photoreceptor cells—the rods and cones—in the retina. It is clear that the mammalian retina is of a different order of complexity altogether from the invertebrate retinae we considered in the previous section.

TABLE 8.1

Cellular constitution of the rat's retina

| *Level* | *Total number of neurons* |
|---|---|
| Rods | 9,180,000 |
| Cones | 120,000 |
| Bipolar neurons | 3,530,000 |
| Optic nerve fibres | 260,000 |

From Lashley K.S. (1952), *S.E.B. Symposium IV.*

Table 8.1 shows that information collected by nearly 9·5 million photoreceptors is condensed into messages transmitted along a mere quarter of a million optic nerve fibres. Clearly a one-to-one representation of the image falling on the retina cannot be communicated, as such, to the brain. In fact it is known that a great deal of information processing occurs before any message is transmitted. Before, however, we can discuss how the retina is believed to select biologically relevant information we must familiarize ourselves with its anatomical structure.

We mentioned at the beginning of the last section that the vertebrate retina is in fact a portion of the brain pushed out to the periphery. Due to this mode of development it is said to be inverted. In other words the photosensitive ends of the rods and cones face inwards away from the incoming light. In fact light has to pass through several layers of nerve cells before interacting with this receptor

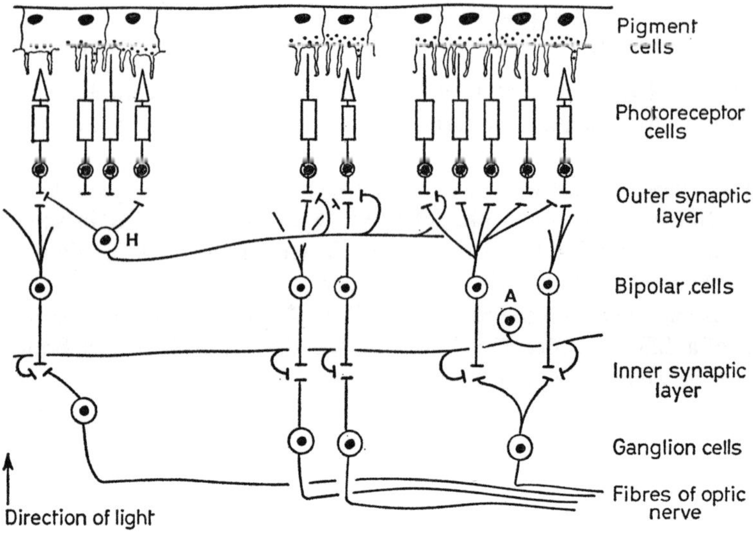


8.9 Vertical section through the mammalian retina.
A = amacrine cell, H = horizontal cell.

region. It is in these layers of nerve cells that the intricacy we have been alluding to is to be found. Fig. 8.9 is a diagrammatic section through a mammalian retina.

The structural complexity of the mammalian retina is very clear from the above diagram. Nevertheless the figure gives only an indication of the real intricacy. For one thing only two dimensions are shown and, of course, the retina is extended in three. For another, not all the neurons which would be present in such a section are in fact shown. For a third, the non-nervous elements—the supporting glial cells, here known as Muller cells—are not included at all. It is small wonder that neurophysiologists faced with such a webwork should have felt it wise to turn, initially, to the simpler retinae of invertebrates.

Fig. 8.9 shows that the bases of the rods and cones form synapses with bipolar neurons which run a short distance through the retina before themselves synapsing with ganglion cells. The latter neurons send axons to the brain and several hundred thousand, or perhaps a million, of these fibres make up the optic nerve.

In addition to this comparatively straightforward pathway from photosensitive outer segment to optic nerve fibre there are, as the figure shows, several complicating factors. Horizontal cells and amacrine cells send processes parallel to the surface of the retina and connect together groups of photosensitive cells or bipolar neurons. Furthermore some amacrines make synapses with *efferent* fibres from the brain. It looks as though the brain can send impulses out to the retina, perhaps to alter its acuity in some way. We shall have more to say about this central control of receptor organs in Chapter 16.

Clearly there are numerous possibilities for a complex interaction in this rich mass of synaptic connections. Clearly, too, the anatomical facts set out in Table 8.1 indicate that some of these manifold possibilities must be realized. The most penetrating investigations of this retinal information processing have been achieved by microelectrode methods. Fig. 8.9 shows that the optic nerve fibres along which the results of this retinal computation are signalled to the brain take their origin from the ganglion cells. Consequently the technique adopted has been to impale these cells on microelectrodes and to record their response when a portion of the retina is illuminated. Let us, therefore, examine some of the characteristics which the electrophysiologist has discovered by means of this technique.

### 8.5 The concept of a receptive field

It is possible to show that a given ganglion cell can be excited by a spot of light falling anywhere on a comparatively extensive area of the retina. A rod or cone cell is seldom more than a few microns in diameter yet a ganglion cell can be activated by light falling anywhere within a roughly circular patch of retina whose diameter may approach one millimetre. This important finding is illustrated in Fig. 8.10.

As Fig. 8.10 emphasizes, this finding indicates the existence of very considerable convergence in the retina. The patch of retinal surface capable of exciting a given ganglion cell is said to constitute that cell's *receptive field*.[1] Fig. 8.11 shows that around the receptive field proper there lies an annulus of retina which, although it does not affect the ganglion cell on its own, is nevertheless capable of altering the response of the cell when its genuine receptive field is illuminated.

[1] The boundaries and extents of receptive fields cannot, in fact, be delineated precisely. They shrink with high background illumination and expand during dark adaptation. Kuffler, S. W. (1953), 'The discharge patterns and functional organisation of mammalian retinae', *J. Neurophysiol.*, *16*, 37–68.

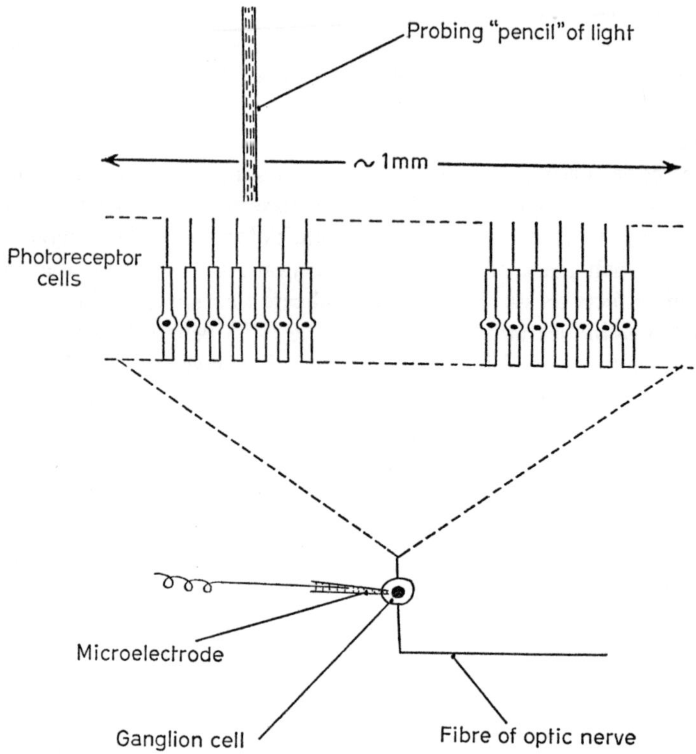


8.10 Concept of a receptive field. For explanation see text.

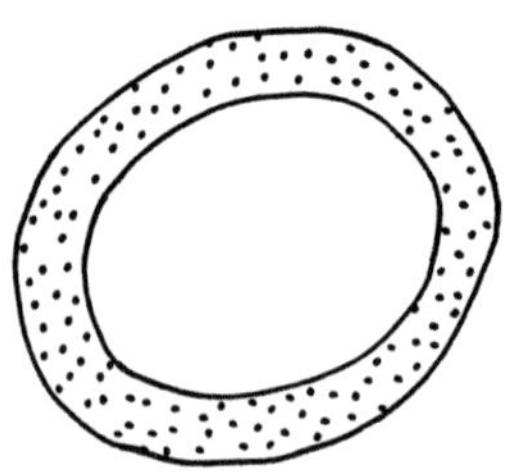

8.11 Surface view of a retinal receptive field and surrounding annulus (stippled).

The initial work on visual receptive fields was carried out on the frog's retina. In this retina H. K. Hartline and others have distinguished three different types of receptive field: *on*, *off*, and *on-off*. Similar, though as we shall see not identical, types of receptive field have been demonstrated in the retinae of other vertebrates including mammals. Let us look, first of all, at the diagnostic characteristics of these three types of receptive field.

Let us begin by considering the *on* field. The characteristic features of this type of field are shown in Fig. 8.12 (a). When a spot of light falls on the field the appropriate ganglion cell begins to discharge. The rate of discharge varies in direct proportion to the intensity of the illumination and the area of the field illuminated. When the light is switched off the ganglion cell is inactivated.

The *off* field is the converse of the above. Its physiology is shown in Fig. 8.12 (b). When the field is illuminated the ganglion cell is inactivated. It remains quiescent until the light is switched off. When this occurs, however, the ganglion cell is activated and fires impulses up its optic nerve fibre to the brain. The frequency of discharge slowly falls off in the dark but is only completely inhibited when the receptive field is illuminated once more.

The *on-off* field combines some of the characteristics of both the former. It is schematized in Fig. 8.12 (c). The ganglion cell is activated both when the light is switched on and when it is switched off. In both cases the response is transient. In steady illumination or lack of illumination the response soon decays and the cell remains quiet.

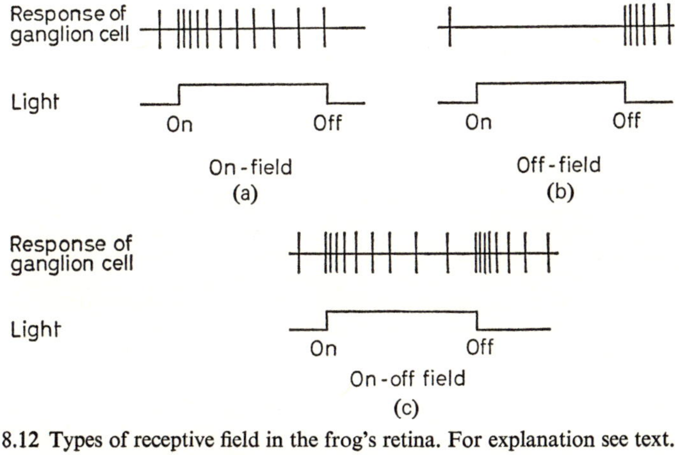


8.12 Types of receptive field in the frog's retina. For explanation see text.

The physiological analysis of *off* and *on-off* fields has been carried a stage further. In both cases it can be shown that there is interaction actually within the field. In the case of the *off* field it can be shown that extinction of a light illuminating the periphery of the field adds to the effect of extinguishing one at the centre. In other words the intrafield interaction is additive. The opposite obtains in the *on-off* field. The intrafield interaction is subtractive. The discharge in response to a light falling on the centre of the field is much reduced if a light is at the same time switched on at the periphery. A similar interaction is found if the lights instead of being switched on are switched off. This phenomenon is shown schematically in Fig. 8.13.

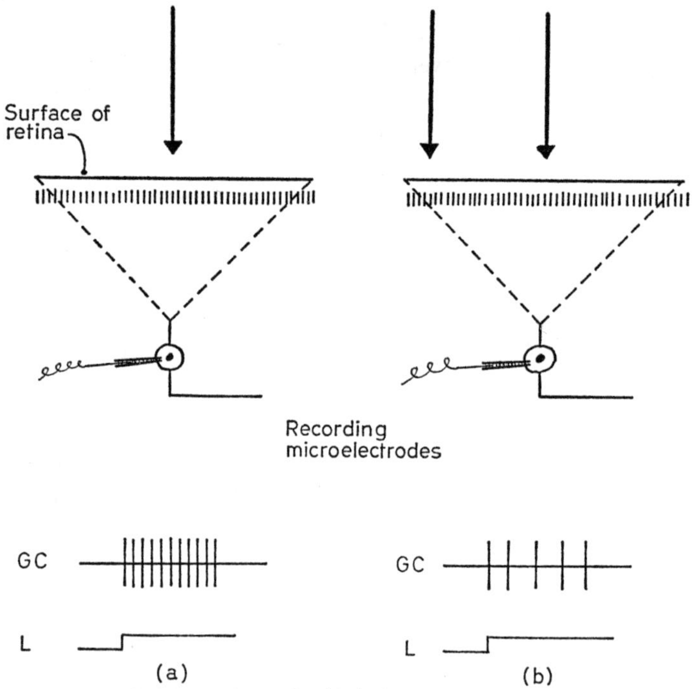


8.13 Intrafield interaction in the *on-off* field. In (a) the response of a ganglion cell (GC) to a light (L) switched on at the centre of the field is shown. In (b) the response of the same cell is shown when two lights are switched on simultaneously, one at the periphery and one at the centre of the field. For further explanation see text.

Fig. 8.13 shows that in the case of an *on-off* field the maximum discharge occurs when there is a maximum difference between the illumination of the centre and the periphery. Such a field is thus adapted, as was the entire retina of *Limulus*, to 'see' edges. For the maximum response occurs when the illumination across the field varies sharply. Not only are edges detected but the movement of an edge is picked up. For when an edge moves across an *on-off* field the light intensity falling on the centre and the periphery will continuously vary. In consequence the ganglion cell will discharge in a characteristic manner. This varying signal will be interpreted in the frog's optic tectum as the signature of a moving edge.

It follows from this analysis of the frog's retina that the optic nerve fibres fall into three main groups. One group, springing from the *on* fields, report where in the retina brightening is occurring. Another group, springing from the *off* fields, report where dimming is occurring. A third group, from the *on-off* fields, keep the brain informed of where boundaries or edges are moving. If the visual pattern remains static and unchanging with respect to the retina there should, according to this analysis, be little or no traffic in the optic nerve. Experiments in which stabilized images are projected on to the human retina (see section 17.3) tend to confirm this deduction.

### 8.6 Receptive fields in the mammalian retina

We have already mentioned that the three types of receptive field distinguishable in the frog's retina are not found universally throughout the vertebrates. Indeed, as Barlow[1] points out, all the vertebrates so far studied have several different types of receptive field, 'but the classes are different in different species'.

Let us therefore glance briefly at the situation found in the mammals. Numerous mammalian retinae have been intensively investigated in the last decade. Perhaps the most intriguing data on intraretinal information processing has emerged from work on the rabbit. In this animal eight different types of receptive field have, so far, been demonstrated.[2]

In addition to *on-off* and *on* fields the rabbit's retina possesses many roughly circular fields with *on* centres and *off* peripheries and vice versa. In fact this type of receptive field seems to be very common

[1] Barlow, H. B., Hill, R. M. and Levick, W. R. (1964), 'Retinal ganglion cells responding selectively to direction and speed of image motion in the rabbit', *J. Physiol.*, *173*, 377–407.

[2] Levick, W. R. (1967), 'Receptive fields and trigger features of ganglion cells in the visual streak of the rabbit's retina', *J. Physiol.*, *188*, 285–307.

in many mammalian retinae. It has, for example, also been shown to exist in feline and primate retinae. A salient feature of this type of field is that there is antagonism between the centre and the periphery. Thus if the centre and the periphery of the field are illuminated simultaneously they cancel each other out at the level of the ganglion cell: the latter cell remains, in consequence, unaffected. Because of this mutual antagonism the region from which *on* effects are obtained is sometimes called the excitatory region, whilst the *off* effect area is called inhibitory. Finally it can usually be shown that there exists between the central *on* (*off*) area and the peripheral *off* (*on*) annulus a boundary region from which *on-off* responses may be elicited. This very common and important type of receptive field is shown in Fig. 8.14.

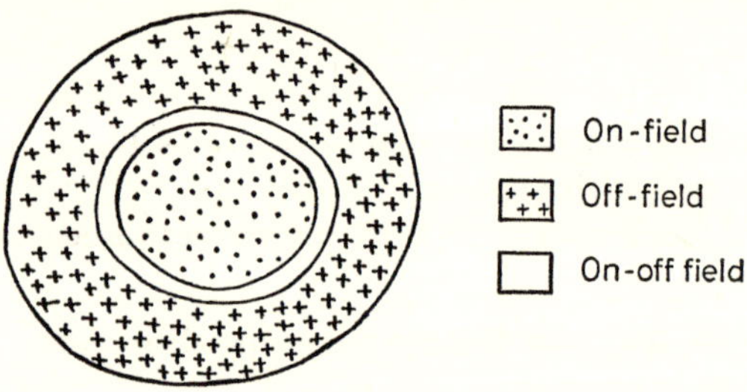


8.14 Surface view of a typical mammalian retinal receptive field. For explanation see text.

The type of receptive field shown in Fig. 8.14 evidently combines some of the features of all three frog fields. It also shares with the frog *on-off* field the important functional characteristic of contrast enhancement. For example, the strongest influence of an *on* centre field on its ganglion cell will be exerted when the centre is illuminated and the periphery in darkness and vice versa. As these concentric fields are of considerable importance in the mammalian retina it is interesting to examine their possible neuro-anatomical bases.

The retina, because of its regular organization, has long been a favourite tissue with electron microscopists interested in neurology. Recently Dowling and Boycott[1] have made a detailed study of the synaptic contacts in a mammalian retina. Fig. 8.15 summarizes their findings.

[1] Dowling, J. E. and Boycott, R. B. (1966), 'Organisation of the primate retina: electron microscopy', *Proc. Roy. Soc. B.*, *166*, 80–111.

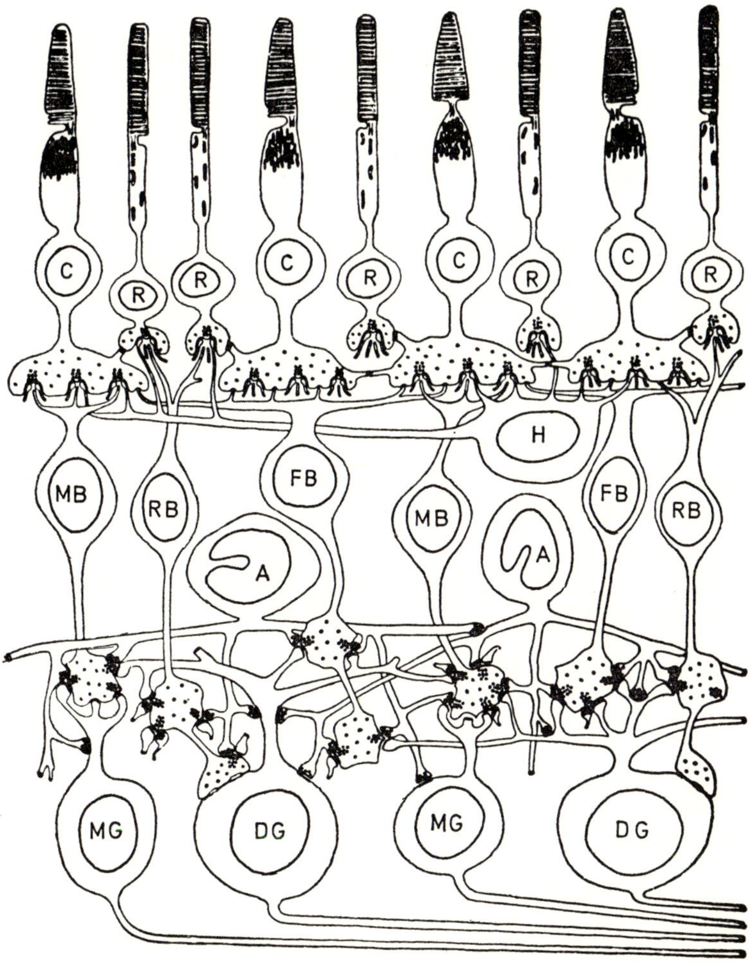


8.15 Summary diagram of synaptic contacts in the primate retina. This is a diagrammatic reconstruction based on detailed electron microscopy. It gives some impression of the ultrastructural complexity of this tissue which, it will be remembered, is embryologically part of the brain. R = rod cell, C = cone cell, MB = midget bipolar cell, RB = rod bipolar cell, FB = flat bipolar cell, H = horizontal cell, A = amacrine cell, MG = midget ganglion cell, DG = diffuse ganglion cell. From Dowling, J. E. and Boycott, R. B. (1966), 'Organisation of the primate retina: electron microscopy', *Proc. Roy. Soc. B., 166*, 80–111.

Fig. 8.15 might be compared with the much more diagrammatic Fig. 8.9 and with the vertical section of the retina shown in Plate XI. It is clear that the structural complexity visible by optical microscopy is only a foretaste of the complexity revealed by the electron microscope. However by a painstaking analysis of their sections Dowling and Boycott have been able to suggest an anatomical basis for the very common concentric receptive field shown in Fig. 8.14. This anatomical basis is shown diagrammatically in Fig. 8.16.

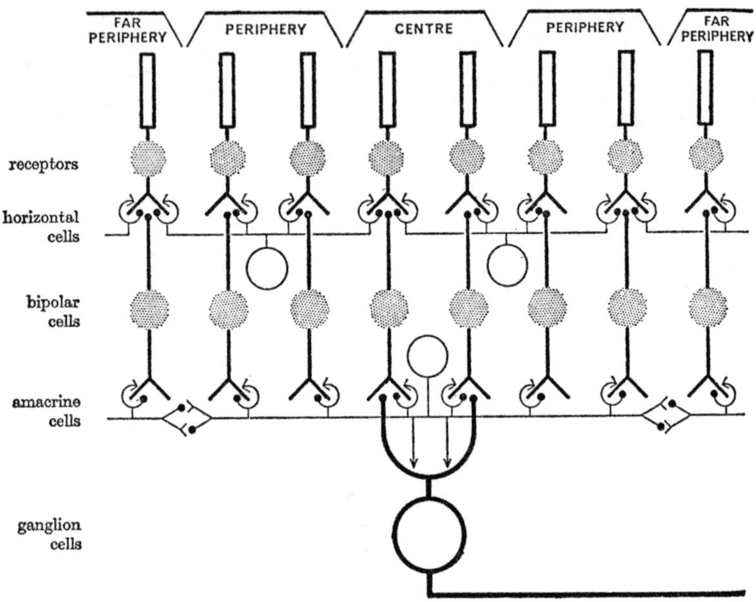


8.16 A 'wiring diagram' for a ganglion cell receptive field in the mammalian retina. ⅄ = excitatory synapse, ↓ = inhibitory synapse, ǐ = dendritic zone. Explanation in text. From Dowling, J. E. and Boycott, R. B. (1966), *loc. cit.*

Dowling and Boycott suggest that this neuronal organization might work in the following way. First let us note that ganglion cells in the mammalian retina show a great deal of spontaneous activity even in the dark.[1] Next we may suppose that for an *on* centre, *off* periphery field excitation of the central rods would lead directly to an excitation of the ganglion cell via the bipolars. Stimulation of the periphery of the field can, however, only affect the ganglion cell via an amacrine. If this cell makes inhibitory synapses with the

[1] Kuffler, S. W. (1953), 'Discharge patterns and functional organisation of the mammalian retina', *J. Neurophysiol.*, *16*, 37–68.

ganglion cell we have the condition necessary for an *off* response. For as soon as the light is switched off at the periphery the ganglion cell is released from inhibition and consequently fires. To account for *off* centre, *on* periphery fields it is only necessary to reverse the synaptic types. The excitation of the central bipolars would then lead to an inhibition of the ganglion cell, whereas excitation of the periphery of the field would result in the ganglion cell being activated. This neuronal wiring diagram also shows how simultaneous stimulation of centre and periphery sum in an antagonistic fashion at the ganglion cell. Fig. 8.16 summarizes these physiological interpretations of retinal fine structure.

Clearly Dowling and Boycott's scheme has much to recommend it. All the synaptic contacts shown in Fig. 8.16 have been detected with the electron microscope. No unknown synaptic events are called for. Excitatory and inhibitory synapses are, as we saw in Chapter 6, nowadays well understood. However, as we also noted earlier in this book, the ability to distinguish between excitatory and inhibitory synapses with the electron microscope is only just beginning to come over the horizon. It will be fascinating to follow the application of this still embryonic technique to the analysis of the retina. We should then be able to determine whether the physiological scheme based on the neuro-anatomy of Fig. 8.15 is valid or is still an over-simplification.

In addition to the fairly simple circular receptive fields discussed above the rabbit's retina possesses, as we have already mentioned, several other more complicated types of field. Indeed it appears that considerably more information processing occurs in the rabbit's retina than in the retinae of the rat, cat, or primate. In fact the types of operation carried out by the rabbit retina are similar to many of those carried out by the feline cortex. This will become apparent when we discuss visual perception in Chapter 14.

One of the more complicated types of receptive field demonstrable in the rabbit's retina seems to be designed to detect the appearance or movement of a contrasting border. It is possible to show that the response of a ganglion cell governed by this type of field is maximal when the image of a small object is brought slowly to a halt within the field and then moved out again. The characteristics of this type of field are schematized in Fig. 8.17.

It can be shown that it is the appearance of a *contrasting* edge, for example the edge of a black object against a white background,

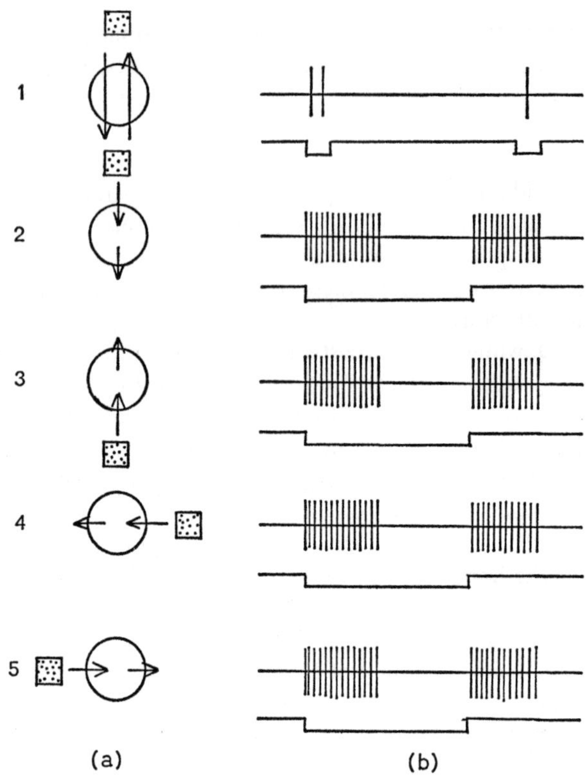


8.17 Local edge detector field in the rabbit's retina. In column (a) the movement of a small object across the receptive field in various directions is shown. The receptive field is represented by a circle. In column (b) the response of the ganglion cell is shown. In record 1 the object is moved rapidly back and forth over the field and the cell shows little response. In records 2–5 the small object is carried *slowly* into the field from various directions and brought to rest within the field. After an interval it is carried out of the field again. The line beneath each pattern of responses indicates the position of the object with respect to the field. The image of the object is present in the field when the line dips. Adapted from Levick, W. R. (1967), 'Receptive fields and trigger features in the visual streak of the rabbit's retina', *J. Physiol.*, *188*, 285–307.

which is particularly effective in activating the ganglion cell. On the other hand if the image of a sharply contrasting border appears in the retinal region immediately surrounding the receptive field at the same time as one appears in the receptive field itself then the ganglion cell is inhibited. Hence it seems that this type of cell is activated by a rather specific stimulus—the appearance of a contrasting edge in its field but not in the inhibitory surround. In consequence this type of receptive field is called a *local edge detector*.

The above example brings out a point which will be emphasized again in Chapter 14. Receptor cells are often sensitive to quite specific stimuli. Moreover these stimuli are often of clear significance to the life of the animal. These specific stimuli, like the localized contrasting edge of the foregoing example, are called *trigger* stimuli. They are the stimuli which cause maximum response in the receptor cell.

Returning to our review of the receptive fields demonstrable in the rabbit's retina it is possible to find ganglion cells responsive to quite a variety of trigger stimuli. In some cases it is the direction, in others the speed of motion which is significant. For example, some ganglion cells give optimal responses to fast movements, whilst others are maximally activated by slow movements. In yet other cases it is the orientation of a slit-shaped patch of light, or of an edge, which is effective. This type of field is called an orientation-selector field. Its essential characteristics are shown in Fig. 8.18.

Fig. 8.18 (a) shows that only when the slit is presented to the field with a certain orientation does a discharge from the ganglion cell occur. Fig. 8.18 (b) shows a possible anatomical basis for this physiological phenomenon. It is easy to see that if a slit-like excitatory centre is surrounded by an inhibitory area then excitation of the ganglion cell will only occur when the stimulus has a certain orientation (X–X). If it has an orientation at right angles to this (Y–Y) then it will fall across so much of the inhibitory surround that any effect on the excitatory centre will be completely cancelled out at the level of the ganglion cell. It is very interesting to find that similar types of orientation-selector units can be detected in the cat's cerebral cortex. These will be discussed in Chapter 14.

The trigger stimulus of another type of receptive field discovered in the rabbit's retina appears to be any spatial or temporal change of illumination. So long as the illumination, or lack of it, remains constant a steady stream of impulses is generated by the ganglion cell. As soon as the illumination changes, either by brightening or dimming, or by the movement of an object into or across the field, the firing rate diminishes or is abolished altogether. In consequence this eighth type of receptive field is called a 'uniformity detector'.

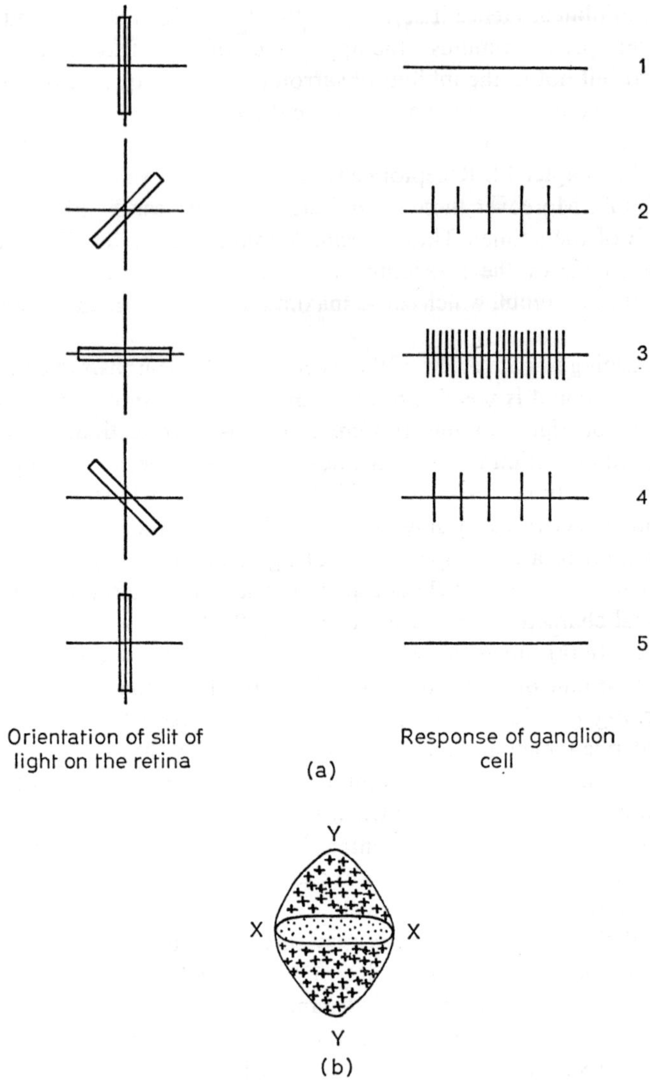


8.18 Orientation selector field in the rabbit's retina. The experimental results are shown at (a). At the left-hand side of (a) a slit-shaped patch of light is presented to the receptive field at various orientations. On the right-hand side of (a) the response of the ganglion cell is shown. The deduced organization of the receptive field is shown at (b). Dots = response of cell, crosses = no response of cell. Further explanation in text. Adapted from Levick, W. R. (1967), *loc. cit.*

There seems little doubt that other types of receptive field await discovery by the neurophysiologist in the rabbit's retina. The brief outline given above indicates, however, that the structural complexity revealed by the anatomist is well complemented by a comparable physiological intricacy. It must however be stressed once more that the receptive fields discussed in the preceding paragraphs are not found in all mammalian retinae. Feline and primate retinae seem, for example, to be much simpler.

It is clear, however, that in general significant information is extracted from the visual scene before any communication is made with the brain. The means by which this preliminary information processing is effected in the mammalian retina are just beginning to be understood. W. R. Levick sums up the flavour of this incipient understanding in the following passage:

'When a rabbit suddenly stops sniffing around in the foliage and lifts its head and eyes above the long grass to study the distant environment, its brain will continue to be bombarded by an irregular roar of activity from the *on* and *off* centre ganglion cells in the retina signalling the contrasts of the new view, but at least one class of unit will at first be completely silent—the local-edge-detectors. Gross movement of the visual field associated with the change of attitude blocks them via the inhibitory surrounds. Soon something in the distance moves against the now steady background; its retinal image will be small and will move slowly; one of the local-edge-detectors therefore starts signalling. It is providing the position information of the most significant event in the environment of the rabbit; it tells where in the tumult of information from the concentric units special attention is required'.[1]

[1] Levick, W. R. (1967), loc. cit., p. 306.

# CHAPTER NINE

# Crystals of Neural Activity

## 9.1 The emergence of a unity of action

In biology we find accentuated one of the features which marks the whole of natural science. This is the property of 'emergence'. In an earlier book—*Molecular Biology: a Structural Approach*—an attempt was made to show how 'wholes' with distinctively novel properties emerged from concatenations of simple elements. Molecules have, by definition, properties quite different from those of their constituent atoms.[1] At a more complex level the cell has the property of being 'alive' which is not predicable of any of its constituent molecules. With the multicellular organism a still further unity emerges. Nowhere is this unity more interestingly displayed than amongst interacting groups of neurons. The individual properties of the neurons are merged in the system; from the interdependent neuronal pool emerges a new character—*a oneness of action.*

In this chapter we shall look at some very simple systems of neurons. In comparison with the vastly complex brains of vertebrates these systems provide an opportunity, as Maynard[2] has pointed out, for studying 'crystals of neural activity'. The phrase reminds us of the crucial importance of protein and nucleic acid crystals in the development of molecular biology. Before, however, getting to grips with these neurophysiological crystals we must briefly consider the nature of biological pacemakers.

## 9.2 The concept of a pacemaker

In the earlier part of this century, perhaps under the influence of Pavlov, the belief grew that animal behaviour was entirely explicable

[1] This is not to say that the properties of molecules cannot, in principle, be predicted from the properties of their constituent atoms.

[2] Maynard, D. M. (1966), 'Integration in Crustacean Ganglia', *S.E.B. Symposium, 20*, 111–149.

in terms of reflex reaction to external stimuli. Perhaps the *locus classicus* for this view is to be found in Watson's book *Behaviour*[1] where he writes (p. 18), '. . . there are no centrally initiated processes. The environment in the widest sense forces the formation of habits'. The idea that behaviours might be internally generated tended to fall into desuetude. More recent analyses, however, have re-asserted the importance of internal motivation. Several interesting examples of such analyses will be set out in Chapter 12.

With the demise, or at least decline, of the concept of animal as reflex automaton increased attention has been paid to the nature and mechanism of the 'internal' forces affecting behaviour. Perhaps the most elementary of these internal 'self-moving movers' are certain types of pacemaker. Probably the best-known physiological pacemakers are those which control the rhythmical movements of hearts and respiratory systems.

In the right auricle of the mammalian heart is a group of several thousand cells which together constitute a region called the sinu-auricular node. This node sets the rate at which the heart beats: it triggers each beat. In other words it acts as a 'pacemaker' for the heart.

The biophysical mechanism underlying this vital activity is at present obscure. If one of the cells of the sinu-auricular node is

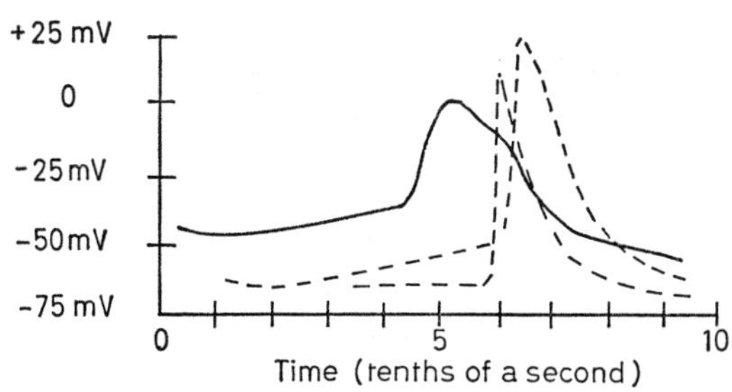


9.1 Biophysics of pacemaker cells in the mammalian heart. Solid line represents variation in the potential of a pacemaker cell, broken lines represent variations in the potential of cardiac muscle fibres. After West, T. C. (1955), 'Ultramicroelectrode recording from the cardiac pacemaker', *J. Pharmac. exp. Ther*, *115*, 283–290. © 1955 The Williams and Wilkins Co., Baltimore, Md. 21202, USA.

[1] Watson, J. B.: *Behaviour, An Introduction to Comparative Psychology*, Holt, Rinehart and Winston, Inc., New York, 1967. (First published in 1914.)

penetrated by a microelectrode it is possible to show that during the relaxation phase of the heart beat (diastole) the cell membrane slowly depolarizes. We may suppose that when this depolarization reaches a certain level it acts like an end-plate potential initiating action potentials in nearby muscle cells. The pacemaker cell membrane is then repolarized during the contraction phase of the heart beat (systole). These events are shown in Fig. 9.1.

The physico-chemical basis of the slow drift in the transmembrane potential of the pacemaker cell is at present unknown. Presumably there is some underlying biochemical process.[1] There are many instances of pacemaker activity within the central nervous system. It seems likely that these sources of internal initiative are based on similar physico-chemical fundamentals. It is clear that within the central nervous system many sorts of interaction between pacemaker potentials, EPSPs and IPSPs are possible.

### 9.3 Elements in the design of neuronal computers

We have already noticed, more than once, that brains and electronic computers are built according to rather different principles. We have also noticed that there are some similarities. We have noticed, for example, that the binary code of electronic computers is in some respects similar to the all-or-none properties of the axon. This on/off digital characteristic also emerges in the sharp division of synapses into excitatory and inhibitory types. There is no middling, halfway type.

This dichotomy of synaptic type is made use of in many neural designs. We have already met it in section 6.4 where it was used to prevent two antagonistic muscles contracting simultaneously (Fig. 9.2 (a) ). However we all know from personal experience that it is quite possible to contract two antagonistic muscles against each other. In this way we customarily stretch and exercise our bodies. It is not difficult to design a neuronal circuit to account for this observation. Such a circuit is shown in Fig. 9.2 (b). In this design an inhibitory neuron from a 'higher centre' synapses with the inhibitor running to the antagonistic muscle.

[1] There is some evidence, especially in invertebrate nervous systems, that the rhythm of pacemaker potentials can be correlated with underlying rhythms in nucleic acid and protein metabolism.

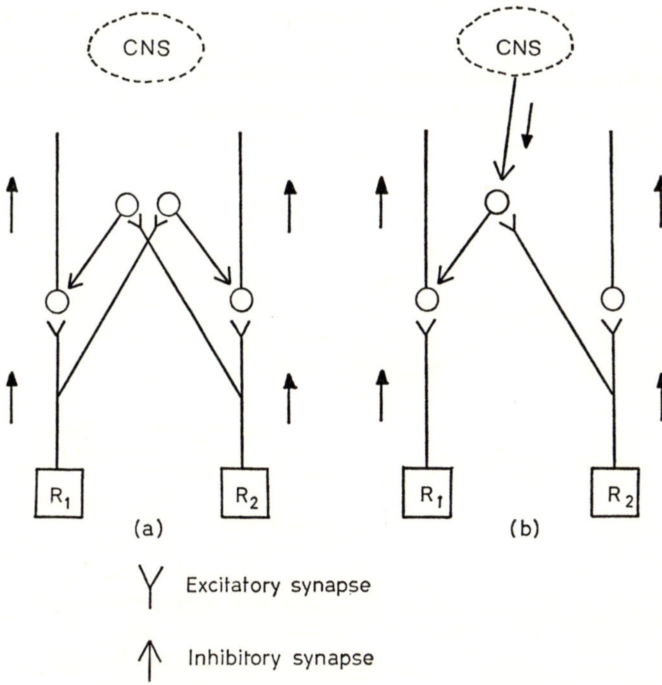


9.2 Two neuronal designs. In (a) stimulation of the receptor, $R_1$, inhibits messages originating in receptor $R_2$ and vice versa; in (b) messages from the CNS may prevent activity in $R_2$ inhibiting messages from $R_1$. Further explanation in the text. After Granit, R. (1966), 'Sensory mechanisms in perception', in *The Brain and Conscious Experience*, edited by J. C. Eccles, Springer-Verlag, Berlin.

Notice that we refer to 'inhibitory neurons'. It appears that all the synaptic contacts of a given neuron are of one type or the other.[1] Hence the dichotomy of synaptic type referred to above is, in fact, a dichotomy of neurons.

Systems of these excitatory and inhibitory neurons may also account for some forms of rhythmical activity. For example, many

[1] Eccles, J. C., *The Physiology of Nerve Cells*, Baltimore, The Johns Hopkins Press, 1957, p. 199. Although neurons appear to be either inhibitory or excitatory it does not necessarily follow that all their terminations produce the same physiological effects. It is possible to demonstrate, for example, that in the sea-hare, *Aplysia*, a common interneuron inhibits one post-synaptic cell but excites another. This is apparently due to a difference in the membranes of the two post-synaptic cells.

behaviour patterns, for instance walking, require the alternate contraction and relaxation of antagonistic muscles. Fig. 9.3 shows a simple pattern of excitatory and inhibitory neurons which could, in principle, control such reciprocating movements.

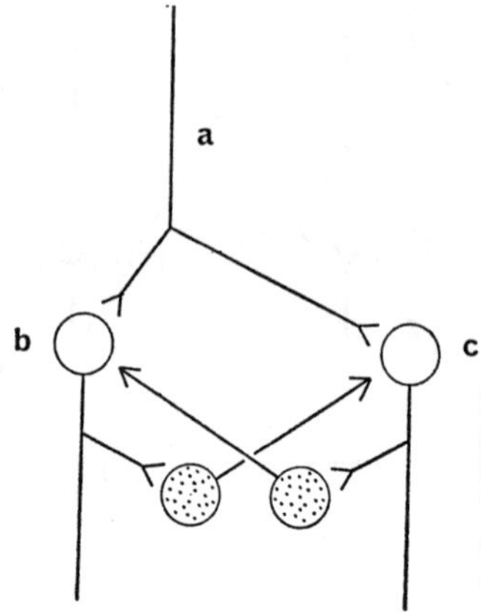


9.3 A neuronal design for recriprocating activity. Synaptic symbolism as in Fig. 9.2. Explanation in text. After Wilson, D. M. (1968), 'The flight-control system of the locust', *Scientific American*, *218*, 5, 83–93.

In Figure 9.3 we suppose, first, that a 'higher centre' commands the onset of the behaviour. This command is expressed in the form of impulses in fibre (a). This fibre innervates the two neurons, or neuron populations, (b) and (c). But (b) and (c) are connected to each other by inhibitory fibres (stippled perilarya). The geometry of the circuit shown in Fig. 9.3 ensures that neuron (b) fires first. This, in turn, ensures that neuron (c) is inhibited. However, when neuron (b) fatigues neuron (c) is released from inhibition and the input along (a) can now affect it. It fires and in so doing inhibits (b). In time it, too, fatigues, neuron (b) is consequently disinhibited and fires, and so on, until the input along (a) ceases. By adjusting the excitability of (b) and (c), their rates of fatigue and recovery from fatigue, different reciprocating frequencies can, in theory, be achieved.

### 9.4 The virtues of crustacean nervous systems

We noticed in Chapter 5 that the development of a profound understanding of the physico-chemical nature of the action potential awaited the discovery of an appropriate biological preparation. A similar situation obtains to some extent today with respect to the central nervous system. And although our understanding of how neurons work together in concert is extremely sketchy when compared with our knowledge of the biophysics of the nerve impulse, several preparations have, in the last few years, begun to show great promise. These preparations are largely based on invertebrate organisms. It is a fascinating and fortunate finding that the Arthropods and, in particular, the crustacea make do with far fewer neurons than vertebrates of a comparable size. Instead of the several billion neurons of a mammalian nervous system that of a comparable crustacean may consist of only several hundred thousand cells. In fact this economic use of neurons is evident throughout the entire organism, the peripheral as well as the central nervous system. Thus the quite complex muscular machinery of a crab's claw is controlled by a mere couple of dozen neurons. In contrast a mammalian limb may be controlled by several tens of thousands of neurons.

The comparatively great simplicity of the crustacean central nervous system has attracted many investigators. It provides the neurophysiologist interested in the co-operative activity of neurons with a preparation in which the neuronal interactions are more easily enumerated. The problems of CNS physiology do not seem so intractable in this group of animals as they sometimes seem in the vertebrates. In consequence we find that several very interesting studies have been made in recent years on nervous systems, or portions of nervous systems, belonging to these animals.

### 9.5 Crustacean cardiac and stomatogastric ganglia: minature central nervous systems

Perhaps the simplest 'crystal of neural activity' is found in the cardiac ganglion of decapod crustacea.[1] This ganglion, consisting of at most a dozen or so cells, controls the rate at which the crustacean's heart beats. This is achieved by means of bursts of impulses directed down fibres leading from the ganglion to the wall of the heart. These bursts cause the heart to contract. Normally they are repeated at regular intervals. If the regularity of these bursts of activity is interfered with the heart contracts in an irregular, incomplete and biologically useless manner.

Physiologists have been able to distinguish two types of cell amongst the dozen or so in the ganglion. Activity seems to begin within four posterior neurons. These neurons, in other words, play

[1] The Decapoda is the order of Crustacea which includes crabs, lobsters, crayfish, prawns, etc.

the part of pacemakers. Activity next spreads from this posterior group of neurons to an anterior group of 'follower' neurons. The activation of the 'followers' appears to be synchronized both by synaptic contacts and also by electrotonic spread. When a certain threshold is reached impulses are discharged down nerve fibres to the heart.

Even in this extremely simple system, however, neurophysiologists are still unsure of the exact means of neuronal integration.[1] Small wonder, then, that the ten billion neuron brains of vertebrates baffle the intelligence of researchers.

Slightly, but not much, more complicated than the cardiac ganglion is the crustacean stomatogastric ganglion. This ganglion consists of about 35 nerve cells and controls the activity of the decapod's stomach. It is obvious that the muscular movements of a stomach are a good deal more complicated than the simple systole/diastole of a heart. This more complicated movement is brought about by the activity of about 25 distinct muscles in the stomach wall. In order to produce physiologically useful movement it is clear that these 25 muscles must contract in a highly co-ordinated fashion. This vital pattern of contractions is initiated by an analogous pattern of impulses in the relevant nerve fibres to the stomach. Now although the stomatogastric ganglion is 'primed' or 'triggered' by the central nervous system, the patterned output is organized within the ganglion itself.

How is this patterning achieved? Clearly the stomatogastric ganglion with its relatively few neurons and its relatively complex output presents a most intriguing problem to the neurophysiologist. There is good evidence[2] that the pattern of impulses in the efferent fibres depends on a fairly intricate interaction amongst the 35 cells of the ganglion. Microscopical study of this miniaturized 'central nervous system' shows that the cell bodies of the neurons lie above a rather intricate neuropil. Synaptic junctions, excitatory, inhibitory and electrotonic, can be shown to occur in this meshwork. The general organization of the ganglion is shown in Fig. 9.4.

[1] Some important progress towards a solution of this problem has recently been made by Hartline and Cooke (*Science*, *164*, 1080 (1969) ). These investigators have shown that it is possible to predict the output along one of the motor neurons from the cardiac ganglion if the input on to that neuron from the pacemakers is known.

[2] Maynard, D. M., (1967), 'Neural co-ordination in a simple ganglion', *Science*, *158*, 531–532.

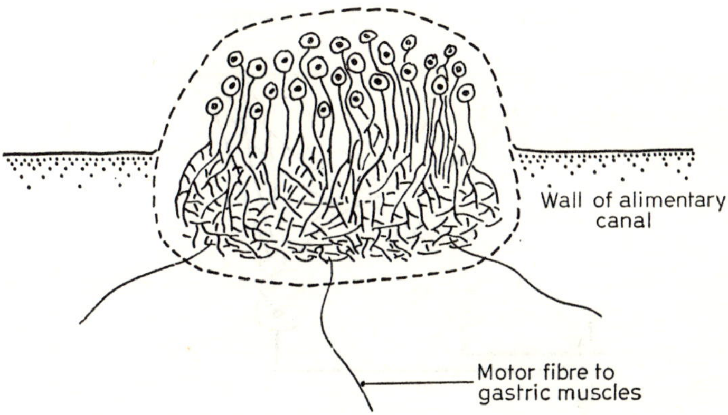


9.4 Decapod stomatogastric ganglion. Perikarya of about 30 neurons are situated above an undergrowth of neuropil. From the neuropil several motor nerves leave to innervate the stomach musculature.

It is an exciting task for the immediate future to work out the synaptic relations in this dendritic undergrowth. If, and when, this is done an explanation of integrative activity in terms of neuron circuits will become possible. We shall, in other words, have at last unravelled a wiring diagram for a 'central nervous system'.

Another fruitful line of approach to this 'wiring diagram problem', a problem which has beckoned like 'Will-o'-the-wisp' to generations of neurophysiologists, is provided by work on the nervous system of the crustacean tail. This very interesting work is outlined in the next section.

### 9.6 'Labelled lines' in the crayfish tail

The principle of neuronal parsimony, which we have said is characteristic of the Arthropods, is well instanced by the nervous system controlling the behaviour of the crayfish's tail. It has, in consequence, proved possible to map the interneurons involved in the movements of this quite large organ. First, on the sensory side Wiersma and his colleagues have been able to show that specific interneurons are activated when certain combinations of sensory hairs on the abdomen are stimulated. It has been demonstrated furthermore that only specific patterns of these hairs are capable of 'firing' a specific interneuron. A diagrammatic representation of these interesting results is shown in Fig. 9.5.

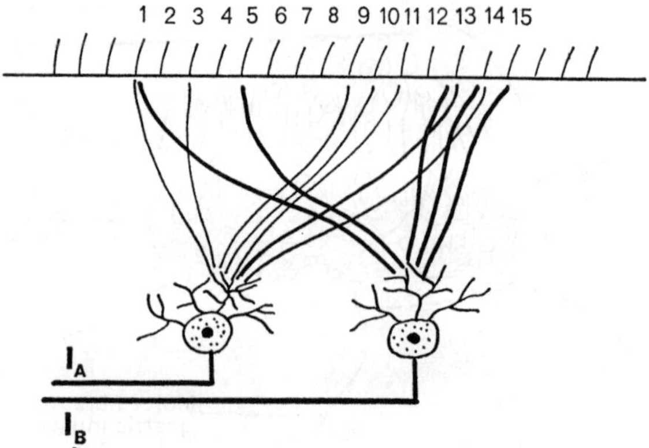


9.5 Schematic diagram to show that in the crayfish certain interneurons are activated by specific groups of sensory hairs. See text for explanation.

In Fig. 9.5 stimulation of hairs, 1, 3, 9, 10, 11, 13, 14 fire interneuron $I_A$, whilst stimulation of 1, 5, 13, 14, 15 fire interneuron $I_B$. It seems that each interneuron, $I_X$, encodes a specific sensory pattern. There is no duplication; each interneuron represents a certain pattern of sensory stimulation.

Second, on the motor side, a similar type of wiring diagram can be elucidated.[1] The posture of the abdomen can be shown to be controlled by muscles acting at each of its five joints. These muscles are arranged in antagonistic pairs—flexors and extensors (Fig. 7.1).

In each segment both extensor and flexor muscles are innervated by the same number of neurons. Moreover the entire tail appears to be controlled by quite a small number, about 120, motor neurons. Hence it has proved possible to identify and examine each fibre. In addition the interneurons, or 'command' fibres, have also been discovered. These neurons activate the motor neurons. It turns out that the motor organization is remarkably analogous to the sensory system described above. Thus stimulation of particular 'command' interneurons causes the activation of specific motor neurons. This in turn results in specific abdominal muscles being activated and, in consequence, specific movements of the abdomen. Stimulation of different 'command' interneurons leads to a different, though still of course specifiable and determinate, type of movement.

[1] Kenney, D., Evoy, W. H. and Hanawalt, J. T. (1966), 'Release of co-ordinated behaviour in crayfish by single central neurons', *Science*, *154*, 917–919.

Thus we see that in the case of the crayfish abdomen, or tail, both sensory input and behavioural output are the predictable outcome of inbuilt neuronal circuitry. How far this is also the case with the far more complex nervous systems of vertebrates must, perforce, remain for the present a speculation (see, however, Chapter 11).

### 9.7 A 'crystal of activity' in the mammalian nervous system

Invertebrates, as we have seen, provide many excellent preparations for studying central nervous mechanisms. The understanding obtained from these simple systems is invaluable in the continuing attempt to explain the functioning of vertebrate central nervous systems. A parallel approach is to subdivide the complex nervous system of vertebrates into small parts and to study the physiology of these 'crystals'. One of the most thoroughly analysed of these subsystems is that which governs the movement of skeletal muscles.

We have already outlined in Chapter 6 some of the control circuits which co-ordinate the contractions of skeletal muscle. The topic was also mentioned in section 3 of this chapter. It is thus already clear that bodily movements are under the control of quite a complex neuronal organization. Indeed neurophysiologists do not, as yet, comprehend all its subtleties. This complexity is also reflected in the commonplace fact that we, each of us, require many years to perfect the control of our own movements so that we can, for example, catch a cricket ball, enunciate a speech or write a sentence.

In section 6.3 the monosynaptic nerve circuit underlying the myotactic reflex was described. It will be remembered that the sensory nerve of this circuit springs from a stretch receptor in the relevant muscle (Fig. 6.2). This stretch receptor, interestingly enough, turns out to lie in a modified muscle fibre (Fig. 9.6).

Fig. 9.6 shows that the specialized muscle fibre (intrafusal fibre) in which the stretch receptor is located is also innervated by motor neurons. The latter neurons are, however, only 3–8 $\mu$ in diameter compared with the 20 $\mu$ axons which innervate the surrounding (extrafusal) muscle fibres. Now it will be recalled from section 5.9 that the girth of an axon is closely related to the velocity with which it can conduct an impulse. Hence the velocity of transmission in these small 'gamma' axons is very much less than that in the large 'alpha' axons innervating the extrafusal fibres. Finally, as Fig. 9.6 shows, the sensory fibre from the stretch receptor is itself an alpha neuron.

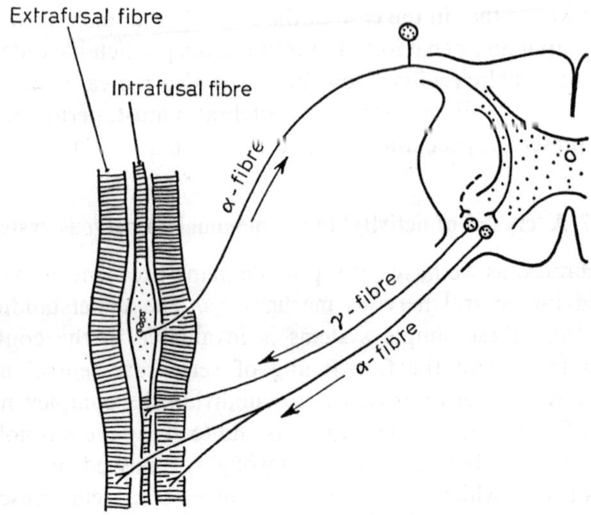


9.6 Control of the contraction of vertebrate skeletal muscle. As with Fig. 6.5 the diagram has been simplified to show only the bare essentials. For explanation see text.

Now what is the significance of this circuitry? We saw in Chapter 6 that when a muscle is stretched the intrafusal stretch receptor is stimulated which, by the monosynaptic myotactic reflex, causes an automatic contraction. Now in life a muscle is seldom passively stretched as it is at the physiologist's work-bench. Instead tension is put across the stretch receptor by an attempted contraction of the intrafusal fibre. This attempted contraction is initiated by impulses arriving down the gamma motor neurons. The tension set up in the intrafusal fibre by this gamma innervation is rapidly signalled to the central nervous system by the large alpha sensory neuron. But this, it will be remembered, synapses with motor neurons running out to the extrafusal fibres. These in consequence contract. It is easy to see that when they contract they relieve the tension on the intrafusal fibres embedded amongst them. It follows that the tension on the stretch receptor is released and that impulses, in consequence, no longer stream up from it to the central nervous system. It follows, in turn, that the monosynaptic pathway to the extrafusal fibres is no longer activated and thus the latter cease contracting.

It is evident from the above outline that the central nervous system can, via the gamma outflow to the intrafusal fibres, set the degree of contraction of the entire muscle.[1] This is, for example, of considerable importance in the control of the postural muscles. Varying gravitational forces as the body bends about its centre of gravity will stress these muscles in many different ways. The 'feed-back' circuits described above ensure that the muscles respond in such a way that their lengths remain invariant. Another case where the value of these servo loops is clear arises when a skeletal muscle is required to contract against a variable resistance. This might occur, for instance, when a weight is picked up or when a lever is pulled. The reflex circuitry ensures that automatic adjustments are made to combat any variations in resistance so that the task is accomplished smoothly, without jerks. Finally the neuronal feed-back automatically compensates for fatigue in the extrafusal fibres when the muscle is required to sustain its contraction over a period of time.

Clearly this comparatively simple servo mechanism relieves the central nervous system of much tedious computation. Instead of having to compute patterns of impulses to be sent out along all the very numerous alpha neurons to the muscles it can exert its control via a relatively small number of gamma fibres. This, however, is not to say that the brain is completely incapable of controlling the discharge of alpha motor neurons. There is evidence to show that the alpha pathway to the muscles is used directly for the control of fast learned movements, for instance rapid typewriting or piano playing. It seems that the cerebellum, in particular, is all the time adjusting and harmonizing the outflow to the intrafusal and extrafusal muscle fibres.

The discussion in the previous paragraphs together with the outline of contralateral inhibition set out in Chapter 6 gives an indication of the type of neuronal organisation which controls muscular movement in mammals. The account, of course, leaves out far more than it puts in.[2] In particular another reflex system based on sense receptors embedded in the tendons exists and works in parallel with the one described. However it is hoped that the discussion sketches the main characteristics of one important 'crystal of neural activity' in the mammalian nervous system.

[1] It is interesting in this connection to remember (p.118) that the smallest fibres in the vertebrate nervous system are believed to be phylogenetically the eldest.

[2] For a more complete exposition reference should be made to *Neurophysiology of Postural Mechanisms* by T. D. M. Roberts, Butterworth and Co. (Publishers) Ltd., 1966.

### 9.8 The template concept and the input control of output

We have looked, in this chapter, at several 'unit processes' in central nervous systems. In examining these 'crystals of neural activity' we are examining the bricks from which the total activity of the system is built. In conclusion let us look at one way in which these units may be welded together to achieve that unity of action which, as we mentioned at the outset, is so marked a character of an animal's behaviour.

The template concept has gained considerable prominence in the hands of molecular biologists. It will be remembered from Chapter 3 that the nucleotide sequences of mRNA are marshalled on a DNA template before being coupled together, and that suitably adapted amino-acids are aligned on a mRNA template during the synthesis of protein. It is possible that this powerful concept may help to crystallize our thinking about the way in which the nervous system governs motor activity.

We shall see in Chapter 12 that students of ethology believe that much of the behaviour of the lower animals may be broken down into sequences of stereotyped units (fixed action patterns). These units are triggered by perceptual 'gestalts' which the ethologists call 'sign stimuli'. We might say, using the template concept, that the pattern of impulses initiated in the sense organ by the sign stimulus fits a specific inbuilt sensory template. When this happens a specific pattern of muscular movements results.

The sign stimuli of the ethologist affect the animal's exteroreceptors. But it is not difficult to see that a similar concept may well apply to the proprioceptive inflow to the central nervous system. Every movement an animal makes initiates a complex pattern of impulses in the sensory nerves from receptors in the muscles, in the joints, over the surface of the body, and elsewhere. It is possible that this complex spatio-temporal pattern is tested for match or mismatch with an inbuilt template.

Experiments on Arthropod locomotion tend to support this conclusion.[1] Let us take for example some work which has been done on the locomotion of the tarantula spider. It is found that the limbs of the spider move in a regular sequence when the animal walks. In Fig. 9.7 legs 1, 4, 5 and 8 move forward together and then, as they move backward, legs 2, 3, 6 and 7 move forward.

[1] See Wilson, D. M. (1968), 'The flight-control of the locust', *Scientific American*, May, 83–90.

Now what happens if legs 1 and 2, and 5 and 6 are removed? If the normal locomotory sequence were to be maintained, legs 4 and 8 would move forward together as would legs 3 and 7. The spider would overbalance on to its side. This, however, does not happen. Instead we find that the pattern of movements is reorganized so that legs 3 and 8 move forward together to be followed by legs 4 and 7. The arachnid thus shows itself fully capable of adapting to its straitened circumstances.

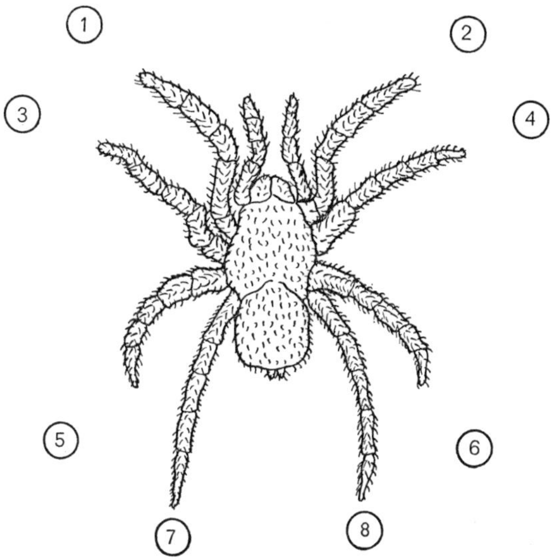


9.7 Locomotion of a tarantula spider. For explanation see text.

Many similar observations confirm the common impression that although the main outlines of the behaviour of the lower animals is stereotyped, it is nevertheless open to considerable adaptive flexibility in detail. It is in the physiological explanation of this adaptive flexibility that the concept of a central 'template' is important.

In the example of Fig. 9.7 we may suppose that there exists in the tarantula central nervous system a template which is fitted only by a particular four-dimensional pattern of sensory impulses. The motor output varies, hunts, until this sensory pattern is most nearly achieved and the template in consequence optimally fitted. In this way the sensory input regulates the intimate details of the motor output.

This template concept is very closely allied to another of the ideas developed in Chapter 12: the concept of internal homeostasis. We shall find in Chapter 12 that much mammalian behaviour is designed to ensure that the main variables of the fluids in which the body's cells are bathed are held constant. The organism's behaviour 'hunts', sometimes literally, until this set of physico-chemical parameters is optimally fitted.

In conclusion, however, it is important to notice that the sensory template concept by no means provides a universal explanation for the control of instinctive activity. It is probably operative in several innate behaviours but very far from all. It has, for example, been shown, especially in the vertebrates, that some quite complex inborn behaviours can proceed in the absence of any proprioceptive feed-back whatsoever. An example of this type of inflexible activity in amphibia is outlined on page 220. Automatic, pre-programmed behaviour of this type has been likened to the playing out of a 'motor tape'. It seems likely that both sensory template and motor tape mechanisms are involved in controlling different parts of the built-in behaviour patterns of the majority of animals.

# CHAPTER TEN

# The Evolution of Vertebrate Brains

## 10.1 The origins of animal brains

As animals evolve, increase in size and complexity, some means of co-ordination becomes essential. Whilst other systems, notably the endocrine system, control the more vegetative activities—growth, reproduction, etc.— it is the system of nerves which governs muscular activity and thus behaviour.

Nerves and muscles are inextricably interfused in animal life. With a few rather unimportant exceptions animals, in sharp contrast to plants, must search out and seize their food. In order to maintain their feelings of inner well-being they must periodically explore their surroundings in search of an appropriate morsel. It follows that one of the primary drives of animal behaviour is hunger; only by satisfying this craving can the internal environment be stabilized in its optimal state. J. Z. Young has likened the brain to the computer of a homeostat: the stratagems engineered by the brain to maintain the glucose content of the internal environment constant provide a striking instance of this concept.

The development of brains is thus tied very closely into the evolution of animal life. And just as the evolution of animals has been diverse and variegated so has the evolution of their brains. Darwin refers to the brain of an ant as the most remarkable speck of matter in the world; Sherrington believed the biology of the future would tend inevitably to centre on the human cerebrum. Both brains carry out many of the same co-ordinative functions; both are deeply fascinating pieces of biological engineering; both are still very imperfectly understood; but, although both consist of neurons and neuroglia, their architectural, principles are widely different. As we pointed out: animal brains are almost as divergent in their morphology as animals themselves.

The comparative study of animal brains is a very fascinating topic. This, however, is not the place to develop it. In this chapter we shall confine ourselves to an account of the brains of that phylum of animals to which man belongs. Indeed we shall restrict ourselves even more closely. The argument of this book is focused on the mammalian brain and, in particular, on the brain of man. Hence only those features of the vertebrate brain which help us to understand the primate brain will be discussed. The primate brain is, however, very large and almost inconceivably complex. Instead of being only a few cubic millimetres in volume as it is in the ant, the brain of a large primate, such as man, averages 1,300 cubic centimetres. It consists of at least thirty billion neurons. It will be remembered, moreover, that each one of these neurons may make up to 60,000 synaptic contacts (section 6.4). It is small wonder therefore that the brain of man offers something of an ultimate challenge to the human understanding.

The neurons of the human brain are arranged in a complicated system of cell masses and fibre bundles. One of the first problems for the neurobiologist is thus to decide the significance of these architectural features. One way, and probably the best way, of making sense of these comparatively large scale features of the brain's design is to examine its evolutionary history. For the brain forms no exception to the rule that each part of our anatomy bears witness to our billion-year pedigree. Thus just as the zoologist recognizes that our finger nails are flat because of our brachiating past, so the neurobiologist derives an explanation for many otherwise puzzling cerebral structures from a knowledge of vertebrate phylogeny.

### 10.2 The ground plan of vertebrate brains

The origin of the phylum Chordata—the great group of animals to which man belongs—is, and will probably long remain, a much debated topic. The fossil record is at best scanty and other evidence can only be indirect. The construction of phylogenetic trees is thus an exercise in zoological ingenuity. Evidence from comparative anatomy, from embryology and from several other disciplines is combined with the sparse and interrupted palaeontological record to obtain a plausible scheme. An understanding of the evolution of a soft, non-fossil-forming organ like the vertebrate brain must *a fortiori* rest on a complex of rather indirect lines of evidence.

One of the most weighty of these lines of indirect evidence stems from Haeckel's so-called biogenetic law. According to this proposition the developmental history of each individual recapitulates the evolutionary history of the group of animals to which the individual belongs. Thus the embryological development of the vertebrate brain, combined with an investigation of its comparative anatomy, is held to illuminate its evolutionary history.

Let us start our account, therefore, by suggesting that the earliest members of the phylum Chordata were minuscule organisms living in the warm surface waters of Cambrian seas some five hundred million years ago. Many authorities believe that these remote ancestors of ours resembled to some extent the larvae of present day Urochordates or sea-squirts. The fact that these primordial chordates populated the sunlit upper layers of ancient seas may well have been responsible for the development of a strip of sensory cells and associated neurons along their dorsal surfaces. Such a strip of nervous tissue is, indeed, the earliest evidence of the developing nervous system in present-day chordate embryos.

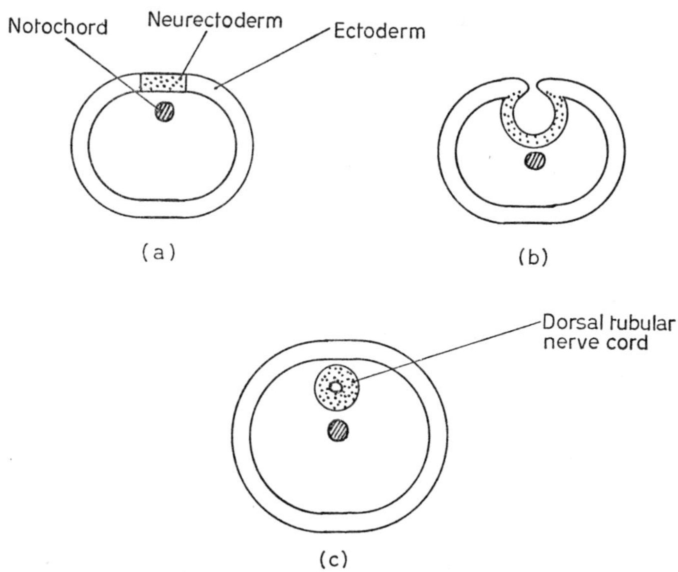


10.1 Formation of a dorsal nerve cord (a) shows the position of the neurectoderm in a very early embryo (T.S.). In (b) and (c) the neurectoderm rolls up and sinks inward to form a dorsal tubular structure. Later it becomes surrounded and protected by the bony arcades of the vertebral column.

In present-day embryos this strip of neurectoderm, as it is called, soon rolls up and sinks into the body of the developing organism (Fig. 10.1). We may imagine that this embryological movement recapitulates a stage in the evolution of the early chordates in which, for safety's sake, the dangerously exposed neurosensory strip invaginates. This step provides the dorsal tubular nerve cord which is so diagnostic a feature of all chordates.

Later on in the evolution of the phylum, and in the embryological development of most of its members, this tubular nerve cord gains further protection by becoming encased in the bony units of the vertebral or spinal column. Accordingly the nerve cord in its protective housing is customarily called the *spinal* cord.

Except in the most primitive members of the phylum Chordata the nerve cord does not long remain a simple undifferentiated tube. Vastly important developments occur at its anterior extremity. The reasons for these transformations are not difficult to find.

The majority of chordates seem, from the earliest times, to have been active, energetic animals. This fact implies that they possessed and still possess efficient and effective sense organs. Now it can be shown that the nerve centres concerned in the analysis of the input of a sense organ tend, during evolutionary development, to move towards that sense organ.[1] This phenomenon has been called *neurobiotaxis*. Now chordates are bilaterally symmetric animals and hence have a definite anterior and posterior end. It follows that sense organs tend to develop most profusely at the anterior end of the animal: for it is this end, after all, which first penetrates new environments and which leads in all the animal's activities. It follows, in turn, from the principle of neurobiotaxis, that this polarization of sense organs is accompanied by a polarization of nervous centres. Thus we would expect from these rather *a priori* arguments to find that the nervous system is most richly developed at the animal's anterior end.

Our expectations are, of course, not disappointed. The anterior end of the nerve cord is greatly developed. Evidence from embryology and comparative anatomy suggests that the aboriginal chordate brain consisted of an expansion or, more accurately, a series of expansions at the anterior end of the tubular nerve cord. Initially, it

[1] Ariens-Kappers, C. U., Huber, G. C. and Crosbie, E. C., *The Comparative Anatomy of the Nervous System of the Vertebrates including Man*, Vol. 1, Hefner Publishing Co., New York, 1960, p. 76 ff.

seems, these expansions were three in number—constituting a fore-, mid- and hind-brain. These three balloonings of the neural tube serve the three main distance receptors. The forebrain (=prosencephalon) is associated with olfaction, the midbrain (=mesencephaplon) with vision and the hindbrain (=rhombencephalon) with equilibrium and vibration. These three 'primary vesicles' are said to constitute the *brain stem* (Fig. 10.2). The vastly more complex brains of higher vertebrates develop by superimposition on this primordial stem.

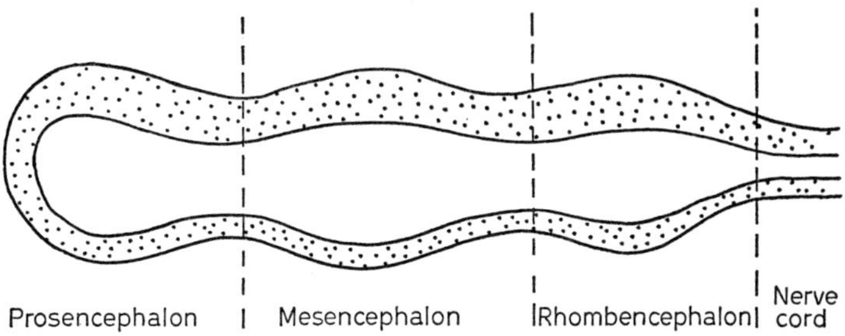


10.2 The three primary vesicles of the brain stem (L.S.).

The first indications of this superimposition are developments in the roofs of all three chambers. From the roof of the forebrain develops a structure which is destined, in the end, to revolutionize life on earth. In the more lowly vertebrates, however, this incipient *cerebrum* is a rather inconspicuous swelling designed to analyse the input from the olfactory organs. The roof of the midbrain enlarges to form the *optic tectum* in which, in the lower vertebrates, fibres from the optic nerve terminate. Finally the roof of the hindbrain gives rise to a structure called the *cerebellum* which, in active animals, is vitally important in co-ordinating muscular movement and balance. These important developments are shown diagrammatically in Fig. 10.3.

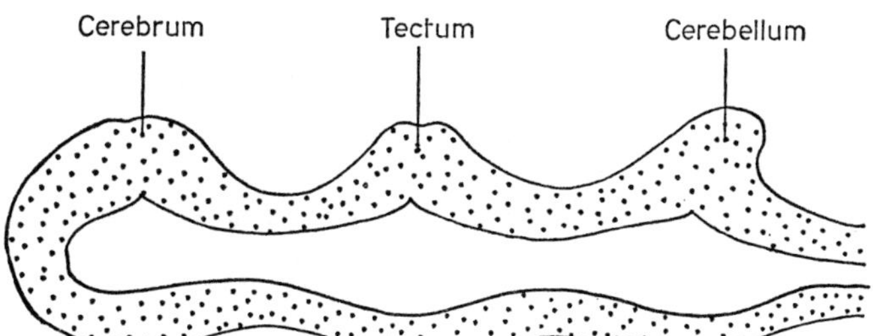


10.3 Major developments in the roof of the brain stem (L.S.).

Fig. 10.3 summarizes the ground plan of the vertebrate brain. Our next task is to consider briefly how this fundamental plan is developed and modified to form the brains of higher vertebrates—in particular, mammals.

### 10.3 The architecture of the spinal cord

In explaining how the brains of higher vertebrates develop from the simple structure of Fig. 10.3 it will be wise to begin at the posterior end, which remains very little modified even in mammals, and work forward to the cerebrum which, in man, has become so gigantic that it rests upon and overhangs everything else.

Most posterior of all is, of course, the spinal cord. The architecture of this part of the central nervous system remains in the mammal very much what it was in the earliest vertebrates. Indeed some of the intricate features of the brains of higher vertebrates can be seen as elaborations of its more primitive structure.

Due to the mode of origin of the central nervous system described in the preceding section the spinal cord is hollow. The cavity in the centre—the central canal—is, however, in the adult very narrow. It continues uninterruptedly into the brain where it is enlarged to form chambers known as ventricles. The grey matter of the spinal cord, consisting of cytons and nerve fibres, is concentrated in the centre immediately surrounding the central canal. Surrounding the grey matter is the white matter which consists of tracts of fibres running up and down the cord.

The grey matter can be shown to be differentiated into several distinct functional regions. The nerve cells in each of these regions are, in the main, concerned with a common function. This organization is shown in Fig. 10.4.

Similarly there is some evidence that the nerve fibres of the white matter are loosely grouped into tracts, or columns, all the members of which have roughly the same function.

In addition to this columnar organization other regions of the spinal cord retain a more primitive tangle of nerve processes and nerve cell bodies. This apparent lack of regular organization is particularly well marked in the vicinity of the central canal. The inextricable tangle of nerve elements in this position is reminiscent of the neuropil of some invertebrate brains. This labyrinthine network

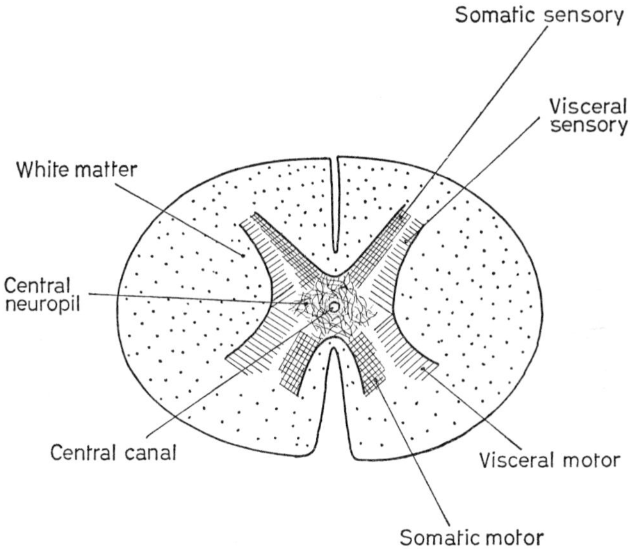


10.4 T.S. of spinal cord. The grey matter of the spinal cord is arranged roughly in the form of an 'H' in the centre of the tissue. The white matter, consisting largely of nerve tracts, is peripheral. Sensory nerve fibres enter the dorsal (posterior) 'horn' of the grey matter; motor nerve fibres leave from the ventral (anterior) 'horn'.

extends anteriorly into the brain itself where it forms the *reticular formation*. In recent years, as we shall see in Chapter 16, many important functions have been assigned to this structure.

Immediately the spinal cord enters the skull it expands to form the hindbrain. We shall see that the most posterior region of the hindbrain—the *medulla oblongata*—retains many of the architectural features of the cord.

### 10.4 The hindbrain

The medulla does not constitute the whole of the hindbrain, or even the major and most important part of it. The primordial rhombencephalon of Fig. 10.3 is divided, for convenience, into two parts. The posterior part is called the *myelencephalon* and it is this which develops into the medulla; the anterior part is called the *metencephalon* and from it develops the cerebellum and associated structures. This rather arbitrary division of the primitive rhombencephalon is shown in Fig. 10.5.

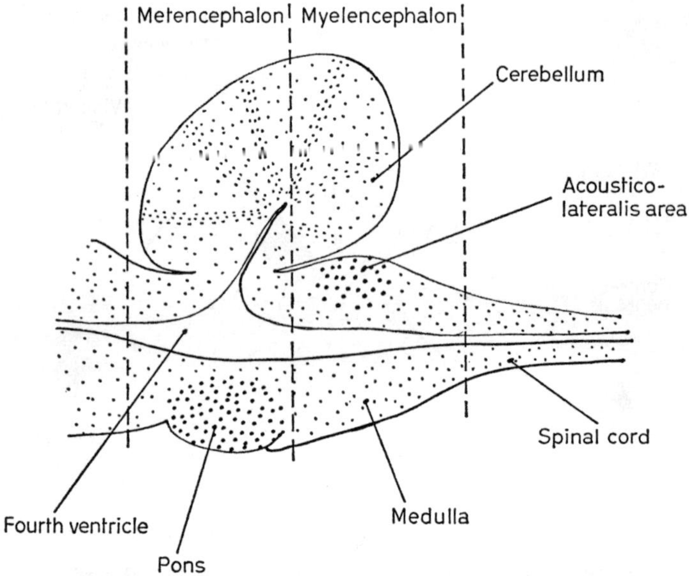

10.5 Differentiation of the rhombencephalon (L.S.).

The medulla itself, although relatively undifferentiated—it still shows the four functional columns of the spinal cord—is of considerable importance in the body's economy. It is from this part of the brain that many of the vital automatic activities of the viscera are controlled. For example, nerve centres in this structure regulate the activity of the heart, lungs and alimentary canal; the calibre of the arterioles in many parts of the body; the metabolism of carbohydrates; the osmotic pressure of the blood. These nerve centres are, however, themselves often governed by centres further forward in the brain.

Immediately in front of the medulla lies the metencephalon. We saw in section 2 of this chapter that the hindbrain originates in association with sense organs able to detect vibration and the orientation of the body. Both these types of sense organ consist, in essence, of mechanoreceptive hair cells (see Chapters 7 and 8). From this type of sensory cell are elaborated accelerometers able to detect movement in space (the semicircular canals), gravity receptors (the utriculus and sacculus) and, finally, vibration receptors (lateral line canals and cochleas). All of these senses are clearly of very considerable importance to an animal.

It follows that the part of the hindbrain devoted to the analysis of all this information—the metencephalon—is, in most vertebrates, very well developed. From its roof (Fig. 10.5) grows the *cerebellum* which in active animals becomes large and elaborate. For it is this organ which, working with the information derived from the equilibrium sensors mentioned above and with information derived from proprioceptors embedded in the muscles and tendons, ensures that the commands travelling down from the higher parts of the brain to the muscles are satisfactorily co-ordinated and result, in consequence, in smooth well-regulated movements. As we stressed in Chapter 9 one has only to meditate on the number of muscles which must be accurately co-ordinated before we can take a single step, much less use a knife and fork, write a sentence or catch a cricket ball, to recognize the vital importance of the cerebellum.

Fig. 10.5 shows that, opposite the cerebellum, on the ventral side of the fourth ventricle, another thickening of the walls of the neural tube develops. This is called the *pons*. In fact it develops in close association with the cerebellum. Nerve fibres carrying messages from the cerebrum to the muscles synapse in this region with fibres running out from the cerebellum. Thus can the logistical operations of the cerebellum impress themselves upon the 'raw' output from the cerebrum, transforming a decision to act in such and such a manner into nicely judged muscular activity (see, also, section 11.7).

Immediately posterior to the cerebellum in the roof of the myelencephalon lies an area concerned with processing the information gathered by the sense organs specialized to detect vibration. In the lower vertebrates a lateral line system capable of picking up rather low frequency vibrations exists in addition to, or in place of, the more familiar auditory organs developed in the mammals. In the fish and amphibia, consequently, a large *acoustico-lateralis* area frequently develops in the myelencephalon. In the mammals this area is much reduced in size although a small centre continues to exist. In both lower and higher vertebrates, as we shall see, information reaching these myelencephalic auditory centres is relayed forward to higher centres of the brain where it is matched up with information arriving from other distance receptors.

## 10.5 The midbrain

In front of the metencephalon lies the midbrain or mesencephalon.

In the lower vertebrates (fish and amphibia) the roof of the mesencephalon is one of the most important regions of the entire brain. It is to this centre that fibres of the optic nerve travel. Terminating in the roof of the mesencephalon they help to form the dominant association area of the brain. Here the visual information is sorted out and correlated with information about the outside world collected by other distance receptors. It is, for example, to this region that information from the auditory centre in the hindbrain is passed. And it is from this region, after appropriate computation, that messages are relayed to the effector organs. Thus in the brains of amphibia and fish the mesencephalon is in command: it is in this centre that the vital behavioural decisions are made.

The greater part of all this important activity as 'head office' of the nervous system is, however, lost in the higher vertebrates. In mammalian brains ultimate decisions are taken in the cerebrum; the mesencephalon is relegated to a very provincial status. The vastly important traffic along the optic nerves from the eyes largely bypasses the roof of the midbrain, or *tectum*, and is displayed instead in the cerebral hemispheres. Fibres from the other distance receptors also give the tectum a miss and converge on the region where the action now is: the cerebrum.

Thus in the mammals we find that the once highly developed optic tectum is reduced to four small swellings in the midbrain roof. These lobes form the *corpora quadrigemina* or, alternatively, they are sometimes labelled as two superior and two inferior *colliculi*. Certain visual reflexes are mediated through the superior colliculi, whilst the inferior pair act as centres for a number of auditory reflexes.

Insignificant as the midbrain may be in the information processing characteristic of the mammalian brain it nevertheless retains some control over behaviour. It is believed (see Chapter 12) that some of the behavioural drives observable in mammals, including men, are initiated in this part of the brain. Thus are the sins of their fish forefathers still visited upon a mankind striving for civilized behaviour.

### 10.6 The thalamencephalon

The most anterior of the three primordial brain vesicles—the prosencephalon—undergoes dramatic development in the higher vertebrates, especially in the mammals. Indeed in the latter animals all the most important functions of the brain tend to be concentrated in this region.

Very early in embryological development this initial 'smell-brain' becomes divided into two. A pair of lobes, probably at first closely involved with olfaction, grow outwards and forwards from the primordial forebrain (Fig. 10.6). These lobes constitute the telencephalon; the region of the forebrain behind the telencephalon is now called the thalamencephalon or diencephalon.

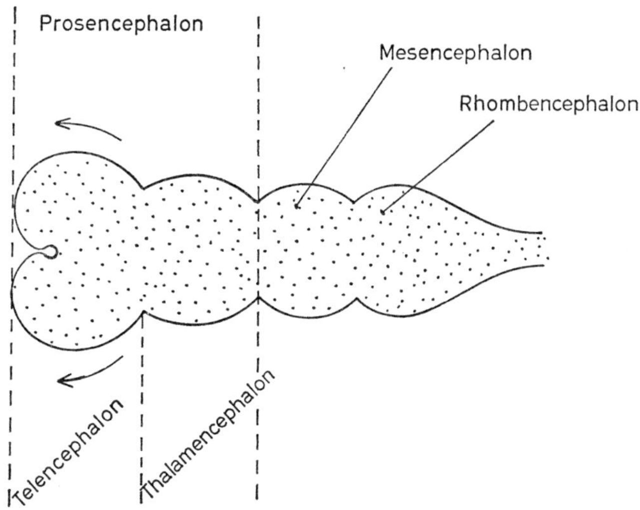


10.6 Origin of the telencephalon. The developing brain is viewed from above. The arrows indicate the direction of morphogenetic movement.

In pursuance of our policy of progressing from posterior to anterior let us begin our account of the forebrain by describing some features of the thalamencephalon.

Like other regions of the brain the thalamencephalon is at the outset tubular in cross-section (Fig. 10.7). The walls of this tube were called by the early anatomists the *thalamus*. This term is derived from a Greek root meaning 'bed' or 'couch'. The conceit was that the thalamencephalon formed a resting-place and support for the greatly developed telencephalon of the higher vertebrates. This idea, as we see, still lies embalmed in neurological terminology.

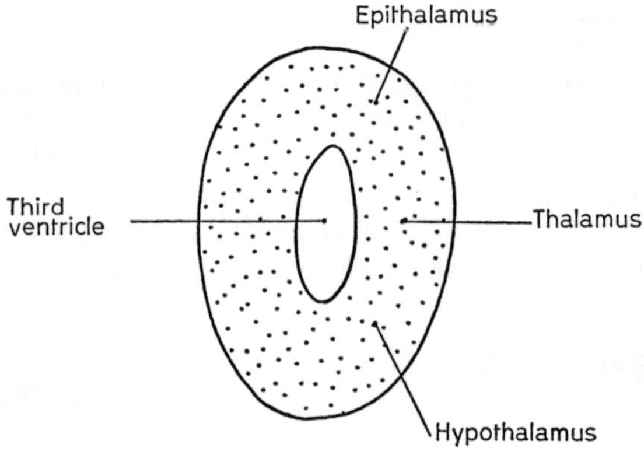


10.7 T.S. through thalamencephalon.

The roof of the thalamencephalon, as Fig. 10.7 shows, is called the *epithalamus*. From it spring two protuberances—the parietal and pineal bodies (Fig. 10.8). In some of the lower vertebrates (cyclostomes, some amphibia and some reptiles) either the parietal or pineal organ develops into a third eye; in the mammals this photoreceptor function is lacking and, although Descartes believed the pineal important enough to act as the seat of the soul, its function has, until very recently,[1] remained obscure.

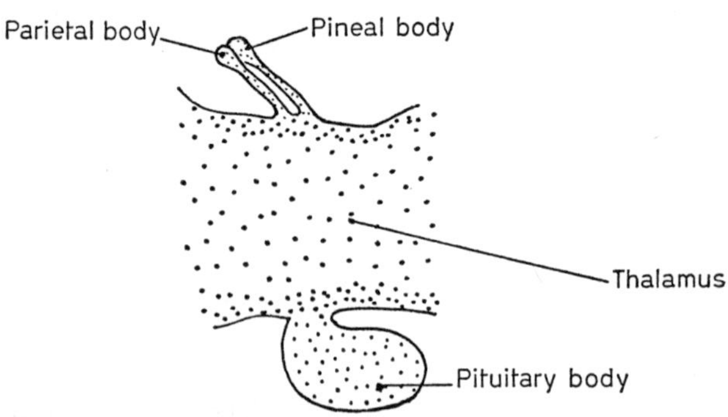


10.8 Positions of parietal, pineal and pituitary bodies. It is usual to find that where the pineal is well developed the parietal is not, and vice versa.

[1] There is some evidence that mammalian pineals are neurosecretory organs which have an influence on reproductive cycles.

The floor of the thalamencephalon is called the *hypothalamus*. It has, as we shall see in this chapter and in Chapter 12, many important functions. Complementing the development of the pineal and parietal from the epithalamus a downwardly directed outpushing develops which eventually unites with an upgrowth from the roof of the pharynx. The composite organ so formed grows into the most important endocrine gland of the vertebrate body: the pituitary.

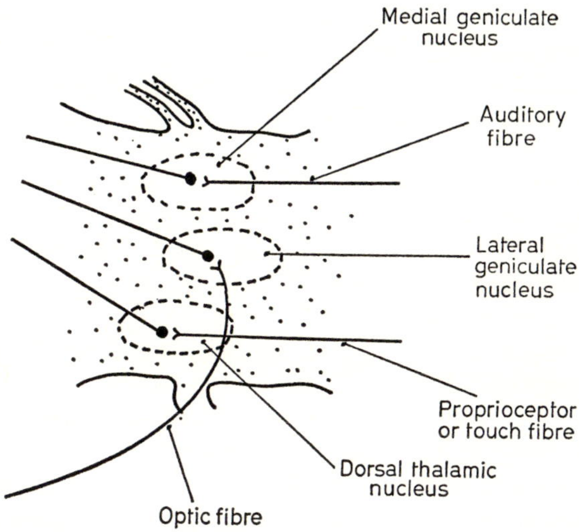


10.9 Some thalamic nuclei. This highly diagrammatic figure shows the thalamus from the side.

In addition to these evaginations from the roof and floor outgrowths of equally great importance develop from the sides of the thalamencephalon. These outgrowths are destined to form the retinae and optic nerves of the eyes.

The floor, roof and side walls of the thalamencephalon left behind by these dramatic developments are, as might be expected, rich with a complex of nerve fibres and concentrations of cytons. These concentrations are called *nuclei*. Several of these nuclei act as staging posts for fibres originating further back in the brain, or arriving in the brain from the distance receptors.

For example, most of the fibres of the optic nerve run first to the *lateral geniculate nuclei* (Fig. 10.9). In these nuclei they synapse with other fibres which relay the visual information to the cerebral cortex.

Similarly fibres from the auditory centres in the hindbrain run to the *medial geniculate nuclei* where, once again, synapses are made with other fibres which run to the auditory area in the cerebral cortex. Yet other nuclei in the thalamus act as staging posts where messages originating in the cerebellum, in touch receptors and in proprioceptors are relayed forward to the cerebrum.

In addition to these thalamic nuclei there are many important nuclei in the hypothalamus. Many of these nuclei are involved in the control of visceral activity. This, perhaps, is not surprising as the hypothalamus can be seen as the anterior terminus of the visceral sensory and motor columns of the spinal cord (Fig. 10.4). Thus we find that these nuclei control many important parameters of the internal environment. The temperature of the mammalian body is, for example, controlled from this part of the brain. The osmotic pressure of the blood and its electrolyte constitution are also governed from this region. In Chapter 12 we shall also find that the hypothalamus is believed to be responsible for several basic behavioural drives. As in the case of the midbrain it seems likely that the existence of thalamencephalic centres governing behavioural repertoires is an evolutionary relic. In the lower vertebrates the telencephalon is only very poorly developed and in these animals the thalamencephalon is deeply implicated in computing appropriate behaviours. In the mammals where this function has been taken over by the cerebrum the thalamencephalon remains, like a grumbling appendix, an unwelcome reminder of a more lowly past.

## 10.7 The telencephalon

The thalamencephalon, as we have just seen, earned its name by appearing to act as a couch on which the cerebrum rests. Clearly the cerebrum has long impressed human anatomists as the major and most important part of the brain. But this is very far from being the case in the lower vertebrates.

In the foregoing section we noted that the telencephalon originated as a pair of forwardly directed outpushings from the archaic prosencephalon. These two outpushings form the two cerebral hemispheres. Initially these hemispheres are concerned in the analysis of impulses arriving from the olfactory organs. This early smell-orientated cerebrum never attains a very great size or organizational prominence. In both fish and amphibia it remains as a pair of swell-

XI Retinae

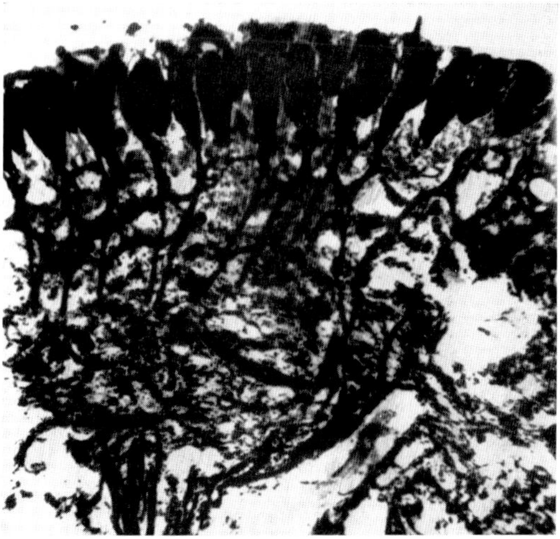

(a) Vertical section through the compound eye of *Limulus* the King Crab. The black masses at the top of the photograph are the ommatidia; emerging from their bases are nerve fibres which go to make the optic nerve. Cross connections between these fibres, believed to be responsible for lateral inhibition, can be seen beneath the ommatidia. (Courtesy of W. H. Miller from Hartline, H. K., Wagner, H. G. and Ratcliff, F. (1956), 'Inhibition in the eye of Limulus', *J. Gen. Physiol.*, *39*, 651–73.)

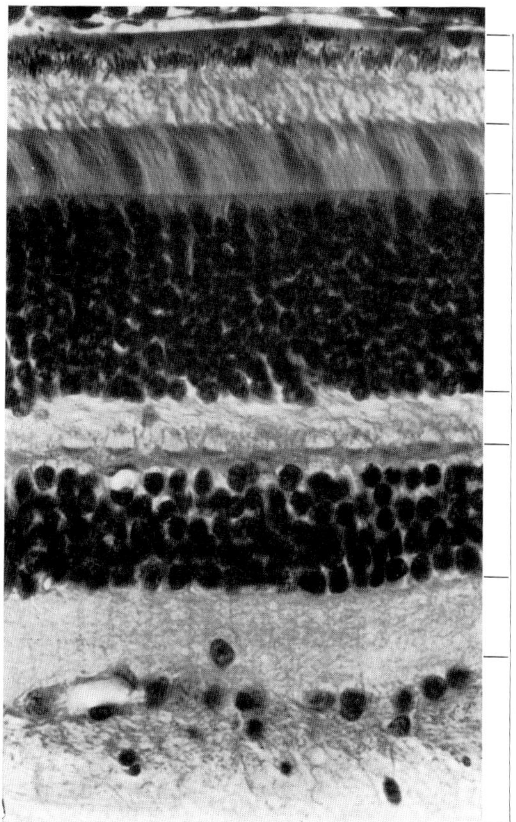


(b) Vertical section through a mammalian retina (×480). Light approaches this retina from the bottom and has to penetrate through the various nervous layers before it can stimulate the outer segments of the rods and cones.

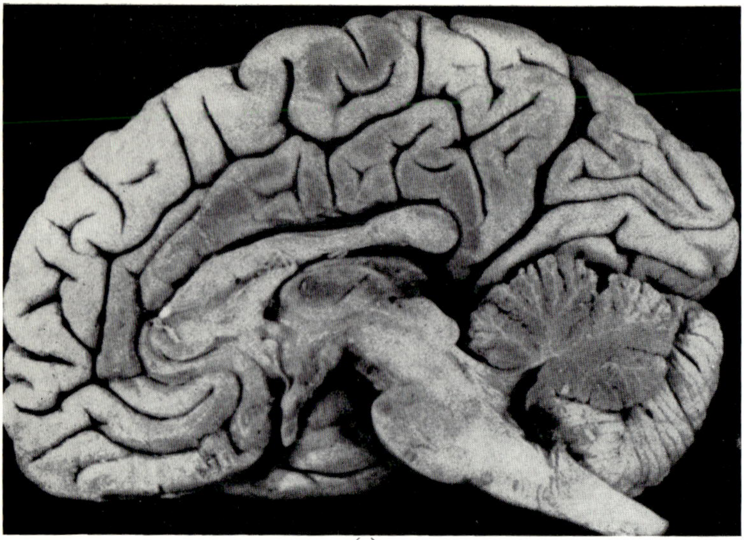

(a)

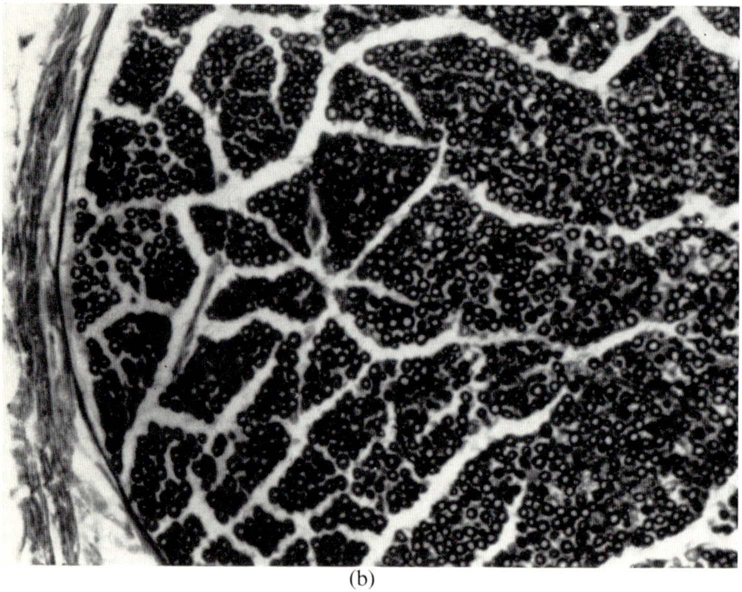

(b)

XII Sections through brain and peripheral nerve

(a) Mid-sagittal section through the human brain. The olfactory bulbs and pituitary body have been removed and the brain is viewed from the medial surface. The parts of the brain may be identified by comparison with fig. 10.10. (From H. Chandler Elliot, *Textbook of Neuroanatomy*, J. B. Lippincott Company, 1963.)

(b) Tranverse section through the sciatic nerve of a mammal (× 120). Only a segment of the nerve can be seen in this micrograph. The small dark-rimmed profiles are myelinated axons.

ings of very modest dimensions. Its comparative unimportance in these lower brains has already been emphasized. It will be remembered that in both fish and amphibia the optic tectum in the midbrain forms the major association area.

With the evolution of the higher vertebrates, however, the cerebrum rapidly assumes a far greater significance. Its relative magnitude is shown in Fig. 10.10 and in Plate XII. This great development is probably to be correlated with the increased part the sense of smell plays in the life of the majority of mammals. It seems probable that olfaction is the dominant sense in many mammalian groups. Hunting, socializing, mating, escaping—all depend to a greater or lesser extent on olfactory cues and clues. The perceptual worlds of most mammals are predominantly olfactory worlds. It is not unreasonable to see in this fact a reason for the re-routing of optic and auditory nerve fibres from the midbrain tectum towards the cerebrum. For it is in this region, as we have suggested, that the crucial sensory information is displayed. It is here, we may imagine, that appropriate behavioural reflexes and postures are assessed. It is thus good design practice for the auditory and optic fibres to terminate in the same neighbourhood. In this way it is possible for the all-important cross-correlation and comparison of information detected by the different sense organs to occur swiftly and efficiently.

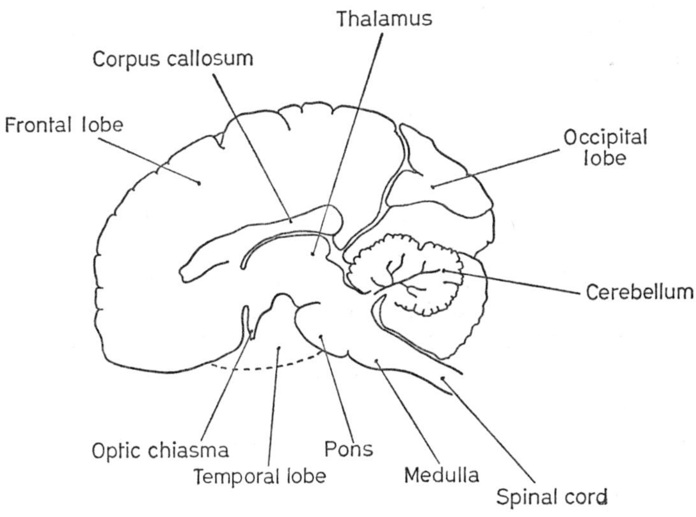


10.10 Mid-sagittal section through the human brain.

If our argument is correct we have in this way an explanation for the cerebrum's great growth in the higher vertebrates.

Almost alone amongst terrestrial mammals the primates somewhat escape the world of scents and savours. There are, of course, good evolutionary reasons for this distinction. The early primates were arboreal animals and in the trees scents hang less heavily than on the earth itself. Moreover an arboreal life puts a premium on good judgement of distance and thus on the development of the eyes. It has often been remarked (see Chapter 14) that the human perceptual world is a visual world. However we have not, of course, lost our senses of smell and taste. Indeed few sensations have such emotional reverberations. It will be remembered that Proust hangs the twelve volumes of *A la recherche du temps perdu* on the sense of taste. So powerful were the memories evoked by a long-forgotten taste that the past itself seemed to have been recovered. Thus we can perhaps glimpse by introspection the psychical correlatives of the instinctive behaviours triggered in non-primate mammals by chemical stimuli.

Thus it is not surprising to find that, although it still exists, the volume of primate cerebrum given over to olfaction is rather insignificant. It is overshadowed by the development of other regions. A detailed discussion of the primate cerebrum is, however, deferred to Chapter 13. In the remainder of this chapter it is proposed to discuss briefly the main architectural features of the cerebrum in higher vertebrates.

The diagrams of Fig. 10.11 trace the evolution of one of the two cerebral hemispheres from a hypothetical primitive condition (a) to the climax reached in the primates (e). Initially the hemisphere, if such it can be called, is entirely olfactory in function. The grey matter in this archetypal cerebrum is central and abuts the ventricle. Its position is thus reminiscent of the position of the grey matter in the spinal cord. One of the first developments in the evolution of the cerebral hemispheres is the migration of this strip of grey matter outwards towards the surface of the brain. Thus does the *palaeocortex* originate. Next (Fig. 10.11 (b) ) the homogeneity of this rind of grey matter is disrupted. The olfactory palaeocortex remains but it becomes sandwiched between the two new regions of grey matter. Dorsally there develops the *archicortex*—an association area— and ventrally another mass of grey matter—the *corpus striatum*—arises. It is in the latter strip of grey matter that, in the lower vertebrates, nerve fibres carrying impulses to the effector organs originate.

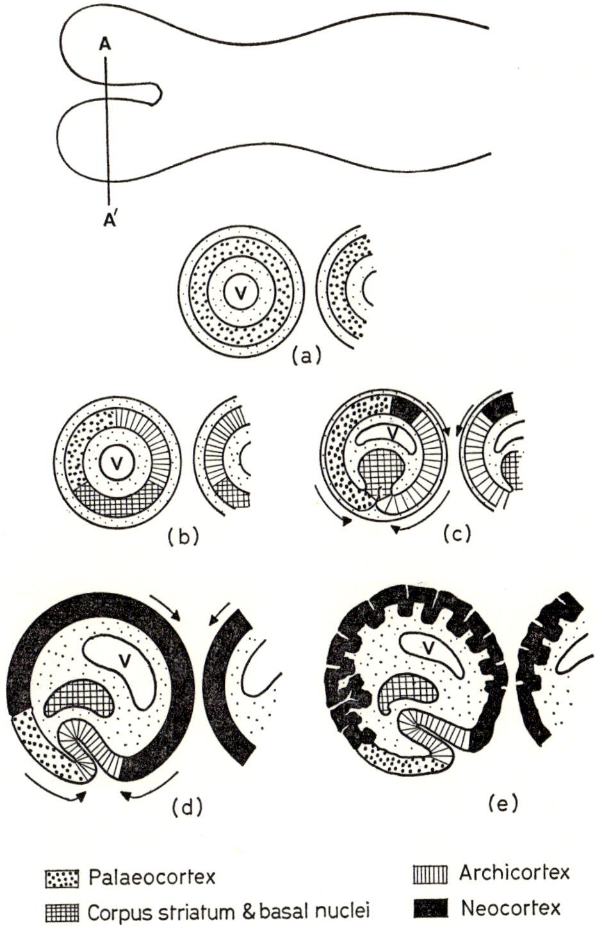


10.11 Evolutionary development of the cerebrum. The top diagram shows the primitive brain from above (see Fig. 10.6) and indicates the plane in which the sections are cut: AA′. V = lateral ventricle. Arrows indicate direction of morphogenetic movement. Explanation in text. Adapted from various sources and in particular Romer, A. S. (1949), *The Vertebrate Body*, W. B. Saunders Company, Philadelphia.

As the vertebrate scale is ascended we find first that the corpus striatum becomes detached from the rest of the grey matter and sinks inwards to form an island nucleus in a sea of white matter (Fig. 10.11 (c) ) and then that a new strip of cortex appears between the palaeo- and archicortices. This is a momentous development. For this rudiment is the beginning of the *neocortex*. It first appears at the level of the reptiles. This new cortex resembles the archicortex and differs from the palaeocortex in being devoted to no single sense modality. From its inception it receives intelligence from all the major sense organs. In Figs. 10.11 (d) and 10.11 (e) it can be seen that dramatic developments occur to the neocortex. These two illustrations are of a cerebral hemisphere in a primitive mammal and in a primate. It is clear that the great growth of the neocortex compresses the archi- and palaeocortices. The archicortex is twisted, so the old anatomists thought, into the form of a sea-horse. Hence this region of the mammalian cortex is known as the *hippocampus*. There are indications that it is involved in memory. The palaeocortex retains its primitive olfactory function although it is forced down into the ventral surface of the hemisphere. Human anatomists know it as the *pyriform* lobe. Fig. 10.11 (e) shows that in a higher primate such as *H. sapiens* the neocortex increases in size still further by developing an intricate series of fissures and folds. The area of both human cerebral cortices ranges between 1460 and 1620 $cm^2$. Each hemisphere contains about $2{\cdot}6 \times 10^9$ neurons.[1] Neurologists believe that the distinctive characteristics of human beings depend on this hypertrophied sheet of tissue.

The evolution of the cerebral cortex may thus be traced through the vertebrates, through the mammalian orders, to a climax in *H. sapiens*. It seems clear that man's dominion over the rest of creation depends on the vast development of this sheet of nerve tissue. Because of its quite outstanding importance it will be considered in detail in Chapter 13.

As we shall see in Chapter 13 the cerebral cortex appears to be essential to speech and thus to symbolic thought or, as Pavlov[2] put it, to a 'second signalling system'. This fact, a fact which Pavlov goes on to point out makes us human, is probably closely related to the

[1] Pakkenberg, H. (1966), 'The number of nerve cells in the cerebral cortex of man', *J. Comp. Neur.*, *128*, 17–20.

[2] Pavlov, I. P., *Selected Works*, Foreign Languages Publishing House, Moscow, 1955, p. 262.

fact that the cortex in the higher mammals is the great end-organ of the exteroreceptors. According to Lenneberg[1] human speech depends on mechanisms for the classification of sensory information which also exist, at a lower level of development, in all vertebrate animals. Thus we can perhaps see that the apparent deep dichotomy between ourselves and animal creation depends only on the increased efficiency of the human cerebral cortex in the analysis of the sensory input.

In other words it seems possible that the processes of perception and symbolic thought are quite closely allied. In Chapter 14 we shall see that perception may be regarded as a process of pattern recognition: an active matching of the incoming sensory signal against a pattern or map of expectations in the brain. In the same way 'thought' might be regarded, to borrow a term from computer science, as *simulation*. As the building of models or analogues of the world. It is the essence of productive thought to match these forming analogues against the data derived from the senses, or the data stored in the memory.

Thus we see that the development of a common organ for sensory analysis in the ballooning cerebral hemispheres has been fraught with still incalculable consequences. Consequences which have ultimately included the conundrum of self-awareness: the reflection of matter on itself.

[1] Lenneberg, E. H., *Biological Foundations of Language*, John Wiley and Sons, New York, 1967, p. 374.

# CHAPTER ELEVEN

# Patterns of Neurons in the Brain

## 11.1 Are nerve pathways inherited?

We have already seen how vastly complex the vertebrate brain has become. We have seen that the human cerebrum consists of over five thousand million neurons. Each neuron in the cerebral cortex may, moreover, make up to sixty thousand synaptic contacts.[1] There is reason to believe that a given cortical neuron will not make more than a hundred or so synapses with any other single neuron and probably far less. It follows, therefore, that a neuron in the cerebal cortex may communicate with at least six hundred others and probably far more.

Another way of gaining some insight into this immense interconnexity is to estimate the number of synapses in the cortex. In the monkey it has been shown that the synaptic density varies from $6{\cdot}2 \times 10^{11}/\text{cm}^3$ in the visual cortex to $9{\cdot}2 \times 10^{11}/\text{cm}^3$ in the motor cortex. It is likely that the synaptic density of the human cerebrum is rather greater than that found in the monkey. Let us therefore take a value of $10 \times 10^{11}/\text{cm}^3$ ($1 \times 10^{12}/\text{cm}^3$) as the average synaptic density in the human cerebral cortex. If we multiply this figure by the volume of the average human cortex (about 500 $\text{cm}^3$) we arrive at the staggering number of $5 \times 10^{14}$ synapses. This is five followed by fourteen zeros. In 1964 there were about 170,000,000 telephones in the world; this is considerably less than one millionth the number of synaptic connections in the cerebral cortex alone.

One question which may strike us when we contemplate this mind-defeating complexity is whether this vast system of connexities is in-

[1] Cragg, B. G. (1967), 'The density of synapses and neurons in the motor and visual areas of the cerebral cortex', *J. Anat.*, *101*, 639–654. The figure of 60,000 synaptic contacts/neuron applies to monkey motor cortex. Other parts of the cortex may have fewer synapses/neuron. On the other hand the Purkinje cells of the cerebellum, as we shall see, may receive over 200,000 synaptic contacts.

built, genetically predetermined, or whether it is merely a random assemblage. Is each nerve pathway exactly specified by the animal's genome or do the pathways achieve their particular routes in the adult brain as a result of the organism's individual experience? Clearly this is a topic of considerable relevance to the interrelated problems of learning and memory.

### 11.2 Morphopoietic movements

The problem of the specificity or lack of specificity of neuronal patterns is a special case of the more general problem of morphopoiesis in the living world. How do cells aggregate to form complex and exquisitely designed tissues and organs? No one can yet say. The phenomenon is, however, striking and has attracted the attention of biologists since the earliest times.

In some cases a chemical mechanism can be shown to be involved. For example, a chemical—acrasin—has been shown to be responsible for the remarkable sight of several hundred individual myxamoebae streaming together and fusing to form the body of the slime mould *Dictyostelium discoideum*. The myxamoebae swim up a gradient of this substance until, on coming together, they unite to form the 'multicellular' body of the mould.[1]

In other cases the concept of 'contact inhibition' has been invoked. It is suggested that embryonic cells move at random until their surfaces make contact with a substrate with a certain submicroscopical structure. Movement then ceases and the cells settle down in this position. This concept has arisen from observations of the reaggregation of disaggregated embryonic cells. Moscona, for example, reports[2] experiments in which dissociated mouse and chick embryonic cells are intermingled in a suspension culture. Now it is possible to distinguish mouse and chick embryonic cells by a marked difference in the sizes of their nuclei. Observations of the growing culture over periods of up to a month showed that cells which would normally have formed one type of tissue—kidney, for example, or cartilage—had regrouped themselves to form primordia of these structures. The

[1] Bonner, J. T. (1947), 'Evidence for the formation of cell aggregates by chemotaxis in the development of the slime mold *Dictyostelium discoideum*', *J. Exp. Zool., 106*, 1–26.

[2] Moscona, A. (1957), 'The development *in vitro* of chimaeric aggregates of dissociated embryonic chick and mouse cells', *Proc. Nat. Acad. Sci.* (*Wash.*), *43*, 184–194.

most striking finding, however, was that chick cells had not grouped themselves with other chick cells, or mouse cells with mouse cells, but that chimaeric structures had been formed. The kidney or cartilage primordia were formed of associations of cells derived from both species. The aggregation of these embryonic cells showed that species specificity was a weaker force than tissue specificity. It looks as if the surface of cells destined to form a particular tissue are mutually adhesive; this stickiness does not obtain to the same degree between cells destined to form different tissues, even though they come from the same animal species. This selective stickiness reminds the molecular biologist of the similar stickiness which exists between enzyme and substrate. This is known to have a physical basis in an exact stereochemical fit between the active site of the enzyme and the substrate molecule. It is perhaps not too wild a speculation to suggest that the globular proteins which are believed (section 3.4) to cover the lipid framework of cell membranes may form the physical basis of this selective stickiness between cells.

Let us return now from this brief sortie into the fascinating field of experimental embryology and examine in its light some of the equally fascinating work which has been done in experimental neuroanatomy.

### 11.3 Wallerian degeneration

Before reviewing some of the experiments which have been tried in an attempt to uncover evidence for or against neuronal specificity it is important to be clear about the nature of Wallerian degeneration. For we shall find that some of the most crucial investigations have depended upon this phenomenon. Quite simply it is found that when the axon of a nerve cell is cut that part distal to the section degenerates (Fig. 11.1). After a couple of weeks there is little left of the axon distal to the cut. When the original axon has more or less disappeared the first signs of regeneration may be found. Minute nerve fibrils begin to sprout from the stump. They appear to grow down the space left by the old axon's demise. Eventually they reach the structure formerly innervated by the original axon. Thus after an accident in which a nerve is severed an individual may lose the power to move certain muscles. If he is fortunate, however, this power will be restored after a year or so by regeneration of the interrupted fibres.

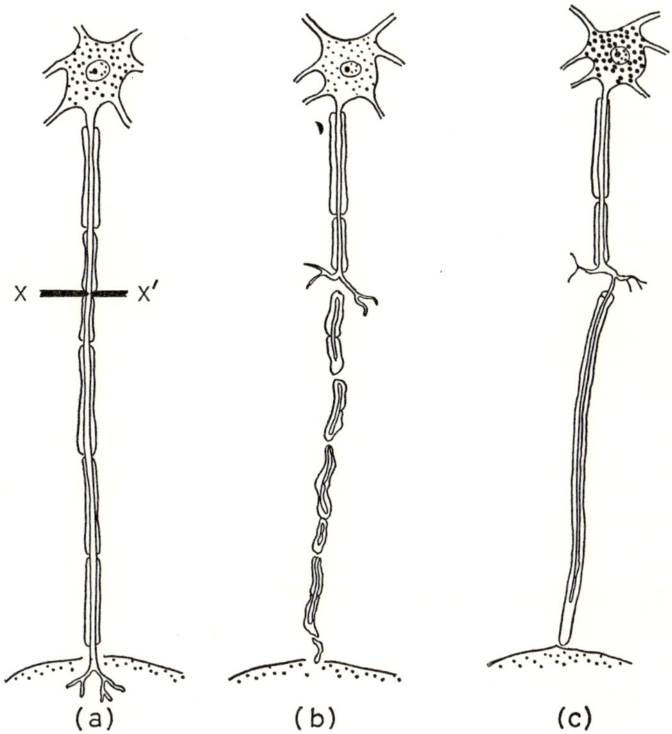


11.1 Wallerian degeneration. In (a) the axon is cut at XX′ and (b) shows that the part distal to the cut degenerates. In (c) the process of regeneration within the remains of the sheath left by the old axon is shown. Note the greatly increased granularity apparent in the perikaryon of the regenerating neuron.

### 11.4 Scrambling the amphibian visual system

Let us now look at some very striking experiments which have been carried out on the visual systems of amphibia.[1] These experiments take their origin from the finding that photic stimulation of the frog's retina causes activity in the midbrain optic tectum (section 10.5). Furthermore it had been shown that stimulation of different parts of the retina resulted in activity in different parts of the tectum. Indeed it was possible to demonstrate that there was a point for point correspondence between the retina and the tectum. In other

[1] Gaze, R. M. (1960), 'Regeneration of the optic nerve in amphibia', *Int. Rev. of Neurobiol., 2*, 1–18.

words there is a faithful mapping of a retinal mosaic on a tectal mosaic.

Now what, we might wonder, would happen if the frog's eye were rotated through 180 degrees in its socket without injuring the optic nerve? The experiment has been tried and it has been shown that the correspondence between the retinal and tectal mosaics is *not* upset. Thus fibres originating from what is now the bottom sector of the retina activate a tectal region which formerly corresponded to the top sector. In consequence the central nervous system is thoroughly confused. The tectum records activity corresponding to the natural and original orientation of the eye, yet the eye is now 'upside down'. It follows that the animal's behaviour in response to visual stimuli is often useless, irrelevant if not downright deleterious to the animal. For example an insect presented on the left-hand side of the frog causes the tongue to be flicked out towards the right.

In parenthesis it may be mentioned that essentially similar experiments have been carried out on higher vertebrates, including humans. In these cases the technique has been to fit the subject with a pair of inverting spectacles. The first experiments were carried out on himself by G. M. Stratton. He found that after about five days he became adapted to his new perception of the visual world. He was able to move around his house and take walks into the countryside. The fitting of inverting spectacles to animals other than primates, however, usually results in their immobilization. It seems, therefore, that the primate and *a fortiori* the human brain possesses powers of adaptation denied to the majority of animals.[1]

Returning to the surgical experiments carried out on amphibia we find that the next step in the analysis involved sectioning the optic nerve. If this is done when the eye is in its normal uninverted position it is found that the optic nerve fibres grow back from the retina to the tectum so that normal vision is ultimately regained. Once again a detailed correspondence can be shown to exist between the retina and the tectum. What happens, however, if the optic nerve is sectioned when the eye has been rotated as in Fig. 11.2? Do the optic nerve fibres grow back to form a physiologically appropriate or inappropriate tectum? When the experiment is tried it is found that the nerve fibres grow back to the tectum in such a way that stimulation

[1] For fuller discussion of these interesting experiments see R. L. Gregory, *Eye and Brain: the Psychology of Seeing*, World University Library, Weidenfeld and Nicolson, London, 1966, 204–210.

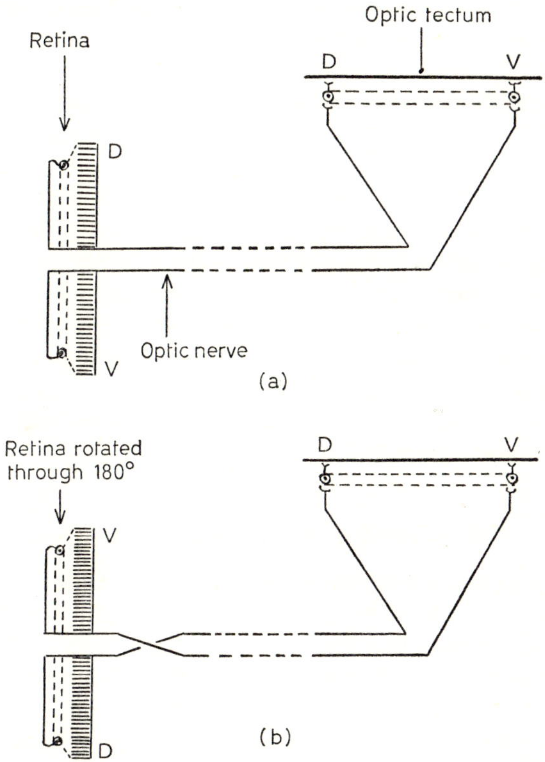


11.2 Scrambling the frog's visual system. In (a) the normal point-for-point correspondence between retina and optic tectum is indicated. Points D and V on the retina correspond to points D and V on the tectum. In (b) the retina has been rotated through 180°. Retinal points D and V, however, still send their messages to points D and V on the tectum. In short the tectal map of the visual world is now upside down. Further explanation in text.

of the original upper (now lower) sector of the retina causes excitation of that part of the tectum corresponding to the upper part of the retina. In other words the inbuilt specificities of the nerve fibres win out. The optic nerve regenerates in an anatomically correct but physiologically incorrect manner. The unfortunate frog reacts to a tempting morsel with the same back to front reflexes.

What conclusions can we draw from this intriguing work? It seems inescapable that each (or at the most small groups of) retinal neuron is in some way different from its neighbours and that this difference is matched by differences in the tectal mosaic. Thus however the retinal neurons may be disarranged, entangled or generally mixed up, each is nevertheless able to find its way back to its correct position in the tectal map. What exactly constitutes the specific difference between neurons is still in dispute.

What straws there are seem to point to a chemical mechanism. Attardi and Sperry were able to show by histological techniques that regenerating optic nerve fibres in the goldfish terminate very exactly on the tectal map.[1] These investigators favour a mechanism based on chemoaffinity between fibre and tectal mosaic. They suggest that the nerve fibre finds its way to its unique destination by following a chemotactic gradient. If this is the case it is clear that the phenomenon is strongly reminiscent of the embryological movements discussed in section 11.2.

### 11.5 Scrambling the amphibian motor system

Next let us consider some cases of neuronal specificity on the motor side. These cases have been intensively investigated by Weiss for many years.[2] Weiss, like Sperry, has used amphibia as his experimental material. He has been concerned to understand how limbs achieve co-ordinated movements after various surgical procedures.

Each amphibian limb is actuated by about forty muscles and is capable of a fairly large but finite repertoire of movements. Each of these movements is the outcome of the co-ordinated and subtly balanced activity of all the forty muscles. It can be shown that these patterns of muscular contractions are specified by the central nervous system. In other words all the proprioceptor fibres from the limb may be cut without grossly changing its co-ordinated movement.

Now it has long been known that it is possible to graft supernumerary limbs into the flanks of amphibia. What, then, would happen if before grafting in a supernumerary limb the nerve plexus to the normal limb is partially transected? The experiment is shown diagrammatically in Fig. 11.3.

The figure shows that nerve fibres grow out from the regenerating

[1] Attardi, P. G. and Sperry, R. W. (1963), 'Preferential selection of central pathways by regenerating optic fibres', *Exp. Neurol.*, *7*, 46–64.

[2] Weiss, P. A., 'Specificity in the Neurosciences', in *Neurosciences Research Symposia Summaries*, *1*, M.I.T. Press, Cambridge, Mass. and London, 1966.

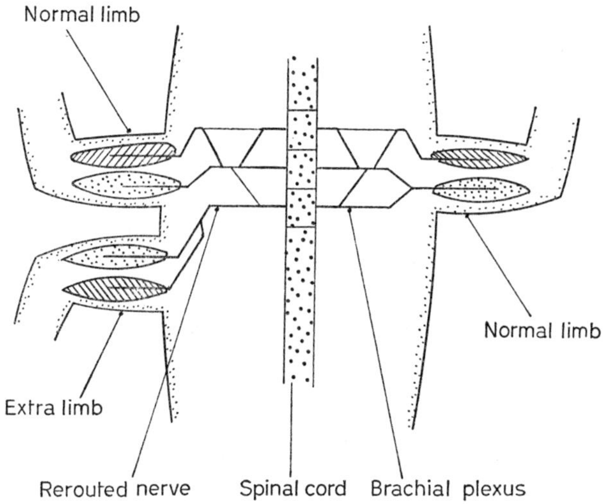


11.3 Innervation of a supernumerary limb. The figure shows that part of the brachial plexus has been rerouted to innervate an additional limb which has been grafted into the animal's flank back to front. For explanation see text. After Weiss, P. (1952), *Res. Publ. Ass. nerv. ment. Dis.*, *30*, 3–23; and Edds, M. V. (1967) in *The Neurosciences* edited by Quarton, G. C., Melnechuk, T. and Schmitt, F. O., Rockefeller University Press, New York.

stump to innervate the supernumerary limb. When regeneration is complete it is found that the two limbs act in tandem. In other words the forty or so muscles in the transplanted limb act in exactly the same sequence and with exactly the same relative force as the muscles in the normal limb. Yet this co-ordination is achieved by means of fibres regenerating from the stump of the partially transected nerve trunk. How on earth is the trick worked?

Subsequent experiments revealed an even more interesting situation. If the supernumerary limb was grafted the wrong way round a result somewhat reminiscent of Sperry's rotated retina experiment was obtained. The limb, though still working in tandem with the normal limb, moved in the opposite sense. Similarly when the animal's own limbs were removed and regrafted in a reversed position they acted in a perfectly co-ordinated manner—but in the wrong direction. The animal presented with a desirable object backed rapidly away; vice versa, presented with a noxious stimulus it ineluctably advanced upon it. This misdirected effort persisted, showing no sign of change through learning. It would seem that the nerve pathways controlling limb movements in amphibia are inbuilt and quite stereotyped.

In order to account for these experiments it has been suggested that the spinal cord at the origin of the limb plexus possesses forty-odd different types of motor nerve cell: one cell type for each limb muscle. The nerve fibre growing out from a particular cell would be adapted in some way to connect with one, and only one, limb muscle. However there is evidence against this type of preordained specificity in amphibian motor nerves.[1] Accordingly we are driven back on another hypothesis: if the specificity is not predetermined then it must be achieved *after* the muscle is innervated.

This concept is somewhat difficult to accept. It suggests that the innervated muscle impresses on the neuron, possibly on the neuronal membrane, its 'name'. This specification then spreads over the whole neuron. If this does indeed happen then this 'modulation', as Weiss calls it, clearly affects the properties of the neuron's dendritic zone. In this way the limb musculature is mapped in the appropriate region of the spinal cord.[2]

The upshot of these experiments is to show that the spinal neurons either by Weiss's modulation or by genetic predetermination represent the amphibian's limb muscles. Weiss likens this representation to the letters of an alphabet. By putting the letters together in different sequences different words can be spelt. Similarly by activating these 'named' motor neurons in different patterns and orders different limb movements can be achieved. The sentences corresponding to instinctive fixed action patterns, and the paragraphs and chapters corresponding to the animal's behavioural repertoire would be put together by higher centres.

These experiments on amphibia seem to show that both the perceptual world and the effector organs are mapped point for point within the central nervous system. However, as Weiss points out, the connections between the sensory map and the motor map are still very much *terra incognita*. The embryological and grafting ex-

[1] Weiss, P. A. (1966), *loc. cit.*, p. 202.

[2] It is interesting to speculate whether the phenomena of phantom limbs, well known to amputees, may also be accounted for in these terms. An individual with an amputated limb may often assert both that he can sense the position of the amputated limb in space and that he can move it. On occasion the patient may complain of severe pain in the missing limb: a pain which seems to have no obvious physical cause.

periments outlined above have so far shed no light on this vital link. Whether the connections are laid down along predetermined pathways, or at random, or whether a mixture of the two, can as yet only be guessed. It is worth while recalling, however, that in the simpler nervous systems of crustacea there is considerable evidence (section 9.6) for genetically predetermined interneuronal pathways which are faithfully replicated in each member of a given species. Wiersma believes[1] that such preordained blueprints also apply to major parts of the vastly more complicated nervous systems of vertebrates. Reflexes and instinctive fixed action patterns which show little variation throughout the members of a given species tend to confirm this view. Wiersma, however, concedes that the brains of 'higher' animals, especially those of the higher vertebrates, may contain uncommitted regions which may be 'specifically' set aside for learning with 'blank' connections awaiting later development.

### 11.6 The 3D geometry of some visual analysers

In the preceding sections of this chapter we have looked at some evidence which suggests that in spite of the vast complexity of central nervous systems the patterns of nerve pathways are to some extent inherited. In some parts of the brains of animals the patterning of neurons has become almost geometric in its clarity. These highly regular regions of neuronal architecture are usually those concerned with analysing the input from major exteroreceptors. In particular the optic nerves of many animals terminate in neuronal lattice-works displaying remarkable symmetries. It has been suggested by many authorities that these three-dimensional grids are concerned in some way with pattern recognition. Some of these intriguing patterns of neurons are shown in Plates XIII and XIV.

The stratified neuronal webwork of vertebrate retinae has already been described (section 8.4). It was also indicated how neurobiologists are beginning to gather an inkling of the functional significance of this intricate design. As we saw in Chapter 10, the optic nerves of non-mammalian vertebrates terminate in the optic tectum of the midbrain. We noticed, moreover, in section 11.4 that this termination is, at least in the frog, very specific. It turns out, if we examine the histology of this region, that, from fish up to birds, the optic tecta of

[1] Wiersma, C. A. G., in *Neurosciences Research Symposium Summaries, 1*, M.I.T. Press, Cambridge, Mass. and London, 1966, p. 221.

vertebrates possess remarkable neuronal organizations. In some respects the tectum resembles the retina itself in being strikingly laminated: layers of perikarya alternate with layers of synapses. The tissue reaches an evolutionary peak, as might be expected, in the birds. Here the information picked up by the highly evolved eyes is processed in a tectum consisting of some fifteen distinct layers. Plate XIII (a) shows that a three-dimensional grid exists with incoming and outgoing fibres running vertical to the surface of the tectum and synaptic processes running mainly in the orthogonal plane. D'Arcy Thomson tells a story of how a nineteenth-century engineer deeply involved in designing the jib of a crane visited an anatomist colleague who happened to be studying a section of the head of a femur. Seeing the tracery of spicules in the femur's head the engineer exclaims, 'There's my crane!' Similarly the present-day computer designer seeing Plates XIII and XIV might make an analogous comment: 'There's my silicon slice!'

Equally interesting neuronal patterns are to be found in the brains

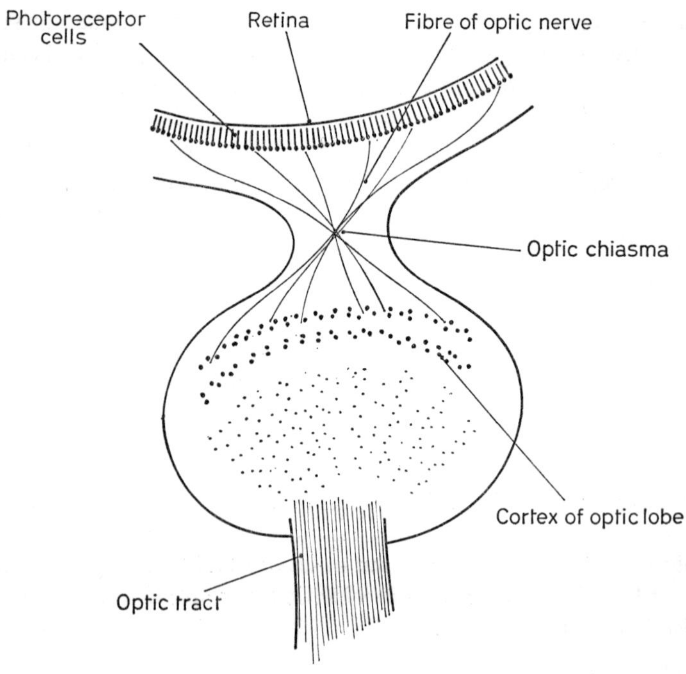


11.4 Optic pathways of a cephalopod mollusc such as the octopus.

XIII Some optic ganglia (i)

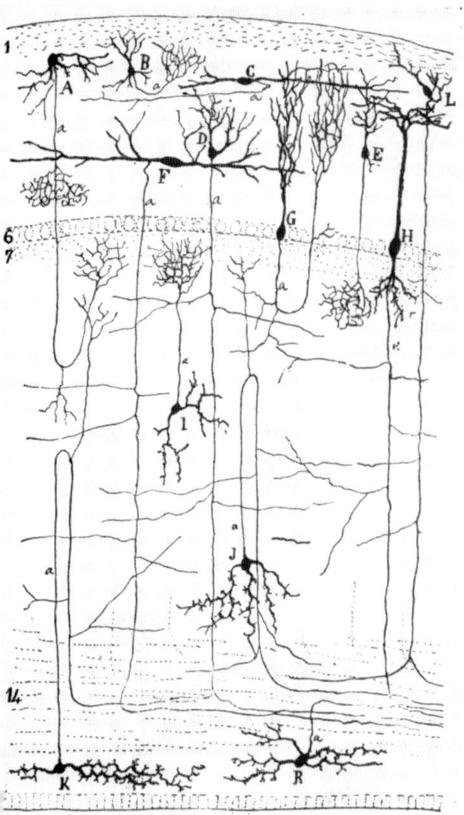


(a) Drawing of a vertical section through the optic lobe of a bird. Some of the fifteen layers mentioned in the text (p. 224) are labelled. (From Ramón Cajal, *Histologie du Système Nerveux*, Paris, 1911.)

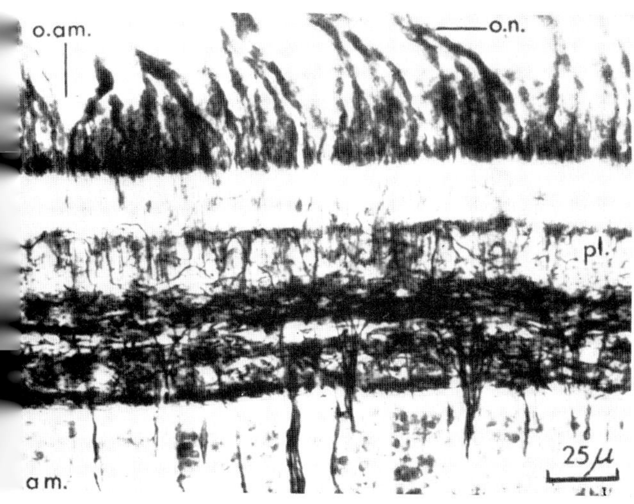


(b) Sagittal section through the optic lobe of *Octopus*. i.a.m. = inner layer of amacrine cells; o.a.m. = outer layer of amacrine cells; o.n. = optic nerve fibres (from retina); pl. = plexiform layer. (From Young, J. Z. (1962), 'The retina of cephalopods and its degeneration after optic nerve section', *Phil. Trans. Roy. Soc. B, 245*, 1–58.)

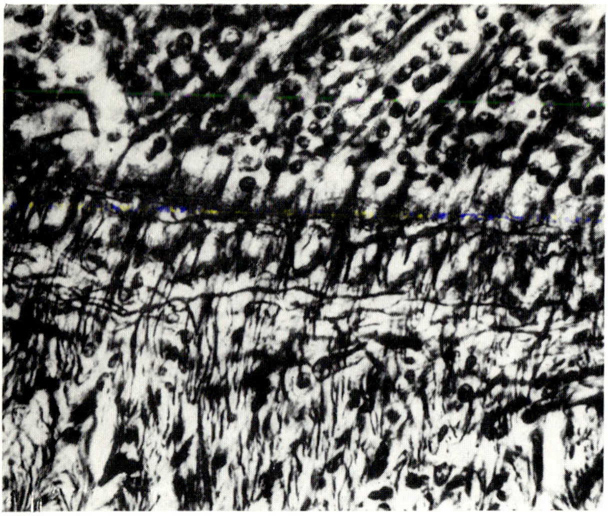

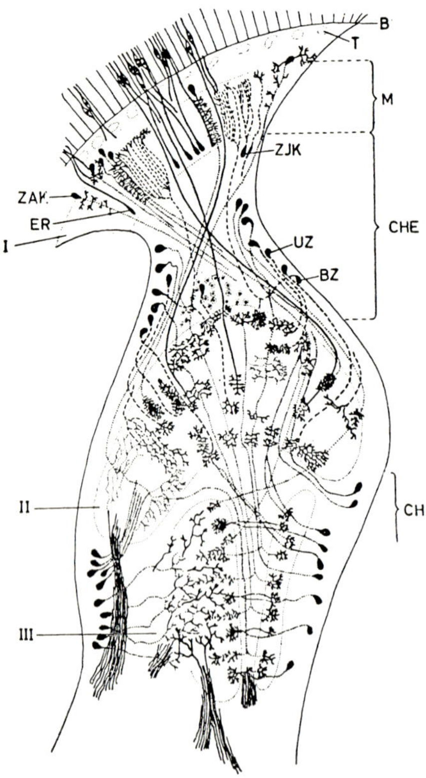


XIV Some optic ganglia (ii)

(a) Vertical section (× 340) through the optic lamina of the green shore crab *Carcinus* (compare Fig. 11.5).
(From Hamori, J. and Horridge, G. A. (1966), 'The Lobster Optic Lamina', *J. Cell Sci.*, *1*, 249–256.)

(b) Optic ganglion of *Calliphora*, the blowfly.

I, II & III = the three optic lamina
B = limiting membrane of the retinula cells
BZ = bipolar nerve cells
CHE = external chiasma
CHJ = internal chiasma
ER = ends of the nerve fibres emerging from the retinula cells
UZ = unipolar nerve cell
ZAK = centripetal nerve cells
ZJK = centrifugal nerve cells

From Cajal, S. R. and Sánche, D. (1915), *Trab. lab. invest. biol. Madrid*, *13*, 1.

of many invertebrates. Plate XIII (b), for example, shows a portion of the optic lobe of the octopus. Again it is clear that a precise geometrical organization exists. The afferent and efferent fibres run into and out of the lobe at right angles to several layers of synaptic junctions. J. Z. Young has shown, moreover, that the dendrites of many of the cells in this lobe are confined to single planes. A similar phenomenon occurs, as we shall see in the next section, in the mammalian cerebellum. In the optic lobe these dendritic planes tend to be orientated at right angles to one another, so that at this level also a rather precise grid is formed. The visual information processed in this lattice-work is passed from the optic lobe to the rest of the brain via the optic tract (Fig. 11.4).

Finally, some remarkable neuronal organizations are developed in the brains of many members of the Arthropoda. In those decapod crustacea which possess well developed compound eyes a whole series of separate regions for analysing the visual information tends to occur (Fig. 11.5).

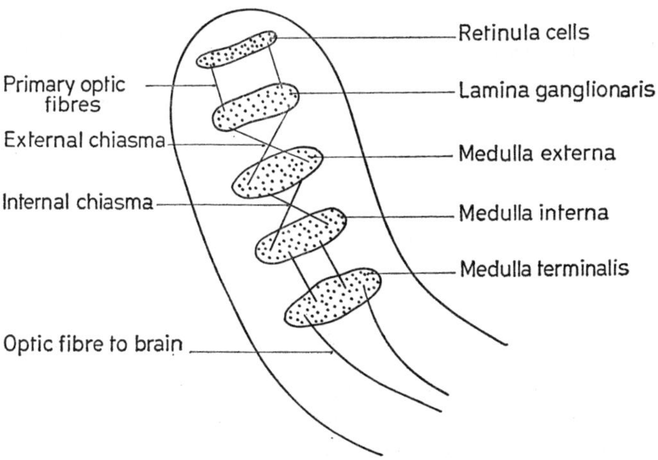


11.5 Optic ganglia in the eye stalk of the Hawaiian swimming crab. Adapted from Waterman, T. H., Wiersma, C. A. G. and Bush, B. M. H. (1964), 'Afferent visual responses in the optic nerve of the crab *Podophthalamus*', *J. Cell. Comp. Physiol.*, *63*, 135–155.

The various laminae and medullae of Fig. 11.5 consist, once again, of regular layers of perikarya and synaptic zones (Plate XIV (a) ). These optic neuropils are, as Fig. 11.5 shows, connected to each other by tracts of nerve fibres which usually form chiasmata.

Insects, also, show some very interesting organizational patterns in their optic lobes. One of the best known of these intricate designs is to be found serving the compound eye of the blowfly (Plate XIV (b)). Similar networks are to be found processing the information picked up by the compound eyes of many other insects.

The physiology of these fascinating neuropils has hardly begun to be worked out. Plates XIII and XIV show that the organization, although regular, is very complicated and, especially in the case of the Arthropoda, the dimensions are minute. Computer engineers hope by progressive microminiaturization to fit useful computers into packs the size of suitcases. The neurobiologist is investigating computers of greater power and sophistication which have the size of a pin head.

The one neuronal computer of which brain scientists are approaching the beginnings of an understanding appears to be the mammalian cerebellum. Accordingly it is to this tissue that the last section of this chapter is devoted.

### 11.7 The functional architecture of the mammalian cerebellum

The 'wiring diagrams' of most parts of the mammalian brain are, as we have more than once emphasized, at present unknown. Their complexity baffles the would-be investigator. In recent years, however, one part of the mammalian brain—the cerebellum—has begun to yield the secrets of its design to the neurobiologist. It is thus appropriate to conclude this chapter with a brief outline of this developing understanding.

The mammalian cerebellum resembles the cerebrum in possessing a cortical rind of grey matter covering a more central mass of white matter and island nuclei. This organization is shown in Fig. 11.6.

We saw in section 10.4 that the cerebellum's job is to co-ordinate the muscular movements responsible for behavioural acts. In order to achieve this function it receives information from proprioceptors distributed throughout the muscular system, from the inner ear and from most of the other major sense organs. It also receives information from higher centres in the brain, in particular from the cerebral cortex, concerning what behaviour is intended. All this information is fed into the cerebellar cortex along two main types of fibre. These two types of afferent fibre are known as *mossy* and *climbing* fibres. Both types are believed to carry mainly proprioceptive information

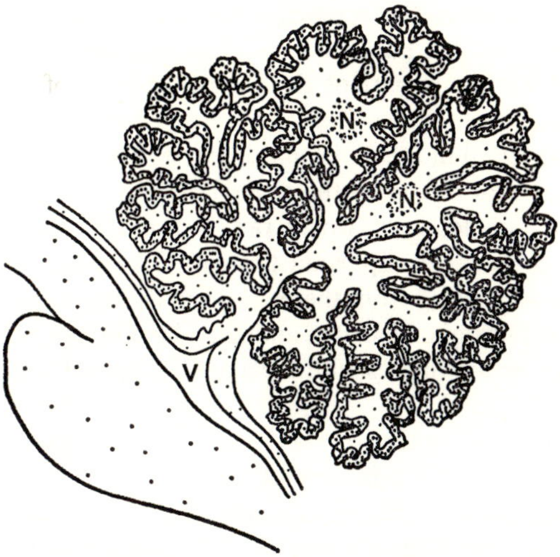


11.6 Vertical section through a mammalian cerebellum to show the distribution of grey and white matter. N = internal nucleus, V = fourth ventricle. Stippled regions represent grey matter.

but whereas the mossy fibres, as their name suggests, branch widely in the cortex, the endings of the climbing fibres remain strictly localized. The output signals from the cerebellar cortex are carried by one type of fibre only: the axons of Purkinje cells.

Purkinje cells (P-cells) possess very large pear-shaped perikarya having diameters of up to 50 $\mu$ in man. Although they have but one axon their dendritic tree is extremely rich and branches profusely. It is, however, intriguing to find that all these branches are rigorously confined to a single plane (Fig. 11.7). Running at right angles to this plane are very large number of small axons. Because these axons all run in the same direction they are called parallel fibres. These axons make very numerous—up to 200,000—synaptic contacts with the dendritic trees of each Purkinje cell in their path.

The parallel fibres originate from smallish perikarya called granule cells which lie between the Purkinje cells and the cerebellar white matter. The granule cells are extremely numerous and very densely packed, there being $2{\cdot}4 \times 10^6$ /mm$^3$ in the monkey cerebellar cortex. These cells send out six or seven short dendrites which synapse with ascending mossy fibres and a single axon which runs up towards the surface of the cerebellum. This axon branches in the form of a 'Y' or

'T' before it reaches the cerebellar surface and continues parallel with the surface as a parallel fibre. The huge numbers of parallel fibres form the major part of the *molecular* layer of the cerebellar cortex.

Also to be found in the molecular layer are numerous stellate cells. These cells, about one-third the size of the Purkinje cells, possess a large number of dendrites which ramify throughout the molecular layer. One of the most important types of stellate cell is the 'basket' cell. Axons originating from these cells run orthogonally to both the plane of the Purkinje dendrites and the plane of the parallel fibres. These axons form synapses with the axon hillocks of twenty to thirty Purkinje cells.

The last type of neuron to be found in the cerebellar cortex is the Golgi cell. These are large multipolar neurons whose perikarya are scattered amongst the granule cells. The dendrites of these cells ramify in all directions throughout the molecular and granular

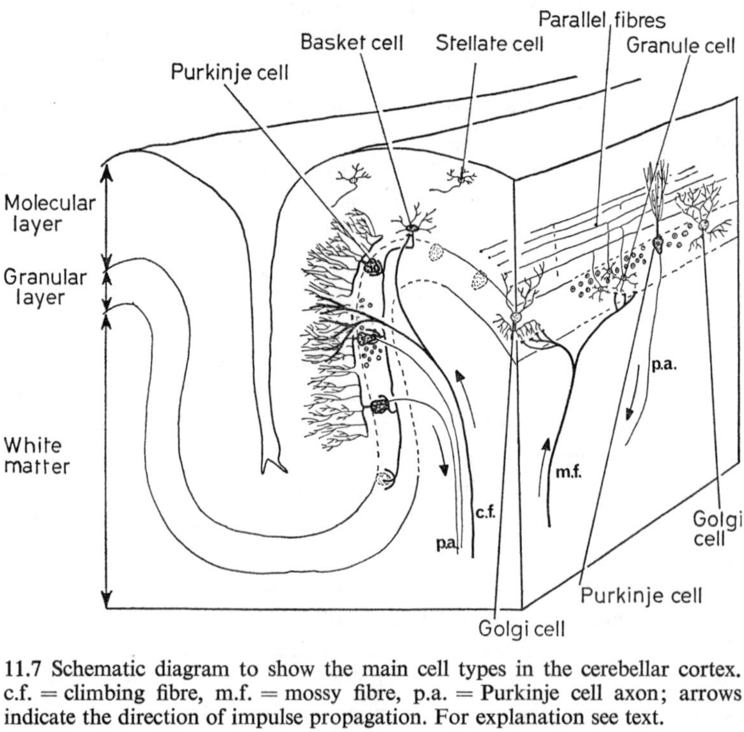


11.7 Schematic diagram to show the main cell types in the cerebellar cortex. c.f. = climbing fibre, m.f. = mossy fibre, p.a. = Purkinje cell axon; arrows indicate the direction of impulse propagation. For explanation see text.

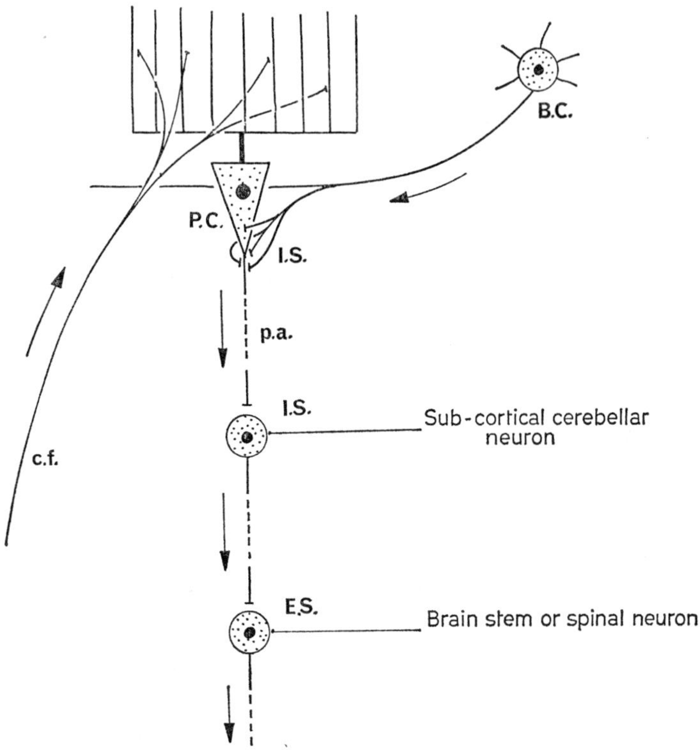


11.8 Output from the cerebellar cortex. B.C. = basket cell, c.f. = climbing fibre, E.S. = excitatory synapse, I.S. = inhibitory synapse, p.a. = Purkinje cell axon, P.C. = Purkinje cell. Arrows indicate direction of impulse transmission. For explanation see text.

layers. The axon after a short run also breaks up into multitudinous branches.

Fig. 11.7 shows the main features of this intricate neuronal architecture.

Now how does the intricate neuronal lattice-work of the cerebellar cortex described above and illustrated in Fig. 11.7 operate? Intensive work by neurophysiologists and neuronanatomists in the last few years is beginning to lead to an incipient understanding. This work has recently been synthesized in a fundamental book by Eccles, Ito and Szentagothai: *The Cerebellum as a Neuronal Machine*.[1] The following very brief resumé is based on this volume.

[1] Eccles, J. C., Ito, M. and Szentagothai, J., *The Cerebellum as a Neuronal Machine*, Springer-Verlag, 1967.

First it can be shown that the output along the Purkinje axons is inhibitory. This output is directed on to cells in the cerebellar nuclei and brain stem. These cells in turn send axons to cells in the spinal cord and elsewhere (Fig. 11.8).

It has been shown that the neurons with which the P-cell axons synapse are normally very active. In the absence of Purkinje cell inhibition they may discharge at rates of up to 80 impulses/second. This on-going activity is inhibited by P-cell discharges. There is, in other words, a sort of negative control. It is not so much that certain groups of muscles are activated as that other groups are inhibited.

Our next question, therefore, must be: How does the cerebellar cortex compute which P-cell to activate? Once again we find that the mechanism is founded on patterns of selective inhibition.

We have already emphasized that the input to the cerebellar cortex is carried by two sets of fibres—the mossy and climbing fibres. The arboraceous terminations of the mossy fibres make synapses with both granule and Golgi cells. Excitation of a group of granule cells necessarily leads to impulse transmission in a band of parallel fibres in the molecular layer. Now the parallel fibres, it will be remembered,

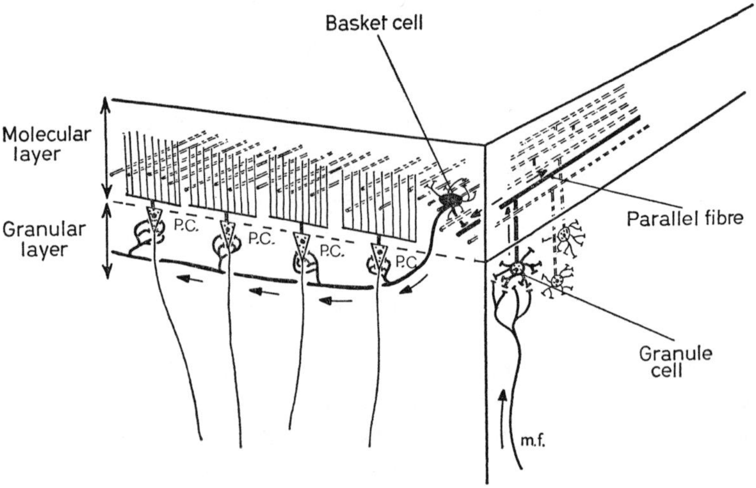


11.9 Schematic diagram to show how a row of Purkinje cells may be inhibited by the action of a basket cell. The basket-cell may be activated by impulses in neighbouring parallel fibres which may themselves be initiated by mossy fibre input on to the granule cells. For further explanation see text. m.f. = mossy fibre, P.C. = Purkinje cell. Arrows indicate the direction of impulse propagation.

pass through, and synapse in passing with, the dendritic trees of the P-cells. These synapses are excitatory. The molecular layer, however, also contains a number of stellate cells and, in particular, basket cells. It will be recalled that the axons of the latter cells run at right angles to the parallel fibres and also synapse with the Purkinje cells. It has been known for some years that these synapses are inhibitory. It follows that excitation of a band of parallel fibres whilst exciting the P-cells in the band also ensures that P-cells adjacent to the band are strongly inhibited (Fig. 11.9).

The edges of the beam of excited P-cells are further sharpened by the focusing action of the Golgi cells. The dendrites of these cells are, as we have seen, distributed widely amongst the parallel fibres. It follows that excitation of the parallel fibres also excites the Golgi cells. The much-branched axons of these cells ramify, however,

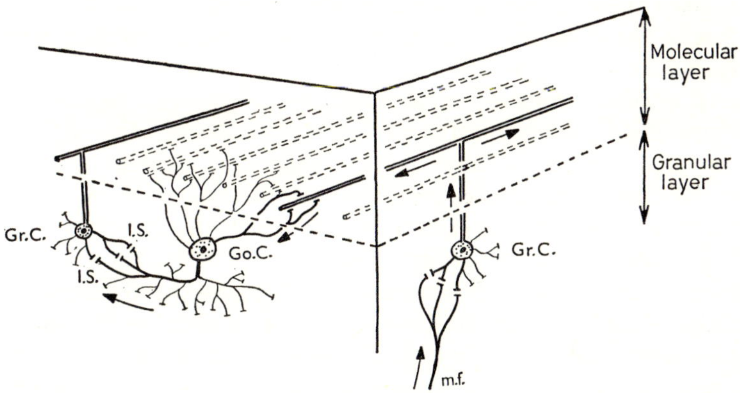


11.10 Schematic diagram to show the way in which activation of Golgi cells sharpens the edges of strips of excited cerebellar cortex. Go. C. = Golgi cell, Gr. C. = granule cell, I.S. = inhibitory synapse, m.f. = mossy fibre. Arrows indicate the direction of impulse propagation. Further explanation in text.

through the granular layer (Fig. 11.7). It can be shown that these axons make inhibitory synapses with granule cells. In consequence feed-back inhibition via the Golgi cells is likely to completely extinguish the weaker mossy fibre excitation to one side or the other of the main beam. This type of 'lateral inhibition', which has some features in common with the simpler case of the *Limulus* compound eye (Chapter 8), is shown diagrammatically in Fig. 11.10.

The cerebellar cortex is subjected to a multitudinous bombardment by the mossy fibres from the body's proprioceptors. It follows that the Purkinje population is subjected to complex and ever-shifting patterns of excitation. The oblongs of Purkinje excitation continually ripple across the cortex interfering with each other in intricate and ever-changing manners. This ravelled ripple is the map of the on-going activity of the body's musculature.

Superimposed on this ripple tank of Purkinje excitation is the climbing fibre input. Unlike the mossy fibre afferents the climbing fibres do not ramify extensively through the granular layer. On the contrary they are believed to innervate just one Purkinje cell. Similarly it appears that each P-cell is innervated by just one climbing fibre. The climbing fibres make excitatory synapses with the P-cells. Even when the Purkinje cell is deeply inhibited by the mechanisms described in the previous paragraphs innervation by a climbing fibre is able to elicit at least one impulse. The less deeply inhibited are the P-cells, the more impulses are given in response to climbing fibre excitation.

The spatio-temporal parameters of the body's musculature dynamically modelled in the cerebellar cortex by patterns of P-cell excitation are, as we have already mentioned, communicated to nuclei deep in the cerebellum, brain stem and spinal cord. Because the P-cell output is inhibitory a sort of 'negative image' of the cerebellar model is projected on to these nuclei. From these nuclei fibres leave to activate the body's musculature. It follows that the representation of the body in the cerebellar cortex—its orientation, its position with respect to gravity, the state of tension in each of its muscles, the positions of its joints, etc.—impresses itself on the spray of outgoing impulses. These impulses are in consequence patterned so that harmonious and balanced sequences of muscle movements result, so that, in short, well-executed behaviour occurs. Eccles draws an analogy between this shaping of the impulse traffic in the motor nerves and the process of sculpturing in stone. 'Spatio-temporal form,' he writes,[1] 'is achieved from moment to moment by the impression of a patterned inhibition upon the "shapeless" background discharges of the sub-cerebellar neurons, just as an infinitely more enduring form is achieved in sculpture by a highly selective chiselling away from the initial amorphous block of stone'.

[1] *Loc. cit.*, (1966), p. 310.

CHAPTER TWELVE

# Motivation

'Reason is, and ought only to be, the slave of the passions'.

DAVID HUME, 1758

## 12.1 Motivation and the 'unconscious'

'Cherchez la femme,' say the French; the less romantic English merely look for a motive. What could have induced the suspect to pull the trigger? The law, of course, assumes that the motive is a mental event though the outcome, the revolver shot, is physical. Clearly this is an important case of the profound mind-matter dualism which becomes increasingly prominent in the last chapters of this book. It will be considered in some detail in Chapter 17.

Not all motivation, however, is conscious. Freud, as is well known, introduced the idea of unconscious motivation, inaccessible to the ratiocinative mind. Freud defines this concept by means of an example. He describes[1] how Bernheim asked a patient under hypnosis to open an umbrella five minutes *after* awaking from his trance. In due course the patient carried out this action though without any idea of why he was doing it. This, says Freud, can only be explained if it is assumed that it occurs on command of part of the mind inaccessible to consciousness—in other words, the 'unconscious'.

Aristotle defined man as the rational animal; since Freud we might more exactly describe him as the rationalizing animal. Many of the reasons we give when taxed with acting in such and such a manner are spurious. They are conscious or unconscious face-savers: justifications after the event. We all live in private worlds built of feeling or affect. The advertising industry has long realized this fact. Citizens are not induced to buy cigarettes or motor cars by appeals to their reason, but by appeals to their feeling, to their emotions. This is no

[1] Freud, S., *Introductory Lectures in Psychoanalysis,* George Allen and Unwin, London, 1929, p. 234.

new discovery. As the introductory quotation puts it: 'reason is . . . the slave of the passions.'

In this chapter it is intended to consider some of the possible anatomical and physiological correlatives of these deeply inbuilt desires and behaviour patterns.

### 12.2 The brain as computer of a homeostat

We are motivated to solve pressing problems, to win bread, to avoid disaster. Success in any of these endeavours tends to restore the *status quo ante*. The most important aspects of the *status quo ante* are the parameters of what Claude Bernard called the 'milieu intérieur': the internal environment. Quite simply the internal environment consists of the fluids in which the cells of the body are bathed. In the mammals many of the characteristics of this fluid—its temperature, its pressure, its pH, its oxygen content, its glucose content, etc., etc.—are kept very constant. The brain can be regarded, in J. Z. Young's phrase, as the computer of this homeostat, as the organ which ensures that the physico-chemical characteristics of the internal environment do not vary greatly whatever the circumstances in which the animal finds itself. Some very striking instances of this concept emerge from Richter's work on the nutritional behaviour of rats.[1]

First Richter was interested to discover whether rats deprived of certain of their endocrine glands would respond with behaviour designed to ameliorate their loss. For example it is known that the cortex of the adrenal gland secretes a hormone which controls the salt balance of the body. This hormone—aldosterone—ensures that sodium ions are reabsorbed from the urine being formed in the kidney. It follows that if the adrenal cortices are removed sodium is rapidly lost from the body in the urine. The body's reserves of NaCl very rapidly become depleted with, of course, fatal results.

Richter studied the dietary proclivities of adrenalectomized rats in comparison with a control group. He showed that if the experimental animals were given access only to the customary stock diet they died within eight to fifteen days. If, however, they were given access to NaCl in addition to the stock diet, in a separate dispenser, they took sufficient to keep themselves alive and free from deficiency symptoms indefinitely.

[1] Richter, C. P., 'Total Self-Regulatory Functions in Animals and Man', *Harvey Lectures* (1942–1943), *38*, 63–101.

Stellar[1] reports a similar instance in *H. sapiens.* In this case a child developed an adrenal tumour very early in life. This has a similar effect to adrenalectomy in rats. Salt continually drains away from the body in the urine. The infant, however, managed to survive by always being at the salt pot. Indeed Stellar reports that the first word the child learnt to enunciate was 'salt'. This story, however, has a tragic ending. In order to cure the child's pathological craving for salt he was taken to hospital for observation. For seven days whilst under observation he was forced to live on a standard hospital diet. At the end of the week he was dead.

In both cases, the experimental rat and the diseased child, it is clear that the behavioural drive to obtain salt emerges for reasons unknown to the organism. The motives impelling African ruminants to trek perhaps hundreds of miles to a salt lick must similarly be, in this sense, motives originating in the 'unconscious'.

Richter developed his researches not only by testing the behavioural responses of rats to the loss of other endocrine glands, but also by examining their ability to select their own diets, cafeteria style, from the unmixed pure ingredients. He was able to show that rats were, in fact, able to do this. They were able to select seventeen different pure constituents of a normal diet so that they grew just as fast, indeed a little faster, than a control group given a pre-mixed diet.

It follows from this wealth of experimental work that the nutritive behaviour of the rat, and by implication that of other mammals, is designed to maintain, as far as possible, the constancy of the 'milieu intérieur'. Nutritive behaviour, like other types of behaviour, is controlled by the central nervous system and, in particular, the brain. Hence we glimpse the validity of Young's concept of the brain as the computer of a homeostat. At the same time it is clear that much of this behaviour must spring from causes unknown to the animal; in other words it falls under Freud's classification of 'unconscious motivation'.

If the brain is acting, as it seems to be acting, as the 'computer of a homeostat' one rather interesting feature emerges. A feature first emphasized by J. von Neumann in his volume of Silliman lectures—*The computer and the brain.*[2] This is that the homeostat is controlled to within very precise limits. The temperature of the blood, for example,

[1] Stellar, E., in *Handbook of Physiology, Section 1: Neurophysiology, Vol. 3,* American Physiological Society, 1960, p. 1501.

[2] Yale University Press, 1958.

is regulated to within $\pm$ 0·2 C; the acidity, glucose content and electrolyte composition are also kept remarkably constant. Yet this regulation is achieved by a 'liquid state' computer whose components —the neurons—are far from being the precise 'on-off' relays characteristic of solid state, metallic, computers. How can such overall precision be achieved by such imprecise components? This question, wrote von Neumann, 'must be emphasized again and again for no known computing machine can operate reliably and significantly on such a low precision level'.

### 12.3 The rôle of the brain stem

Next in our investigation of the physiological bases of behavioural drives and motivation we must inquire whether it is possible to localize control centres in the brain. In fact the last two decades have seen much progress in this line of inquiry. Many of the behavioural drives identified by psychologist and layman have turned out to be the responsibility of quite localized groups of cells situated in the brain stem. The most important region of all appears to be the hypothalamus. This, perhaps, is hardly surprising for we saw in Chapter 10 that the hypothalamus can be regarded as the anterior end of the visceral sensory and visceral motor columns of the spinal cord. In other words it acts as head office for that part of the nervous system —the autonomic nervous system—which directly controls the internal environment. It is a logical feature of the brain's design that the centres controlling behaviour intended to equilibrate the 'milieu intérieur' should be situated in the part of the brain most closely concerned with this milieu. Let us, therefore, examine briefly some of the enlightening work which has been carried out on this part of the brain.

### 12.4 A technique for investigating behavioural 'drives'

The pioneering work which opened up this important field of physiological research is largely due to W. R. Hess. The technique which Hess perfected consisted in the implantation of electrodes into the hypothalami of experimental animals. Hess showed first that after recovering from the operation the animals were still able to move about their cages quite freely. If the electrodes were attached to a suitable stimulator by a flexible wire (Plate XV (a)) the brain could be stimulated as and when the experimenter desired. At the end of a series of experiments the animals were sacrificed and it was then possible to tell by histological investigation of their brains exactly where the electrodes had been inserted.

Using these techniques Hess was able to demonstrate a number of different behavioural responses to stimulation of different parts of the hypothalamus in fully conscious animals. Perhaps the most striking of these responses were those concerned with feeding and drinking behaviour, with 'fight/flight' responses, with sleep and with sexual behaviour.

In addition to electrically stimulating the hypothalamus it is also possible to destroy small regions by electrocoagulation. The behavioural defects resulting from such lesions have also been most instructive in the attempt to delineate 'centres' concerned with drive and motivation.

Hess's techniques have proved extremely useful in analysing the behavioural functions of the hypothalamus. Before founding any firm conclusions on this work a powerful criticism has, however, to be taken into account. This is that at present we have no means of knowing whether the regions of the hypothalamus stimulated or destroyed by the probing electrode are in fact genuine control centres, merely 'way stations' or simply tracts running to and from yet to be discovered centres.

## 12.5 Hunger and thirst

The first drive to be localized in the manner described above was the 'hunger drive'. It can be shown that after the destruction of a pair of nuclei lying towards the centre of the hypothalamus—the ventromedial (VM) nuclei—the experimental animals were transformed into 'compulsive eaters'. This characteristic has also sometimes been observed in humans suffering from a tumour in this region.

Some time after the discovery of these 'satiety' centres their opposite numbers—'hunger' centres—were discovered. Destruction of these centres which are located on each side of the VM nuclei stopped the experimental animals eating. If they were not forcibly fed they were liable to starve to death even in the midst of plenty.[1]

These findings suggest that the hypothalamic centres concerned with feeding are related in the way indicated in Fig. 12.1.

[1] Anand, B. K. and Brobeck, J. R. (1951), 'Hypothalamic control of food intake in rats and cats', *Yale J. Biol. Med.*, *24*, 123–140.

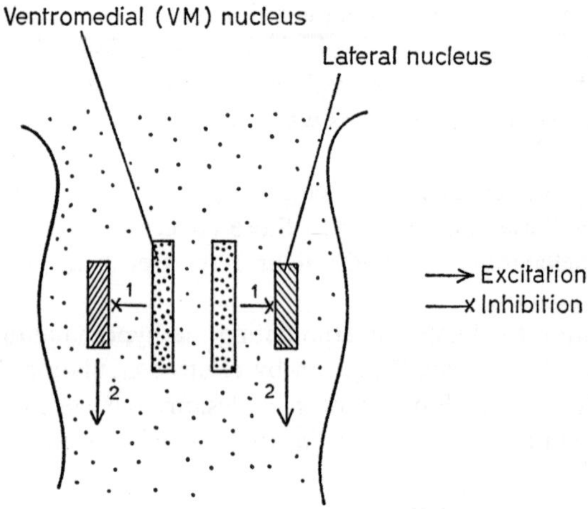


12.1 Schematic view of the hypothalamic centres concerned with feeding behaviour. The hypothalamus is drawn as seen from above or below. Explanation in text.

The figure shows that the VM nuclei normally inhibit the lateral nuclei (reaction 1). When the glucose content of the blood falls below a certain threshold this inhibition is cut off. The lateral nuclei then discharge through pathways (reaction 2) which activate food-seeking behaviour and food intake. It is clear that a scheme of this type would nicely explain the experimental findings described above. It would also account for Hess's additional finding that stimulation of the lateral hypothalamus causes cats to eat voraciously.

Very close to, or perhaps intermingled with, the cells controlling the hunger drive are cells controlling drinking behaviour. Electrocoagulation and/or stimulation of the lateral and ventromedial hypothalamus frequently affects drinking in the same way that we have seen that it affects feeding.

## 12.6 Fight or flight

The hypothalamus has long been known to be deeply implicated in the fight or flight responses of animals faced with an emergency. This is to be expected on anatomical grounds as these responses are largely caused by the discharge of the sympathetic nervous system. This system forms one of the two main divisions of the autonomic nervous system (the other being the parasympathetic nervous system) and as such is strongly connected with the hypothalamus.

The fight or flight responses which we can observe in animals and in our fellow human beings are, of course, experienced by ourselves as the emotions of anger and fear. At the human level these feelings may or may not be accompanied by appropriate motor discharge. It is frequently the case that modern man, striving to live in close communion with his fellows, finds it necessary to dissemble. These powerful emotions, denied behavioural expression are, as the saying is, kept 'bottled up inside'.

With experimental animals it is relatively easy to show the part played by the hypothalamus in aggressive or submissive behaviour. Removal of the cerebral cortex results in an animal liable to show 'sham' rage. The word 'sham' is really a misnomer. Decorticate dogs and cats respond with extreme rage—biting and clawing. There is nothing sham about this. The fraudulence comes in the stimulus to which this extreme reaction is given. These stimuli can be quite trivial: stimuli which the normal animal would hardly notice. It looks as though the removal of the cerebral cortex removes a restraining or inhibitory influence from the brain-stem.

Similar effects can be achieved by stimulating animals in appropriate regions of the brain-stem. A few observations have also been made on human patients undergoing surgery. Electrical stimulation of the amygdala, which are closely related to the hypothalamus, has resulted in patients reporting feelings of anxiety, or even acute fear.

Carrying the analysis to a yet finer level it has been possible[1] to detect cells in the midbrain which fire only when the experimental animal—in this case the cat—displays anger at the behavioural level. Vice versa, stimulation of these cells results in an angry, hissing, spitting, animal.

## 12.7 Sleep

Sleep is yet another behavioural phenomenon which is believed to be influenced by centres in the hypothalamus. It is believed that two centres—excitatory and inhibitory—exist. In this respect the central control of sleep resembles the control of eating and drinking discussed above. An inhibitory centre, causing wakefulness, seems to be situated in the posterior part of the hypothalamus, whereas an excitatory centre appears to exist in the anterior region. This neural mechanism, indicating that sleep and wakefulness are caused by an

[1] Adams, D. B. (1968), 'Cells related to fighting behaviour recorded from the midbrain central grey neuropil of cat', *Science, 159*, 894–896.

interplay of inhibitory and excitatory influences, suggests that somnolence may not be merely a running down of the machine's batteries, but possibly an alternative state of cerebral activity. A fuller discussion of sleep, which has been the subject of a good deal of interesting research in recent years, is, however, deferred to Chapter 16.

### 12.8 Reproduction

A fourth major motive which is strongly influenced by regions of the hypothalamus is the reproductive urge. Destruction of both sides of the anterior hypothalamus leads to a loss of sexual interest and potency in several species of mammal. Similar observations have been made on humans who have suffered damage to the anterior hypothalamus.

As in the case of the other hypothalamic centres the experiment can be done the other way round: instead of destroying the centre it can be stimulated. Several interesting observations have been made when this second approach has been used. For example if a pipette is implanted into the anterior hypothalamus of a female rat and minute quantities of testosterone (the male reproductive hormone) injected, vigorous and prolonged male sexual behaviour is elicited.[1] The female rat will pursue and mount other females and will continue the attempt whilst the hormone lasts. This, perhaps, suggests that the neural pathways responsible for male reproductive behaviour are built into the female rat's nervous system and only require activating by the appropriate hormone in the appropriate place.

Another piece of work which shows the importance of the anterior hypothalamus in the governance of reproductive behaviour has used the domestic cat as the experimental animal. It is well known that female cats are only willing to accept the advances of a male during a short period of the oestrous cycle. This receptive period may be correlated with the build-up of oestrogen secreted by the ovaries. It follows that if the ovaries are removed the female cat is never willing to accept the advances of the male. If, however, a pipette containing oestrogen is embedded in the anterior hypothalamus of a castrated female the animal, whilst the hormone lasts, remains perpetually receptive to males. Implantation of similar pipettes into other parts of the brain has no such influence on female receptivity.

[1] Fisher, A. E. (1964), 'Chemical stimulation of the brain', *Sci. Amer., 210*, (June) 60–68.

### 12.9 Ethology and the analysis of the reproductive instinct

The reproductive drive has also been studied in great detail by the ethologists. The approach of these investigators has been somewhat different from the essentially laboratory investigations described above. A strong emphasis has been laid on studying the animal in its natural environment. This has resulted in a great deal of meticulous observation of the habits of animals such as herring gulls, grey lag geese and certain species of fish and insect in their customary habitats. In more recent years similar approaches have been made to the study of the behaviour of many other animals including several species of anthropoid ape. Clearly this 'natural history' approach complements the laboratory studies of neurophysiologists and experimental psychologists.

Tinbergen, in the nineteen-forties, investigated the reproductive behaviour of the three-spined stickleback.[1] In this now classical study he was able to show that this instinctive behaviour was organized in a rather precise hierarchical fashion. The behaviour was initially triggered by an increasing photoperiod. This, presumably, alters the hormone balance of the 'milieu intérieur'. The fish, in response, swims until it finds itself in warmer, shallower, reedy waters. The male fish prepares a nest. The next stage in the behaviour pattern is dependent on a female fish, in a suitably gravid condition, entering the male's field of vision. The female fish, when ready to mate, possesses a swollen abdomen and assumes a striking posture in the water. This characteristic form and posture constitute, according to the ethologists, a *sign stimulus*. One can construct quite grotesque models of female sticklebacks and as long as this particular gestalt is faithfully represented the next stage of the male's reproductive behaviour is triggered. Tinbergen, in fact, suggests that the sign simulus actuates an *innate releasing mechanism* (IRM) which 'unlocks' the 'nervous energy' necessary for a particular instinctive act. Returning to the stickleback example we find that the instinctive behaviour released in the male on being vouchsafed the view of an appropriate female is a peculiar type of erratic swimming known as a 'zigzag dance'. This is said to be an example of a *fixed action pattern*—a complex sequence of movements given by all members of a species when presented with a particular sign stimulus. The zigzag dance of the male acts, in turn, as a sign stimulus for the

[1] See Tinbergen, N. S., *The Study of Instinct*, Oxford University Press, 1951.

female. In consequence one of the female's repertoire of fixed action patterns is released. This, once more, leads to a further instinctive behaviour on the part of the male and so on until the female is induced to spawn in the nest and the male, in a final consummatory act, fertilizes the eggs.

Ethologists thus see the reproductive behaviour of the three-spined stickleback as a chain of action and reaction on the part of the two participants. Each step is necessary if the subsequent steps are to occur; the nervous machinery for each step is built into the nervous system of the stickleback and is actuated only when the correct sign stimulus is presented to the exteroreceptors. The biological function of this system is clear. It ensures that the fertilized eggs are deposited in the correct position; that only members of the same species attempt intercourse.

The ethologists although they have analysed in similar terms numerous instinctive behaviours in numerous animals do not, in general, attempt to explain their findings in terms recognizable by neurophysiologists. Sign stimuli, innate releasing mechanisms, fixed action patterns, nervous energy must, presumably, have correlatives in the animal's nervous system, but what exactly these correlatives are has not usually interested the ethologist. Indeed Tinbergen and others have developed an intricate 'hydrodynamical' model which, like the Ptolemaic astronomy, 'saves the appearances' but has not been capable, so far, of development in terms of action potentials and synaptic transmission.

When a physical theory of the brain is at last put together the observations of the ethologists will, no doubt, find a 'deeper' explanation as did the Ptolemaic epicycles in the heliocentric elipses of Kepler. Indeed we can, perhaps, see signs of this development already. In Chapter 11 we noted how analysis of the control of amphibian limb movements had led to the concept of labelled neurons in the spinal cord representing the different limb muscles. Fixed action patterns might well have their neurological bases in certain inbuilt, inherited, connections between groups of these 'named' neurons. Similarly sign stimuli might find an explanation emerging from the neurophysiology of perception which is discussed in Chapter 14. There we shall find that it has been possible to show that certain neurons in the visual cortex respond maximally to particular geometrical configurations presented to the visual field. It seems a short step from this to the firing of inbuilt patterns of neurons in response

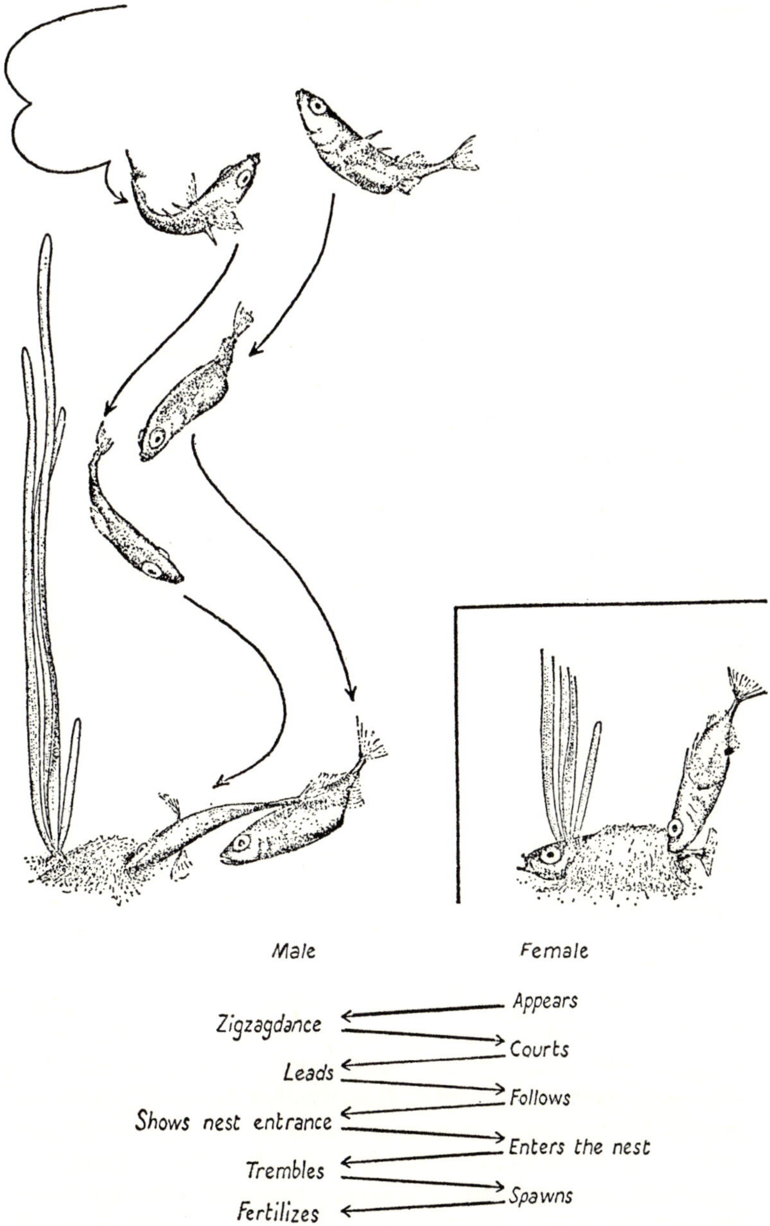


12.2 Mating behaviour of the three-spined stickleback. At the bottom of the figure is represented the chain of relations obtaining between male and female during the process of 'courtship' leading up to fertilization of the eggs. From Tinbergen, N. (1951), *The Study of Instinct*, Oxford University Press.

to the presentation of certain perceptual gestalts. Finally it is not difficult to imagine some form of neuronal 'wiring diagram' whereby the activation of a particular group of neurons by a specific sign stimulus would cause the discharge of a certain pattern of motor neurons in the cord. This *hypothetical* neurology would thus account for one of the major ethological findings: the linking of sign stimulus to fixed action pattern.

### 12.10 The remote control of animal behaviour

Moving back from the field towards the laboratory we meet at something like a halfway stage experiments in which the brain is stimulated in the relatively unhampered animal. Electrical stimulation of the brain by the methods developed in Hess's laboratory required, as we saw earlier in this chapter, that the implanted electrodes be connected by flexible wires to the stimulator. Now some of the important technological 'spin-offs' from the space race have been a number of microminiaturized electronic devices. In consequence it has become possible to attach minute radio receivers to experimental animals and thus to activate implanted electrodes by remote control. Thus the experimenter can examine the effects of brain stimulation on the behaviour of freely moving animals.

These remote control experiments have tended to confirm the findings made with the Hess technique. Thus, for example, stimulation of the postero-ventral region of the hypothalamus causes an animal to display aggressive behaviour. Indeed one animal can be 'driven' to fight another by remote controlled stimulation of this region.

Delgado[1] reports an experiment in which a small cat with electrodes implanted into its hypothalamus is introduced into a cage inhabited by a larger animal. At first relations between the two cats are amicable; radiostimulation of the hypothalamus of the small cat, however, soon alters the situation. It unsheathes its claws, growls and attacks its larger companion. The latter retaliates and the fight continues until the stimulus is switched off. The smaller animal then desists but, not altogether surprisingly, amicability does not rise to its pre-hostility level. The large cat continues to regard its smaller visitor with some suspicion and apprehension.

[1] Delgado, J. M. R. (1964), 'Free behaviour and brain stimulation', *Int. Rev. Neurobiol.*, *6*, 349–449.

Not only can aggressive behaviour be initiated by these means, it can also be inhibited. Stimulation of the basal nuclei of the cerebrum (Fig. 13.4) can be shown to have this effect. It is found that even normally ferocious animals like bulls can be rendered docile and approachable by this technique. Perhaps, however, the most sinister observation is one reported by Delgado in 1963.[1] He relates how electrodes were inserted into a basal nucleus of the boss monkey of a monkey colony. The energising circuit was so arranged that it could be switched on by pressing a lever within the monkey cage. In time other monkeys of the colony came to learn how to control the aggressiveness of their one-time boss by pressing this lever. It was not long before the 'pecking-order' in the colony was up-ended.

Aggressive behaviour is, of course, frequently very stereotyped. In the human case we speak of the angry individual 'losing control of himself'. By this we imply, presumably, that instinctive, inbuilt, behaviour takes over. Revealingly we assert that the individual is no longer responsible for his actions. It is interesting to find that behavioural sequences we should not have thought to be stereotyped in this way can, in some cases, be shown to have this character. Thus Delgado reports that radiostimulation of one of the basal nuclei of the monkey's cerebrum results in the following sequence of actions: 'interruption of existing activities, change in facial expression, turns to the right, standing up on two feet, walking with erect posture around the cage, climbing the wall and then descending to the floor'. When the stimulation was switched off 'the monkey vocalized once or twice, stood on all fours with a threatening attitude, opened its mouth, flattened both ears, raised its tail, looked menacingly at a particular monkey in the group, and then resumed its normal activities'.

Delgado found that this repertoire of activities could be elicited each time the stimulus was given. In one case an animal responded in this way some 20,000 times over a period of two weeks. This sequence of activities is, of course, the outcome of a complex integration of a great number of muscles in all parts of the body. It is, moreover, not an isolated instance. Other behavioural repertoires can be elicited by stimulation of other parts of the monkey brain.

[1] Delgado, J. M. R. (1963), 'Cerebral heterostimulation in a monkey colony', *Science*, *141*, 161–163.

### 12.11 Self-stimulation of the hypothalamus

Finally, in this very brief discussion of some of the neurophysiological bases of motivation, mention must be made of the very interesting work which has been done on the self-stimulation of the brain. We saw in the last section that it is quite possible to get animals to do their own stimulation by wiring the energising circuit to a switch inside the cage. When the electrodes are inserted into certain parts of the hypothalamus some very interesting observations can be made.

It can be shown, for example, that once an animal has learnt to depress a lever to stimulate a certain part of its own hypothalamus it becomes very difficult to deter it from continuing such self-stimulation. Indeed rates of up to five thousand lever depressions per hour have been recorded. Moreover it has proved possible to induce rats to scramble across an electrified grid with the pedal as their sole reward; similarly rats starved for twenty-four hours will sooner actuate the self-stimulating circuit than run to a life-preserving meal.[1]

These and similar experiments seem to show that there is a region in the anterior hypothalamus where electrical stimulation causes a pleasurable sensation. This rather ill-defined region has, indeed, been said to constitute a 'pleasure centre' in the brain. Conversely regions of the posterior hypothalamus are sometimes regarded as aversive centres. Rats stimulated in these regions will work quite hard in order to turn the stimulus off.

Understanding of the way in which these 'pain' and 'pleasure' centres are related to the more precisely defined centres controlling the drives mentioned earlier in this chapter is at present not very far advanced. Attempts to localize the centres anatomically have so far failed. Thus we might conclude this section by re-emphasizing the caution of section 12.4. Whether the electrophysiologist's probe is actually penetrating a definite nerve 'centre' or whether it is merely interfering with nerve pathways, afferent or efferent, leading to and from other parts of the brain is a crucial point which has not yet been decided.

### 12.12 The influence of 'higher' centres on the brain stem

In concluding this chapter it is worth while reminding ourselves that the many drives and instinctive behaviours we have considered are all

[1] Olds, J. (1967), 'Emotional centres in the brain', *Science Journal* (May), 87–92.

highly integrated and adaptive activities. Although there is evidence, as we have seen, that they originate in the hypothalamus or the basal nuclei of the cerebrum they are played out against the varying background of the animal's environment. The behaviour patterns, although in their main outlines stereotyped, are very variable in detail. There is a great deal of flexibility and responses are modified to suit different environmental conditions. This suggests that higher regions of the brain are also involved. The complex interplay between these higher regions, the brain stem and the internal environment is summed up in Figure 12.3.

Figure 12.3 shows that the cerebral cortex has an important influence on the hypothalamic centres we have been discussing. In Chapter 10 (section 10.7) we saw that the neocortex undergoes a huge development in the mammals and particularly in man. Somewhat left behind by this great expansion are the older parts of the

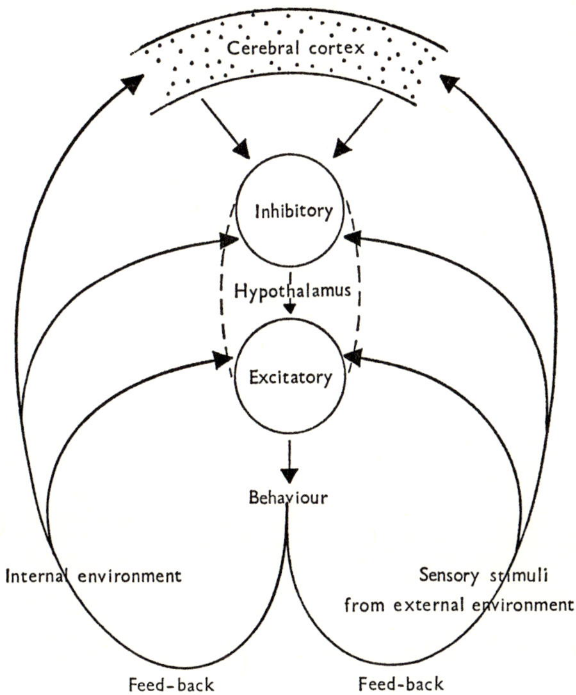


12.3 Schematic diagram to show how the hypothalamic centres motivating behaviour are subjected to feed-back resulting from that behaviour.

cortex. These regions, however still retain their old links with the thalamencephalon and midbrain. Indeed these ancient areas of the cortex—the hippocampus, the pyriform lobe and the cingulate gyrus (above the corpus callosum in Fig. 13.4)—together with some of the basal nuclei, for example the amygdala, are said to form a functional unit called the limbic system. The word limbic is derived from limbus meaning edge or border. Thus the limbic system is conceived as standing at the border between the telencephalon and the thalamencephalon—in limbo, as it were. It follows that it is strategically placed to influence the hypothalamic centres we discussed above. Indeed some authorities like to regard it as the 'visceral brain' and it is often suggested that activity in this system forms the neural basis of our emotional experience, or, as the Americans so graphically phrase it, of our 'gut reactions'. It is thus appropriate that this chapter, which started with a reference to Freudian theory, should end with an allusion to this half-submerged substratum of the emotions.

# CHAPTER THIRTEEN

# The Primate Cerebral Cortex

## 13.1 The human cerebrum

In the last chapter we reviewed evidence which suggests that motivation, drive, perhaps the neurological correlatives of emotion, are largely matters of the brain stem and of the deep nuclei of the cerebral hemispheres. And the brain stem, we saw in Chapter 10, is a structure of vast antiquity. It cannot surprise us therefore to recognize in other, more lowly, vertebrates the same drives—fear, hunger, aggression, sex—which move men and form the roots of our own psychical lives.

Where, however, humans differ from other animals is in their greatly increased powers of ratiocination. Compared with other mammalian orders, compared even with other primates, humans have broken through on to a completely new plane:

> 'Sole judge of truth, in endless error hurled;
> The glory, jest and riddle of the world.'

Teilhard de Chardin refers to this new plane which humans inhabit as the 'noosphere'. Certainly the mutation which has led to the origin of man is as portentous as that which, billions of years ago, led to the emergence of a biosphere on the surface of the cooling planet. The origin of life is nowadays seen as an event in geochemistry: as the result of certain physical conditions acting on certain concatenations of atoms. The origin of a noosphere is also the result of a fortuitous concatenation of material entities: in this case nerve cells and, in particular, nerve cells situated in the cerebral cortex.

Whilst chemists are beginning to understand how living organisms may have arisen *de novo* from such simple inorganics as methane, ammonia, water and carbon dioxide, neurobiologists remain, surprisingly enough, almost completely mystified about the possible origins of symbolic thought—the essence of the noosphere. Certainly it is easy to show that the cerebral cortex becomes larger and more complexly wrinkled as it is traced through the mammalian groups, through the primates, to a climax in man. Certainly, too, it is not difficult to think of behavioural hypotheses: the development and interconnection of hand and eye during arboreal life, the use of tools and weapons by races of apes deprived of their former sylvan existence—a tool, after all, is a means to an end, an end which must, presumably, be in some way symbolically present. Yet when we try to look deeper, when we try to discern a basis for symbolic thought in the detailed structure of the cerebrum, we are baffled. Sheer size seems to be no criterion. R. L. Holloway[1] refers to a pair of Bantu brothers whose cranial capacities were less than 561 mls., well below the upper limits of some pongid brains, who could nevertheless speak and behave in a recognizably human way. Often quoted, too, are the brains of Anatole France and Turgenev, the former of some 1,000 mls. and the latter over 2,000 mls., yet both brains of great intellectual brilliance. Other physical parameters are similarly unrevealing. Some animals have more cells in their cerebral cortices than humans, and some animals have a higher dendrite to perikarya ratio than humans. Some comparative data are given in Table 13.1.

It seems possible, therefore, that the crossing of the cerebral Rubicon, as it is sometimes called, the emergence of humanity from the animal world, is based upon some qualitative change in synoptic connexity due, perhaps, to an alteration in the brain's developmental rate. Let us therefore look first at the histology of the cortex.

## 13.2 Histology of the cerebral cortex

If we look at a relatively low power micrograph of the cerebral cortex (Plate XVI (a) ) we can see that it appears to be stratified. The cells seem to be arranged in layers. There has been much acrimonious debate as to the reality of these layers. Closer inspection of the tissue using the higher powers of the microscope tends to suggest that the laminar structure so obvious to a cursory examination may, like the canals of Mars, be illusory. In spite of this neurohistologists traditionally recognize six layers of cells in the human cerebral cortex.[2]

[1] Holloway, R. L. (1968), 'Evolution of the primate brain: some aspects of quantitative relations', *Brain Res.*, *7*, 121–172.

[2] Brodman, K., *Vergleichende Lokalisationslehre der Grosshirnerinde*, Leipzig, 1909.

TABLE 13.1

Comparison of some mammalian brains

| | *Man* | *Chimpanzee* | *Macaque* | *Indian Elephant* | *Cat* | *Rat* | *Mouse* |
|---|---|---|---|---|---|---|---|
| Veight of entire rain (gms) | 1400[a] | 435[b] | 80 | 4717[c] | 25 | 2·4 | 0·2 |
| atio of brain veight to body eight | 0·02[d] | 0·007 | 0·05 | 0·0015 | 0·008 | 0·005 | 0·015 |
| rea of the cortex f one cerebral emisphere ($mm^2$) | 90,172 | 24,224 | 6940 | | | 16 | |
| tio of the area f cerebral cortex f one hemisphere weight of body nm²/gm) | 0·8 | 0·4 | 0·23 | | | 0·04 | |
| umber of cells mm³ of cortex | 10,500[e] | | 21,500 | 6,900 | 30,800 | 105,000 | 142,000 |
| olume of largest yramidal cells etz cells) ($\mu^3$) | 113,400 | | | | 24,112 | | |

Information derived principally from Blinkov and Glezer, *The Human Brain in Figures and Tables*, Basic Books Inc., 1968.

[a] This is an average value. Some human brains are very much smaller. Nanocephalic dwarfs, for example, always have extremely small brains. This type of dwarf remains perfectly proportioned though seldom attaining a height of more than three feet. In consequence their brains never exceed about 400 gms in weight. These individuals are nevertheless able to master the rudiments of human speech, an accomplishment no pongid has so far achieved.

Microcephalics, like the Bantu brothers mentioned in the text, grow to a normal adult stature whilst retaining very small brains. Clearly these individuals possess a very low brain to body ratio. Once again, however, rudimentary speech and other social accomplishments are developed.

[b] The largest pongid brain yet recorded is that of a gorilla weighing some 750 gms (Holloway, 1968).

[c] The largest brain of all is that developed by the blue whale *Balaenopterus musculus*. This weighs some 6,800 gms. It is, however, situated in a body weighing about 5,800 kgms and thus the brain/body ratio is rather low.

[d] This is probably not a very significant parameter as different animals are built of rather different proportions of fat, connective tissue, bone, etc. The ratio will also vary considerably with the age of the animal.

[e] This number provides an indication of the volume of cortex remaining for the ramifications of nerve cell processes.

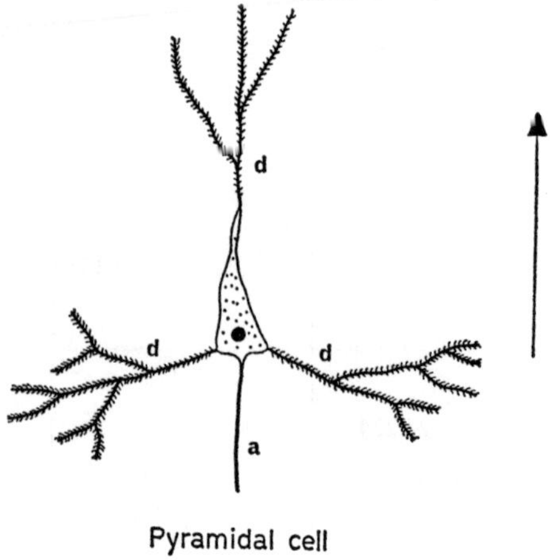


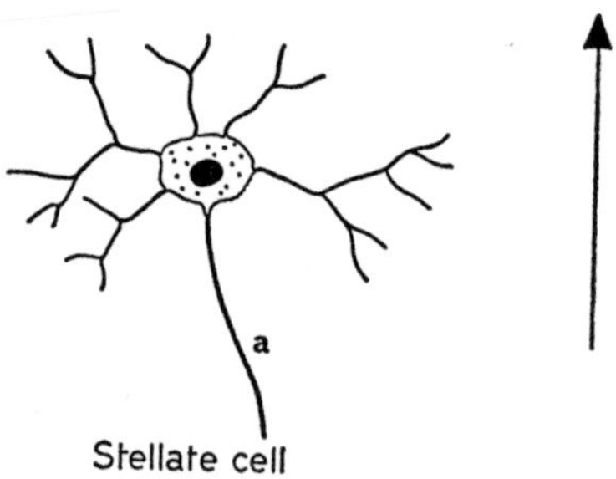


13.1 Two principal types of neuron found in the cerebral cortex. a = axon, d = dendrite. The arrow indicates the direction in which the surface of the cortex lies. Note the spines on the pyramidal cell's dendrites.

The cells are of many different types. The famous histologist Lorente de No recognized at least sixty different types of neuron in the cortex of the rat. D. A. Sholl[1] introduced a very considerable simplification (some authorities say oversimplification) by reclassifying cortical neurons into only two main classes. The first of these classes consists of neurons with conical perikarya which are in consequence called *pyramidal* cells. The second class consists of cells with nearly spherical perikarya from which radiate numerous processes. Accordingly these neurons are called *stellate* cells. These two main types of cortical neuron are shown in Fig. 13.1.

[1] Sholl, D. A., *The Organisation of the Cerebral Cortex*, Methuen, London, 1956.

Sholl subdivided his class of pyramidal cells into four main subgroups depending principally on the nature of the axon's branches. Similarly he recognized three varieties of stellate cell, again distinguished by axonal differences. In general the pyramidal cells seem to occupy the outermost and innermost cortical layers with the stellate cells sandwiched between.

One subgroup of stellate cells seems to be of very considerable neurophysiological importance. In this type of neuron the axon bifurcates shortly after it leaves the perikaryon to form a number of lengthy horizontal processes. These processes end as closely knit 'basket-works' surrounding the perikarya and axon hillocks of pyramidal cells (Fig. 13.2).

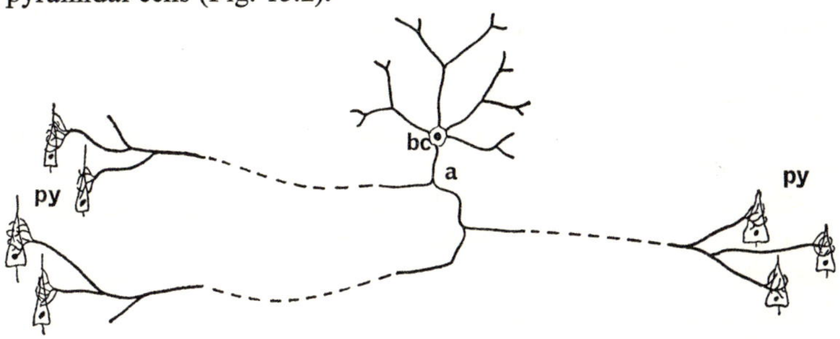


13.2 A basket cell. The axon branches and ends in basket-works which surround and inhibit pyramidal cells. a = axon, bc = basket cell, py = pyramidal cell.

We have already met similar sorts of cell when we discussed the cerebellar cortex. It will be remembered that in this tissue they are called 'basket cells' and have been shown to have an inhibitory function. Basket cells have now been shown to exist in all parts of the cerebral cortex. It is very interesting to note that the basket cells of the hippocampal cortex have also been shown to have an inhibitory function.[1] In other words activation of the cell shown in Fig. 13.2 inhibits the pryamidal cells, and there may be several hundreds of these, around which the basket-like terminations of the axons entwine. It is a fair assumption that the basket cells in other parts of the cerebral cortex are also inhibitory.

If this is in fact the case it has important physiological consequences. We shall see in Chapter 14 that there is good evidence to show that the sensory areas of the cerebral cortex are organized into

[1] Anderson, P., Eccles, J. C. and Lyning, Y. (1964), 'Location of post-synaptic inhibitory synapses on hippocampal pyramids', *J. Neurophysiol.*, *27*, 592–619.

a mosaic of functional columns. These columns, which, so far, have been demonstrated only by electrophysiological techniques, are packed together with their long axes at right angles to the surface of the cortex.

The best known instance of this columnar organization is found in the visual cortex of the cerebrum's occipital lobe. Here neurons concerned with information derived from one particular area of the retina are all organized into a single column. The histological basis of this functional organization has, so far, remained obscure. The demonstration that basket cells exist in all parts of the cerebral cortex suggests, however, a way in which this columnar organization might be achieved. We can suppose that excitation of the pyramidal cells in any part of the cerebral cortex leads by way of their richly branching dendritic trees to an excitation of neighbouring basket cells. Excitation of these cells leads, as Fig. 13.2 shows, to inhibition of adjacent pyramidal cells. Thus excitation is confined to a more or less narrow column at right angles to the surface of the cortex.

What the significance of a columnar organization in non-sensory areas of the cortex might be is not at present clear. It does, however, seem that the entire neocortex consists of a mosaic of overlapping functional columns.[1]

### 13.3 Lobes, sulci and basal nuclei

The great growth of man's cerebral cortex has thrown it into extensive lobes, convolutions and fissures (Plate XVII). In the smaller, less advanced mammals this is not the case. The cerebral cortices of insectivores like the hedgehog and shrew are smooth. The extensive wrinkling of the cerebral cortex in the higher primates seems to be almost entirely due to the physical strains and stresses of its growth in the confined space of the cranium.

Why, we might ask, does the cortex not increase in size in the third dimension—as does the thalamus in, for example, the birds? The answer to this question may lie in the columnar construction of the cerebral cortex described in section 13.2. If this construction is basic to cortical function then the only way to increase its potential as the body becomes larger and behaviour more complex is to increase the number of columns. This can only be done by increasing

[1] M. L. Colonnier (1966), 'The Structural Design of the Neocortex', in *Brain and Conscious Experience*, edited by J. C. Eccles, Springer-Verlag, p. 18.

the area of the cortex. But the only way in which this can be accomplished in a closed cranium is by bending, folding and fissuring the tissue.

Whatever the functional reasons may be, anatomists have long realized that the fissures and lobes provide important and convenient landmarks. Accordingly names have been assigned to all the fissures, or sulci, and lobes. The most important lobes are named after the skull bones beneath which they are situated. Fig. 13.3 shows the positions of the more important of these lobes and sulci.

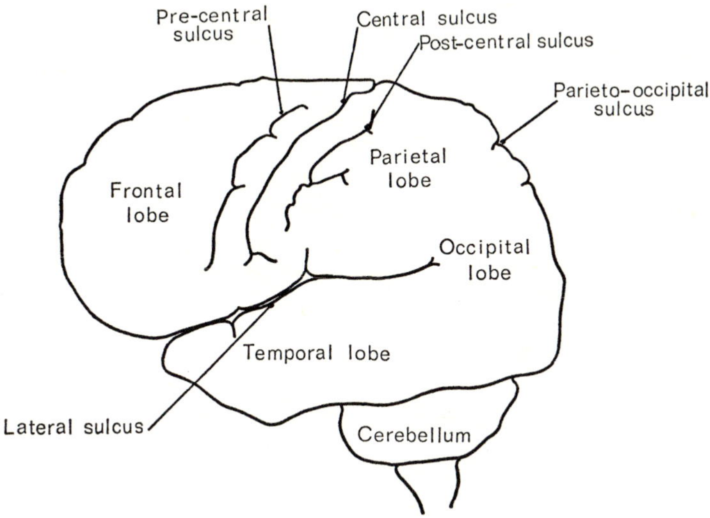


13.3 Principal lobes and sulci of the human cerebral cortex. The left-hand side of the brain is shown. The figure should be compared with Plate XVII.

The figure shows that the human cerebral cortex is divided into four principal lobes. The frontal lobe forms the anterior part of the cortex having as its posterior margin the central sulcus. Behind the central sulcus is the parietal lobe and this is bounded posteriorly by the parieto-occipital sulcus. Behind this sulcus lies the occipital lobe. The ventral part of the cortex below the lateral sulcus forms the temporal lobe.

In addition to these lobes and sulci neurologists recognize and name many subsidiary features. The eminences between the smaller sulci are called gyri, or convolutions. Thus in Fig. 13.3 the precentral gyrus lies between the central sulcus and the pre-central sulcus and, likewise, the post-central gyrus lies between the central and the post-central sulcus. These two gyri are, as we shall see, of considerable functional importance. The interested reader can find the names of other gyri and sulci set out in anatomical text-books.

The two cerebral hemispheres are separated from each other by a deep median cleft called the longitudinal cerebral fissure. The magnitude of this fissure is shown in Fig. 13.4. This figure also shows the relationship of the cerebral hemispheres to the thalamencephalon on which, as we saw in Chapter 10, they rest.

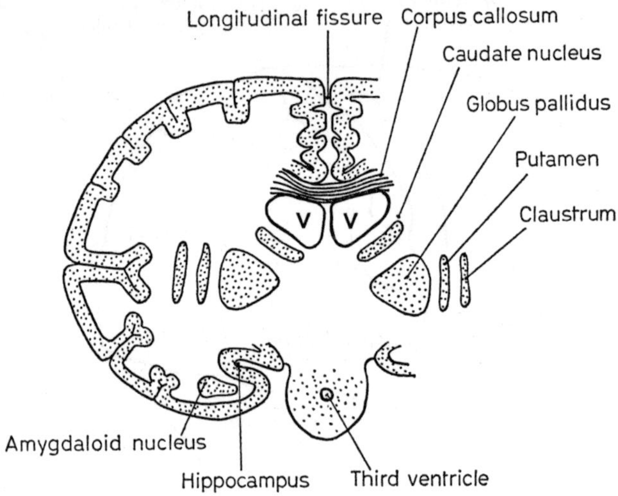


13.4 Schematic coronal section through the human cerebrum to show the principal basal nuclei. For explanation see text. V= lateral ventricle.

Fig. 13.4 shows that although the two cerebral hemispheres are divided from each other by the deep crevasse of the longitudinal fissure they are, nonetheless, united at its base by a prominent tract of fibres—the corpus callosum. This tract of fibres ensures that the left-hand side of the cerebrum knows what the right-hand side is doing. In Chapter 15 we shall mention the very interesting results of some experiments wherein this tract of fibres is sectioned. In fact the corpus callosum is not the only means of communication between the two hemispheres. Another, smaller, tract of fibres—the anterior commissure—also connects the two hemispheres.

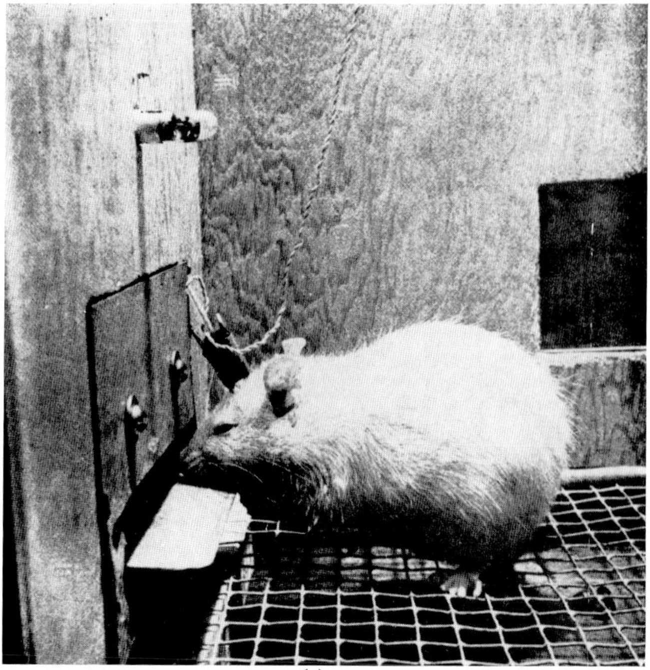

(a)

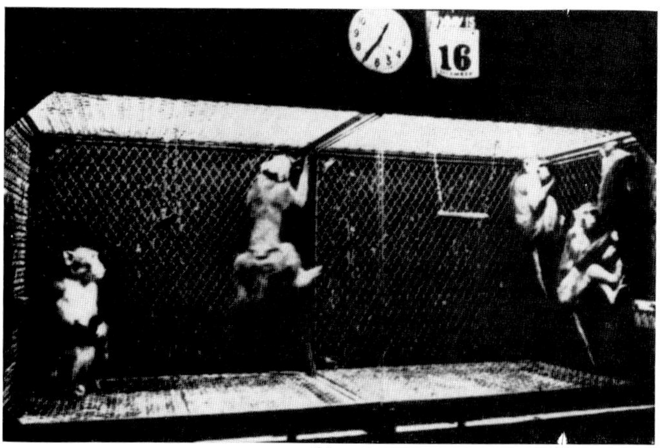


(b)

XV Stimulation of the brain

(a) The white rat has electrodes implanted into a defined region of its brain. By appropriate wiring the rat can stimulate its own brain by pressing the lever shown in the illustration.
(From Olds, J. in *Electrical Studies on the Unanaesthetised Brain,* edited by Ramey, E. R. and O'Doherty, D. S., Paul B. Hoeber Inc., New York, 1960,

(b) Monkeys with chronically implanted electrodes may be caused to act out a precise sequence of walking-jumping-hanging-walking back to starting place. See text for further explanation.
(From Delgado, J. M. R. in *The Physiological Basis of Mental Activity* edited by R. Hernández-Péon, Elsevier, Amsterdam, 1963.

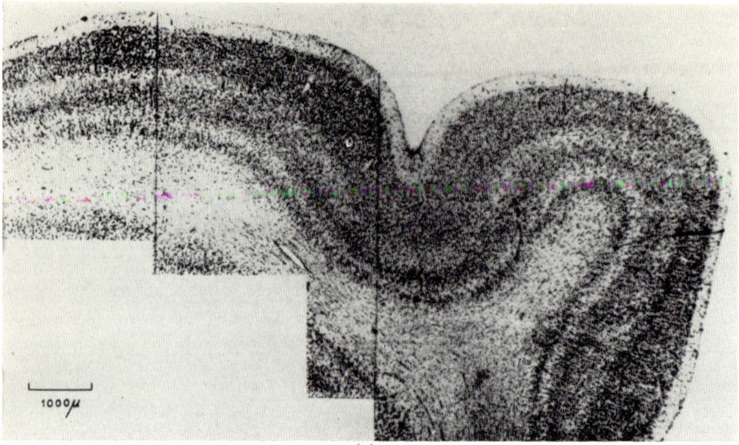


(a)

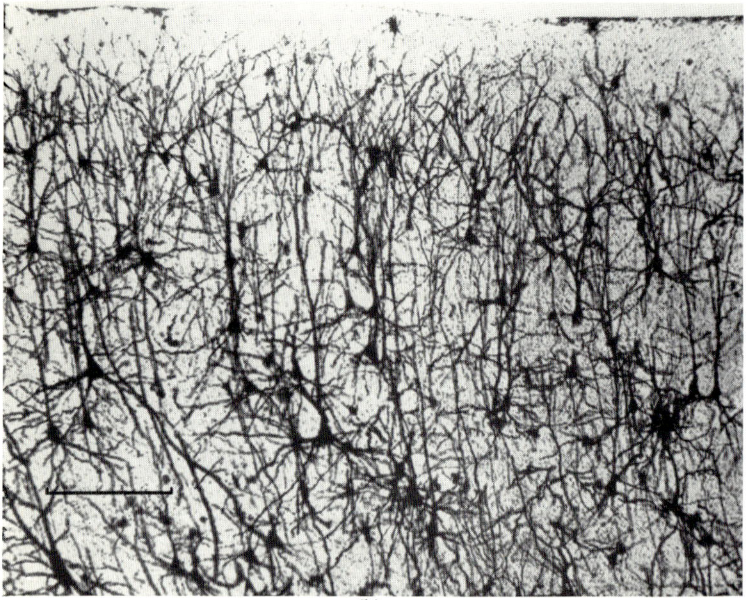

(b)

XVI Fine structure of the cerebral cortex

(a) The characteristic six-layered structure of the neocortex is well shown in this plate. In more primitive regions of the cerebral cortex, for example the hippocampal cortex, only four layers can be recognised.
(From Sholl, D. A., *The Organisation of the Cerebral Cortex*, Methuen and Co. Ltd., 1956.)

(b) Pyramidal and stellate neurons in the cat's cerebral cortex. Only about 1·5% of the neurons present in the preparation are visible in this photomicrograph. Scale marker = 200 μ
(From Sholl, D. A., *The Organisation of the Cerebral Cortex*, Methuen and Co. Ltd., 1956.)

Fig. 13.4 also shows the positions of some of the basal nuclei of the cerebrum. It will be remembered (Fig. 10.11) that these nuclei develop by an inward displacement from the developing cortex. They are islands of nerve cell bodies surrounded by myriads of fibres. The three most important basal nuclei in the human cerebrum are the *corpus striatum* (consisting of candate nucleus, globus pallidus and putamen), the *claustrum* and the *amygdaloid body*.

The functions of some of these nuclei will be mentioned in later chapters of this book. Here it suffices to say that, in general, they act as relay stations for nerve fibres leaving the motor areas of the cerebral cortex. It is also believed that in addition to this purely junctional function the basal nuclei may also regulate and co-ordinate motor commands initiated in the cerebral cortex. In this way their activity is somewhat reminiscent of that of the cerebellum (section 10.4).

### 13.4 The life support system of the brain

Cabined within the capsule of the skull the brain relies upon the blood coursing up the carotid and vertebral arteries for its supply of nutriment and oxygen and for the removal of its wastes. Perhaps the most important single factor in this life support system is the continuous supply of oxygen. The brain stores oxygen sufficient for only about ten seconds' normal activity; if fresh supplies are interrupted neurons suffer irreversible damage. Thus in order to ensure that each part of the brain is provided with ample supplies of oxygen a very complicated network of blood vessels has developed. This network is well shown in the illustration serving as the frontispiece to this book.

Whilst the concentration of oxygen is probably the most critical factor in the brain's molecular environment the concentration of other molecules is also of considerable significance. We have already noticed in section 6.8 the influence of hallucinogenic molecules. Linus Pauling points out[1] that the brain seems to be more sensitive to small changes in the chemical constitution of its fluid environment than any other of the body's organs and tissues. Pauling believes that many mental diseases, in particular schizophrenia, may be caused by a chemical deficiency in the bathing blood. He believes, in other words, that mental disabilities are at root similar to conditions like scurvy and pellagra which were shown at the beginning

[1] Pauling, L. (1968), 'Orthomolecular Psychiatry', *Science, 160*, 265–271.

of this century to be due to the lack of very small quantities of certain vitamins. Cure for certain types of mental disease may thus be achieved by ensuring that the blood coursing through the brain contains an optimum mix of the appropriate molecules. Pauling names this approach to the cure of mental disease orthomolecular therapy.

Not only does the vascular system provide the brain with a carefully balanced solution of vital molecules but it also ensures that the physico-chemical parameters of the cerebral environment are delicately adjusted. In Chapter 12 we noticed how the brain may, in one of its aspects, be regarded as the computer of a homeostat. It can be shown that the organ which this homeostat is principally designed to cosset is the brain itself. It is the brain which is principally affected when any of the parameters of the internal environment escapes its preset limits. Without doubt we have all experienced the delirium, hallucinations and general mental confusion accompanying a fever; accompanying, in other words, a rise in blood temperature beyond the appropriate limits. Similarly with the other parameters of the internal environment. To take just one example of what is, in fact, a large and fascinating topic in physiology, let us consider the regulation of the blood pressure. Clearly the distribution of oxygen and nutriment to the entire brain depends on the maintenance of an appropriate blood pressure in the vessels supplying the brain. The most important of these vessels are the two common carotid arteries which ascend each side of the neck (large vessels in frontispiece). At the angle of the jaw each of these common carotids splits into two. One branch, the internal carotid, carries blood to the brain whilst the other, the external carotid, supplies the outside of the skull and face. In the wall of the common carotids, just before they divide, are to be found receptors sensitive to blood pressure. If the pressure of blood in the common carotids falls these receptors immediately signal intelligence of this fact to a nerve centre in the medulla. This centre—the vasomotor centre—regulates the blood pressure by controlling the rate of heart beat, the diameters of billions of arterioles all over the body and the amount of blood stored in 'reservoirs' such as the spleen. On receiving intelligence that blood pressure is falling this centre immediately acts to counteract the fall. Blood pressure in consequence mounts until the monitoring receptors at the top of the carotid are satisfied. It is, however, possible to fox these carotid receptors. If the neck is squeezed just beneath the angle of the jaw they signal the increase in pressure to the vasomotor centre. This centre accordingly acts in such a way that the blood pressure falls. The brain bleaches and we feel faint.

Bleaching of the brain may occur in response to more permanent causes than transient pressure increases on the carotid receptors. It may be that one or more of the arteries shown in the frontispiece becomes blocked so that blood cannot pass. It follows that the part of the brain which the artery normally serves is cut off from its vital supplies of oxygen and hence dies. Arterial blockade may occur by the development of a clot of blood in the artery (cerebral thrombosis), by a rupturing of the artery walls (cerebral haemorrhage), or, finally, by a progressive narrowing of the artery due to arteriosclerosis. Clearly the larger the artery that is blocked the greater the extent of the brain which is cut off from its supplies and the more catastrophic are the consequences. Individuals who suffer these vascular catastrophes are said to suffer a stroke.

By carefully mapping the territories supplied by the main cerebral arteries it is possible to draw some conclusions about the functions of the various lobes of the cerebral cortex. For it is possible to correlate the behavioural irregularities shown by man and experimental animals after a vascular occlusion of this sort with the territory of the brain put out of action. For example an occlusion of the middle cerebral artery which runs along the lateral sulcus (Fig. 13.12) puts out of action large areas of the temporal and parietal lobes. It is found that patients who survive such an event frequently suffer a continuing speech defect, often amounting to complete aphasia. Accordingly it may be concluded that the territory of the middle cerebral artery includes that part of the brain responsible for speech. The 'speech cortex' will be considered further in section 13.7.

## 13.5 The primary projection areas

Analysis of the functions of the various lobes and convolutions of the cerebral cortex has been carried out by a variety of techniques. Chief amongst these have been close observation of the behavioural effects of injury and of electrical stimulation. In experimental animals portions of the cortex may be removed, or electrodes may be inserted on a semi-permanent basis. In the case of humans, and the human cerebral cortex is, of course, of paramount interest, clinical observations of the behavioural effects of injury or of surgery may be made. In addition, as we shall see in section 13.7, the behavioural correlatives of electrical stimulation of the human cortex may be examined. A note of caution should, however, be sounded here. It is the same caution as that sounded in some parts of Chapter 12. Behavioural effects consequent upon destruction or stimulation of a part of the nervous system by no means necessarily locate the centre controlling the missing or evoked effect in that part.

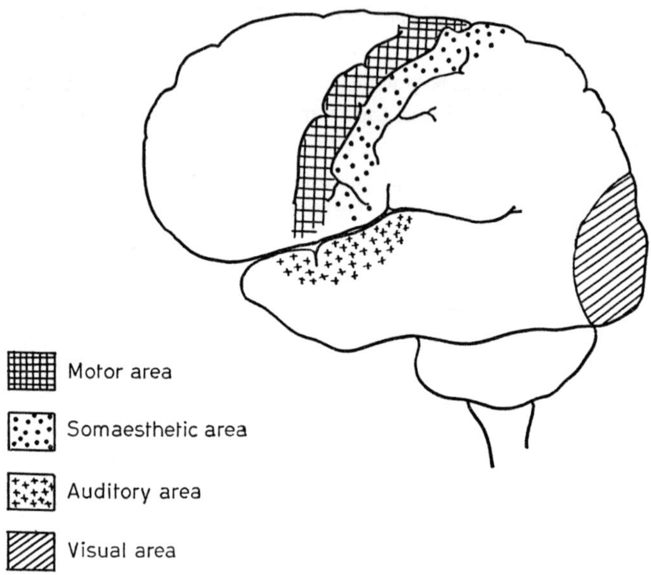


13.5 The primary projection areas on the human cerebrum. For explanation see text.

It seems likely, however, that this proviso is less important when considering the main cerebral 'projection' areas than during the discussion in Chapter 12 of the hypothalamic centres controlling motivation. Evidence is much stronger than the 'buck' really does stop in the cerebral cortex than that it starts in the hypothalamus. The primary projection areas are regions of the cerebral cortex on to which are projected information picked up by the body's sense organs. It is in these areas that the map or model of the animal's environment, both internal and external, is set up. In addition to these sensory (afferent) areas there is also a well defined motor (efferent) area. The positions of the primary sensory and motor projection areas on the human cerebral cortex are shown in Fig. 13.5.

The figure shows that there are four primary projection areas on the cerebral cortex. Three of these are concerned with the 'display' of information picked up by receptor organs and one acts as a marshalling area for outgoing motor impulses.

Visual information is collated in the occipital lobe. It follows that lesions in this area cause blindness even though the eyes and optic nerves are in perfect working order. Moreover it can be shown that the projection of the visual scene, as picked up by the retina, on to the visual cortex is very precise. Localized lesions of the cortex produce local, and predictable, blind spots in the retina. A more detailed discussion of the visual cortex will be found in Chapter 14.

The primary auditory area lies just below the lateral sulcus in the temporal lobe. Again there is a precise mapping of the sense organ—in this case the cochlea—on to the cortex. Now it will be remembered from section 8.2 that tones differing in frequency cause maximal stimulation at different points along the cochlea's length. Low frequency tones have a maximal effect towards the apex whilst high frequency tones stimulate the base. Thus the mapping of the cochlea on to the cortex has considerable functional significance. It means that tones differing in frequency activate different regions of the temporal cortex. In the dog, for instance, it can be shown that each octave is represented by a 2 mm. strip of the auditory cortex. Much the same can be shown in the primate. The situation is, however, much more complicated than is shown in Fig. 13.6. There are, in

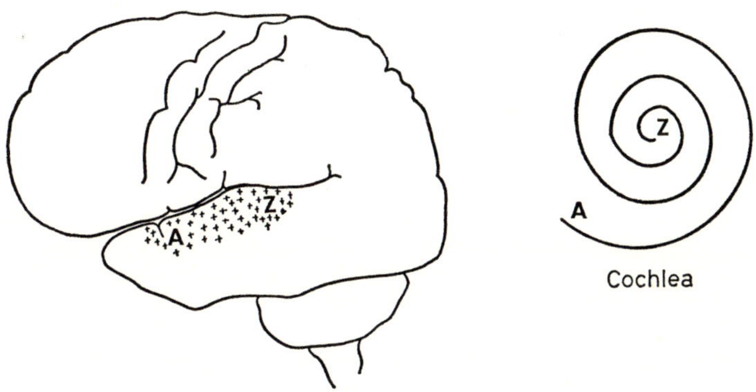


13.6 Projection of the cochlea on to the temporal lobe of the cerebral cortex. The figure shows that high frequency vibration (A) is mapped towards the back of the lobe and low-frequency vibration (Z) is mapped towards the front.

fact, several auditory areas in the human temporal cortex and it seems that the map is reversed and inverted in intricate ways in successive areas. Thus Fig. 13.6 shows only very diagrammatically the major auditory area in the human temporal lobe.

Similar rather precise mapping is to be found in the somaesthetic, or general sensory, area of the post-central gyrus. This is shown in Fig. 13.7 where the somaesthetic 'homunculus' is drawn over a coronal section of the cerebrum in the region of the post-central gyrus.

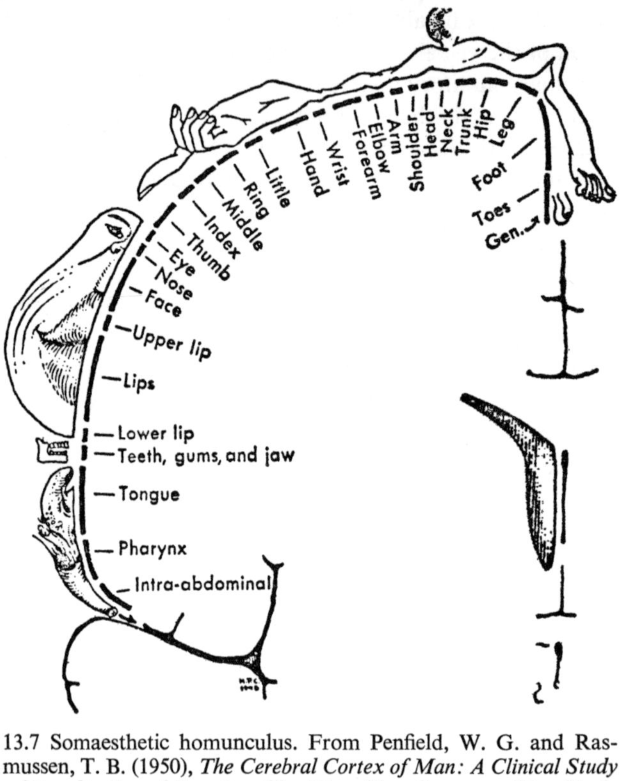


13.7 Somaesthetic homunculus. From Penfield, W. G. and Rasmussen, T. B. (1950), *The Cerebral Cortex of Man: A Clinical Study of Localisation of Function,* The Macmillan Company, New York.

The dimensions of the various parts of the homunculus indicate the relative area of the post-central gyrus devoted to the sensory input from that part. The information received by the cortical neurons of the post-central gyrus relates principally to temperature and touch, and to muscle, joint and tendon senses.

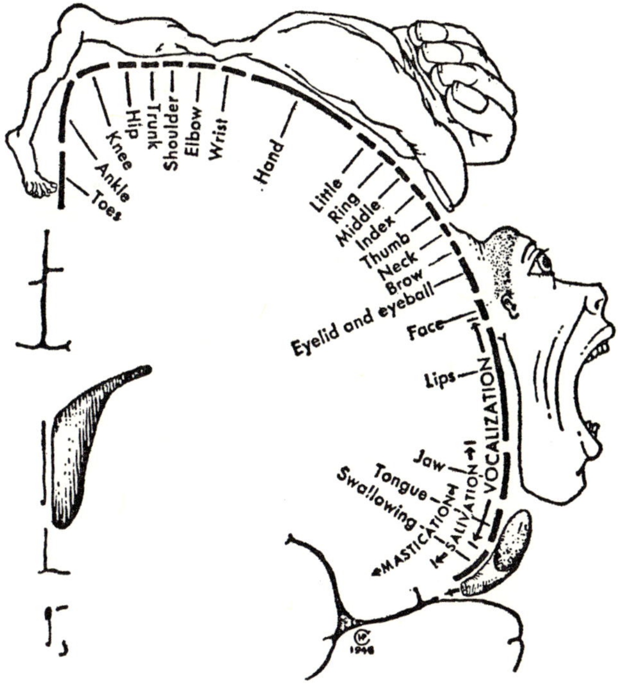


13.8 Motor homunculus. From Penfield, W. G. and Rasmussen, T. B. (1950), *loc. cit.*

Immediately in front of the central sulcus, in the pre-central gyrus, are to be found cortical neurons concerned with the initiation of muscular movement. This area is consequently known as the general motor area. Its topographical organization, as Fig. 13.8 shows, is very similar to that of the general sensory area discussed above. The areas of the pre-central gyrus concerned in the control of different parts of the anatomy vary in size in approximately the same way as did those of the post-central gyrus. It should be noted that the nerve cells of both pre- and post-central gyri are connected with the opposite sides of the body. Thus stimulation of the *left* pre-central gyrus causes movement of appropriate muscles on the *right* side of the body.

### 13.6 Nerve pathways to and from the pre- and post-central gyri

Visual and auditory perception will be discussed in detail in Chapter 14. In that chapter an outline of the pathways taken by the sensory

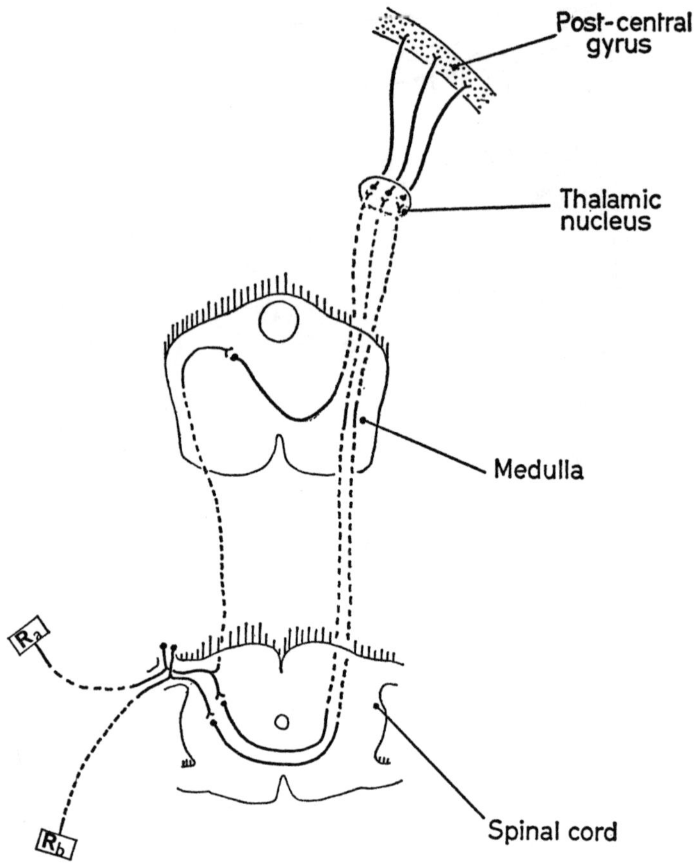


13.9 Sensory pathway to the somaesthetic cortex.

$R_a$ = pain/temperature receptor, $R_b$ = touch/pressure receptor. The broken lines between the section of the spinal cord and the section of the medulla represent the somaesthetic nerve fibres running up the white matter of the cord.

fibres from the sense organs to the visual and auditory cortices will be given. In this section we shall confine ourselves to a description of the nerve pathways connecting the general sensory and motor areas with the periphery.

Fig. 13.9 shows that information reaches the post-central gyrus via a chain of three neurons.

Similarly a chain of three, or sometimes only two, neurons conducts messages away from the pre-central gyrus to the voluntary muscles. The 'wiring diagram' of this pathway is shown in Fig. 13.10.

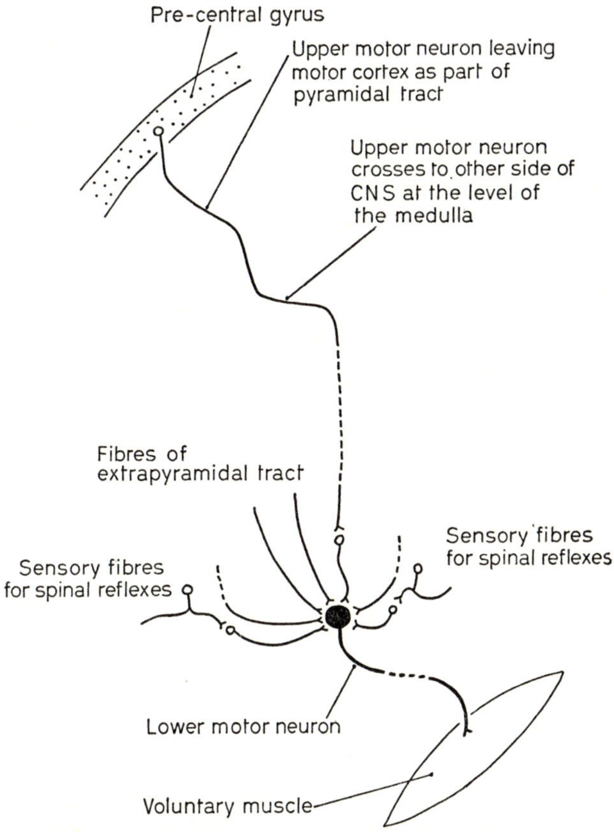


13.10 Motor pathway from the pre-central gyrus. The figure emphasizes that the lower motor neuron is exposed to nerve impulses originating in many different locations. Not only do fibres originating in the precentral gyrus and descending in the pyramidal tract affect it but it is also influenced by fibres of the extrapyramidal tract originating in the cerebellum and elsewhere. In addition to these central influences the lower motor neuron is also exposed to impulses entering the spinal cord in the sensory fibres of the spinal nerves. These multitudinous influences are all integrated on the soma of the lower motor neuron. The axon of this neuron is consequently often referred to as the final common path.

The figure shows that the nerve fibres leaving the pre-central gyrus descend in the white matter of the brain's core—as the cortico-spinal tract—and cross over in the medulla. A few fibres escape this decussation. In general these neurons (the upper motor neurons) synapse with an interneuron and this in turn contacts the lower motor neuron. There are some exceptions to this organization: sometimes the upper motor neuron synapses directly with the lower. In all cases the lower motor neuron, as Fig. 13.10 shows, runs out to innervate the effector organ. However, Fig. 13.10 also shows that the soma or dendritic zone of the lower motor neuron is also exposed to many other influences. Not only are synaptic contacts made by sensory fibres responsible for spinal reflexes, but also the perikaryon and dendrites of the lower motor neuron are invested by the endings of fibres belonging to the extrapyramidal system. These fibres originate in subcortical regions of the brain including the cerebellum. They are responsible for adjusting the output along the lower motor neuron in the light of the ongoing activity in other parts of the body's musculature. There is, in other words, a complex interplay of EPSPs and IPSPs on the soma of this terminal motor neuron. The integrated result of this flux of electrochemical activity either initiates or inhibits an impulse along the axon. The axon of the lower motor neuron is thus sometimes said to constitute the 'final common pathway'. It is along this pathway that the behavioural 'print-out' from all this intricate neuronal computation is finally transmitted to the effector organs.

## 13.7 Speech and interpretative areas

In addition to the primary projection areas discussed above mammalian cerebral hemispheres possess areas committed to neither motor nor sensory function. Wilder Penfield has pointed out that compared with other mammals the cerebrum of *H. sapiens* is lavishly provided with these uncommitted areas. This is largely due to the great development of the frontal, parietal and temporal lobes in the human cerebrum. Penfield and his colleagues have shown that the uncommitted areas of the last two of these lobes are devoted to speech, perception of the body image and spatial relationships. Fig. 13.11 shows the relative areas of the 'uncommitted cortex' in the rat and man.

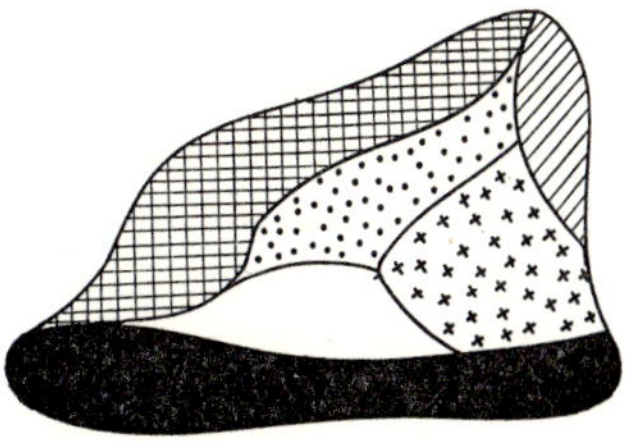

(a)

13.11 Relative areas of 'uncommitted' cortex in (a) the rat and (b) man. The primary projection areas are shaded in the same way as in Fig. 13.5. In addition the olfactory cortex is represented by plain black and the 'uncommitted cortex' by plain white. Adapted from Penfield, W. (1966), 'Speech, perception and the uncommitted cortex' in *Brain and Conscious Experience*, edited by J. C. Eccles, Springer-Verlag, Berlin.

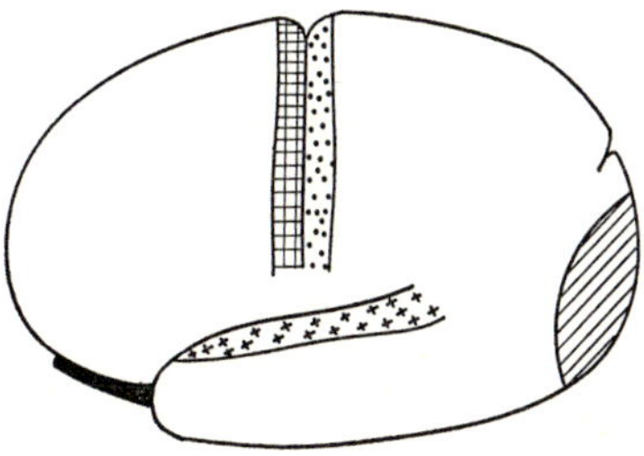

(b)

Penfield and his colleagues at Montreal have carried out many fascinating studies on the uncommitted cortex of the temporal and parietal lobes. These investigations are summarized in a long paper published in 1963.[1] All these studies were carried out on patients undergoing surgery for epilepsy.

Epilepsy is the disease which was known in the ancient world as 'the sacred disease'. To the contemporaries of Hippocrates it must have seemed that the sufferer was indeed smitten by the gods. In its most spectacular form the epileptic 'fit' consists of a sudden loss of consciousness so that the victim falls to the ground often uttering a cry. This is succeeded by powerful convulsions of the body's musculature. In most cases a characteristic 'aura' precedes the attack. In other words the patient is warned of an impending seizure by a rather specific sensation: it may be a visual, auditory or olfactory memory, or it may be merely a feeling of nausea or of numbness. It is not difficult to understand why the ancients believed there to be something supernatural about this 'falling sickness'.

[1] Wilder Penfield and Phaner Perot (1963), 'The Brain's Record of Auditory and Visual Experience—A Final Summary and Discussion', *Brain*, *86*, 595–697.

Hippocrates, however, in the work quoted in the Introduction, argues strongly that epilepsy is no more due to supernatural intervention than any other of 'the ills the flesh is heir to'. He maintains that the disease is due to a malfunctioning of the brain in the same way that other diseases are due to malfunctioning of other parts of the human organism. Hippocrates, we therefore see, is an early exponent of the point of view supported in this book. The brain is a mechanism no more and no less 'supernatural' than any other part of the material world. The advance of our understanding in the two and a half millennia since the Hippocratic treatises were written merely allows us to pinpoint more exactly the nature of the malfunction causing epilepsy. The disease appears to be due to localized regions of abnormally active brain tissue. These act as foci from which the widespread neuromuscular seizure may spread. However our understanding even today is very far from being complete. The causes of the abnormal activity are often obscure. One way, however, of treating epilepsy is to remove the suspect region of the brain; to remove, in other words, the epileptogenic tissue. It is during operations designed to do just this that Penfield and his colleagues at Montreal have been able to make their important observations.

First Penfield was able to show that patients whose temporal or occipital lobes were electrically stimulated reported rather crude ill-defined sensations. Stimulation of the occipital lobe, for example, caused patients to experience flashes of coloured light, whilst stimulation along the lateral fissure called up rather meaningless buzzings.

Stimulation of the posterior regions of the temporal lobes and of parts of the parietal and frontal lobes had, however, a very different outcome. At first it seemed that these areas were 'silent', that there was no experiental correlative to electrical stimulation. On the other hand it had been known since the nineteenth century that injury to, or disease of, the upper temporal lobe resulted in speech deficiencies. Indeed major lesions cause complete loss of speech (aphasia). Thus Penfield thought to show his subject a familiar object, for example a butterfly, whilst stimulating this region of his cortex and found that the patient was completely unable to say what the object was. However, as soon as the stimulating electrode was withdrawn the patient was immediately able to give the correct name and explained with relief that he 'had tried to get the word "butterfly" and then had tried for "moth" '. Use of this technique has allowed Penfield to map the cortical speech areas (Fig. 13.12). The technique is also of considerable surgical importance as it ensures that excision of epileptogenic cortex does not result in an aphasic patient.

The speech cortex develops in one cerebral hemisphere only—the dominant hemisphere. In most human beings this is the left hemisphere. If, however, destruction of the speech cortex in the left hemisphere occurs before the age of ten or twelve it is possible for the non-dominant hemisphere to take over the speech function. In this case the child is aphasic only for a year or two. If destruction occurs in the adult aphasia is permanent. These observations are very similar to some experiments on the cat visual cortex which are discussed in section 14.7.

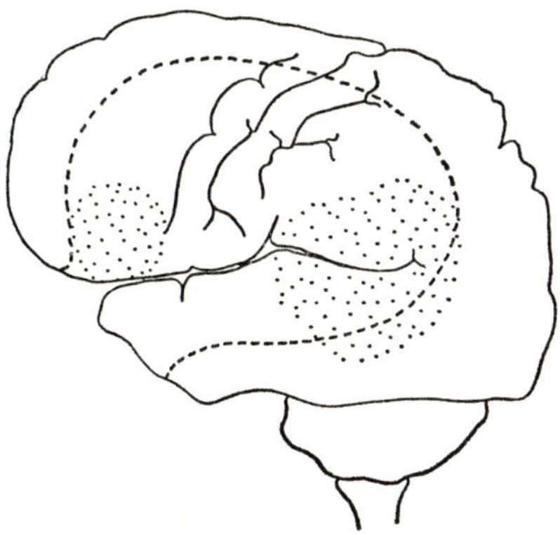

13.12 Major speech areas in the human cerebral cortex. The stippled areas indicate the positions of the anterior and posterior speech areas. In addition there is another small area (not shown in the figure) on the dorsal surface of the cerebrum immediately in front of the precentral sulcus. The broken line encloses the approximate territory of the middle cerebral artery. After Penfield, W. and Perot, P. (1963), 'The brain's record of auditory and visual experience—a final summary', *Brain*, *86*, 595–697.

The homologous area to the speech cortex in the non-dominant hemisphere does not, however, remain functionless. It can be shown that this area is concerned with interpretation of spatial relationships and of the body image. Penfield describes a case where a bullet had scarred this area producing epilepsy. Removal of the scarred tissue cured the epilepsy but left the patient unable to orientate himself. As soon as he turned the corner at the end of his street so that his home was out of sight he became hopelessly lost.

A great deal more may be learnt about this part of the non-dominant hemisphere by careful mapping with electrodes. It is found, for example, that stimulation of this area often causes a detailed recall of times past. We must be careful in our interpretation of these results for the evidence suggests that electrical stimulation of these cortical areas initiates impulses to other parts of the brain. Indeed excision of regions where stimulation causes vivid hallucinations does not remove the memory.[1]

[1] Penfield, W. and Perot, P. (1963), *loc. cit.*, p. 689.

In the paper already referred to Penfield and Perot give many examples of the intense experiental recall associated with stimulation of these areas of the cortex. The experience is usually accompanied by a feeling of familiarity, a feeling of *déjà vu*. The vivid memory may be of a song or of an orchestra playing; alternatively it may be of a visual scene—a gymnasium in the patient's school, or men fighting.[1] Strangely enough, however, no experiences other than auditory or visual memories have been summoned by the surgeon's electrode. But, as Penfield points out, man's life is filled with a multiplicity of non-auditory, non-visual experience. He does mental arithmetic, he eats, he drinks, he defecates, he makes love. So far none of these facets of man's existence has been reported when the cortex is stimulated.

The conclusion which Penfield arrives at from the evidence of over a thousand brain operations is that stimulation of the cortex activates a random strip of the patient's memory. The past stream of consciousness tapped in this way is, however, very restricted. It is restricted to 'times of watching or hearing the action and speech of others and times of hearing music'. The detail of the memories called forth in this way are hallucinatory in their intensity—they are far more profuse than those evoked in voluntary memory. The remembered experience, moreover, appears to unfold at its original tempo.

We may imagine that the interpretative cortex, like the speech cortex in the dominant hemisphere, is labile and uncommitted in the infant. Penfield and Perot suggest that whereas the speech cortex makes words and phrases available when speech is intended, so the interpretative cortex makes past experience available for comparison with incoming current experience. The interpretative cortex, in other words, holds a map or model of the world against which the world sensed by the sense organs is matched. We have already met this general concept of a map or model in the brain in previous chapters, and we shall examine it in more detail in the later chapters of this book.

[1] By means of this technique the neurosurgeon hopes to localize the cortical region responsible for the epileptic seizure. Hopefully, correlation between the electrode's position and the patient's statement that he is aware of the particular experience which customarily heralds an impending seizure allows the surgeon to localize his excision.

# CHAPTER FOURTEEN

# Perception

'To perceive: to take in with the mind or senses; to apprehend with the mind; to become aware of; to observe; to understand'

*Shorter Oxford English Dictionary*

'To common sense it seems obvious that what we perceive are "things" '

BERTRAND RUSSELL, *An Enquiry into Meaning and Truth,* Pelican Books, Harmondsworth, Middlesex, 1962, p. 110.

'. . . we never come to an act of perception with an entirely blank mind, but are always in a state of preparedness or expectancy, because of our past experience'

ABERCROMBIE, M. L., *The Anatomy of Judgement,* Hutchinson, London, 1960, p. 54.

## 14.1 Towards a definition of perception

These propositions suggest that when we arrive at the topic of perception we have left the solid ground of physiology behind and are beating about in the more dubious realms of metaphysics and introspective psychology. What can the physical theory of the brain which we have been piecing together in the earlier chapters of this book have to say about 'observing', 'understanding', 'becoming aware of' or having 'an entirely blank mind'? On the other hand if it is not capable of treating these properties it is a poor thing. For these are some of the most characteristic and important features of higher brains. It is these characteristics we think of first when we ask for an explanation of how the brain works; if our physical theory fails here it fails altogether.

It is clear that in the last chapters of this book where we discuss perception, memory and consciousness we come increasingly against the great schism which shatters the unity of the modern world view. The Cartesian schism which separates *res cogitans* from *res extensa*, that divides mind from matter. We can, however, temporarily avoid the pressure of this problem by lumping all our questions and investigations on to the *res extensa* side of the chasm. This is the approach of behaviourism. It is, however, only a temporary expedient. We are, all of us, conscious beings: this fact is insuppressible. The relationship of mind to matter is not solved, only shelved, by the behaviourist approach. It will be considered further in Chapter 17.

The attitude of behaviourism is well epitomized by the title of an important book published in 1921: *Psychology of the Other One.*[1] What we have to account for is the *behaviour* of other organisms—animals or men. The behaviourist believes, and most physiologists with him, that this behaviour is explicable in terms of the neurophysiology we have been reviewing in the previous chapters of this book. In other words there is no need for 'strange' concepts like 'mind' or 'consciousness'.[2] These things, if they are things, have never yet been detected by the anatomist's scalpel or the physiologist's electrode. They are unnecessary 'occult' causes and hence, in the best scientific tradition, superfluous.

Our programme is thus to redefine 'perception', 'memory', 'consciousness', etc. in terms of the organism's behaviour. Once this is done the physiologist can search in his customary manner for the machinery responsible for the behaviour. Let us therefore see if we can come at a definition of perception which will in this way open the topic to physiological analysis.

We noticed at the outset of this chapter that what we commonly believe ourselves to perceive are 'things'. We also commonly use the notion of perception when we talk about perceiving relationships between things. What, then, do we mean by 'things'? Most of us would be inclined to agree with Wisdom[3] when he defines a thing as a bundle of characteristics related in a unique and enduring fashion. F. G. Worden puts it another way when he writes '. . . receptor organs extract from the fluctuating (environmental) energies certain invariant patterns which signify objects and relationships'.[4]

The important concept here is 'pattern'. To perceive is to recognize a pattern, whether it is a pattern of properties which characterize a 'thing' or a pattern of relationships between things. Now this is an

[1] Meyer, M. F., *Psychology of the Other One,* Columbia Mo., Missouri Book Co., 1921.

[2] See also in this connection Gilbert Ryle, *The Concept of Mind*, Hutchinson's University Library, London, 1949.

[3] Wisdom, J., *Problems of Mind and Matter*, Cambridge University Press, 1963.

[4] Worden, F. G. (1966), 'Attention and auditory electrophysiology', *Progr. in Physiol. Psychol., 1*, 45–116.

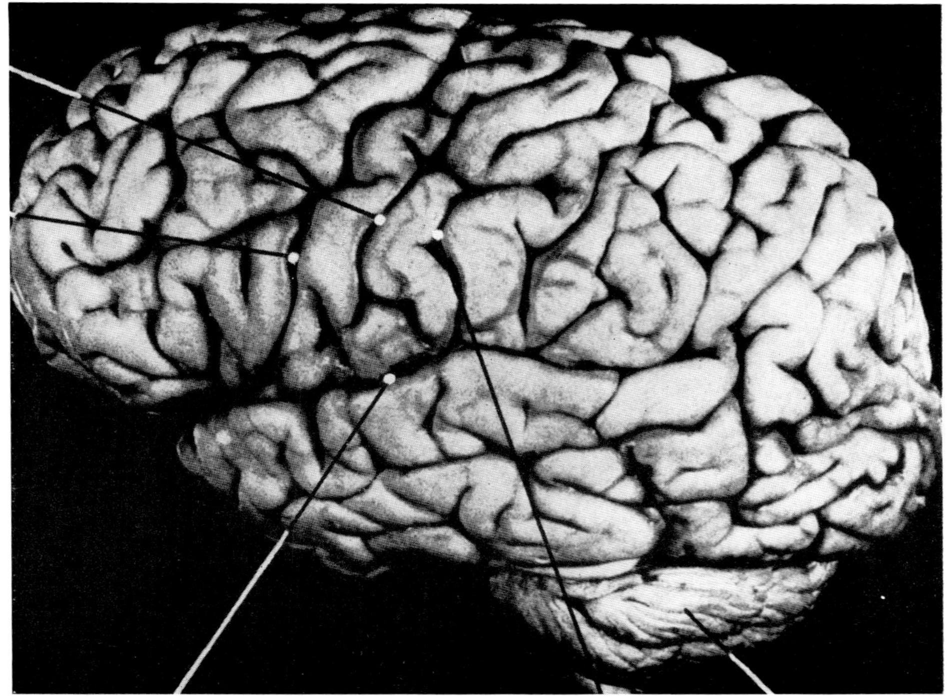


XVII Lateral surface of the human brain

The brain is viewed from the left side and is tilted slightly towards the viewer. (From H. Chandler Elliot, *Textbook of Neuroanatomy*, J. B. Lippincott Company, 1963.)

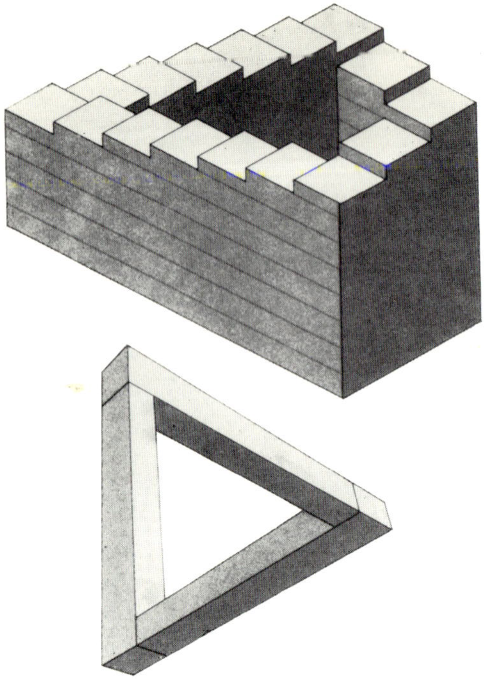

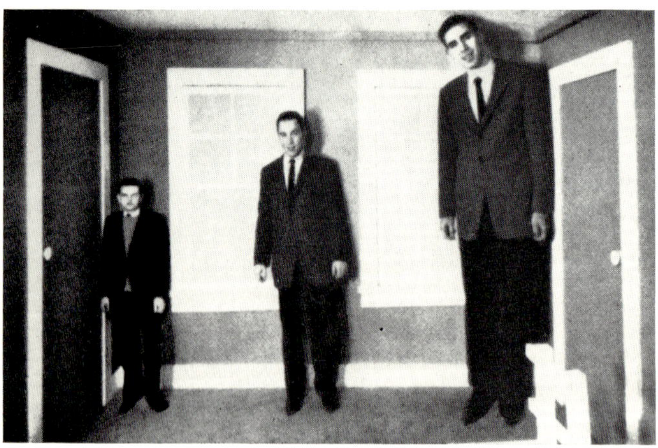

XVIII Some 'impossible' figures

(a) Drawings of three-dimensional figures which could not exist in the 'real' world.
(From Gregory, R. L., *Eye and Brain*, Weidenfeld and Nicolson, 1966.)

(b) The observer 'expects' the room to be rectangular and its roof to be parallel with the floor, etc. Hence he has the illusion that the sizes of the figures differ absurdly.
(From Ittelson, W. H., *The Ames Demonstrations in Perception*, Princeton University Press, 1952.)

attractive equation for the behaviourist. We have all heard nowadays of artificial pattern recognizers: most of us will know, for example, that the odd-looking figures inscribed on our cheques are 'read' by the bank's computer. And we certainly don't have to import 'ghostly' factors like minds or consciousness into the fairly simple machinery used by banks. Our task, therefore, in trying to understand the physiology of perception is the task of trying to understand how the cerebral computer recognizes patterns.

### 14.2 Tactile perception

According to Aristotle the fundamental sense in man and animals is the sense of touch. 'All the other senses,' he writes,[1] 'for example smell, sight and hearing apprehend through media; but where there is immediate contact the animal, if it has no sensation, will be unable to avoid some things and take others and so it will find it impossible to survive'. This belief, of course, has persisted into our own times. We are persuaded that the final test of reality is the test of touch. We habitually believe ourselves able to distinguish between a person and his 'ghost', between a dagger and a 'dagger of the mind' by the sense of touch. If we cannot touch it we incline to believe our percept to be 'a false creation, proceeding from the heat-oppressed brain'.

Yet recent experimental work has cast doubt on this hoary belief. It is possible to show that, in man, vision is the dominant sense. Instead of touch educating and confirming vision, as Berkeley and many others have believed, there is considerable evidence to show that, in fact, matters are quite the other way about. In experimental situations in which the subject's sense of touch is at variance with what he sees as, for example, when he wears various types of distorting spectacles, then his ultimate decision is to believe what he sees rather than what he feels. The visual perception captures and dominates the subject's attention.[2]

Tactile perception can nevertheless be very elaborate. Anyone who has watched a blind person examining an unfamiliar object will be aware of this fact. A good idea of this complexity is given by Lord

[1] Aristotle, *De Anima*, 434$^{b}$15, translated by J. A. Smith, Encyclopaedia Britannica Inc.

[2] Rock, I. and Harris, C. S. (1967), 'Vision and Touch', *Scientific American*, May, 96–104.

Adrian in the following passage. 'The wide dispersion and intermingling of the terminal branches of the sensory fibres', he writes,[1] 'means that a touch on the skin will send messages to the spinal cord along many paths. Where these terminate there will be a focus of activity corresponding to the point touched and a zone of declining activity around it. Thus the pattern of excitation of the skin will be reproduced more or less faithfully and if one or other of the sensory fibres were put out of action it would not seriously affect the reproduction of the pattern. The pattern is both spatial and temporal. Indeed the temporal aspect may be the most important for recognition. The important sensory surfaces never behave as static receiving screens. In the intact animal a touch which differs from the expected range of contacts will immediately arouse exploratory movements by which the object can be felt, as, for instance, when something put in the hand is moved about, so that the pattern which is available to the brain is compounded of signals from the tactile receptors and from those which show movement and position of the fingers. Such qualities as roughness and smoothness, softness and hardness, could only be judged by a combination of temporal and spatial analysis'.

This passage brings out several important points about perception in general and tactile perception in particular. The incoming information, for example, is matched against a pattern of expectations. Perception is an active process. This general characteristic of perception was alluded to by Abercrombie in the passage quoted at the beginning of this chapter. The pattern of expectations is derived from past experience. The question as to its physical nature is a question as to the physical nature of memory: as such it is deferred to the next chapter. Another general feature of sense perception brought out by Adrian is that the spatial pattern of excitation at the sense organ is mapped or modelled in the brain. The map and the excitatory pattern are not, as we shall see more fully in the next sections, necessarily isomorphous. Features of biological importance take up larger areas of the map than they do in reality. The map is thus a map of the biological significance of the stimulus pattern. It is comparable to those demographic maps which greatly distort the facts of geography in order to bring home to the demographer those aspects in which he is particularly interested.

[1] Adrian, E. D. (1950), 'Sensory Discrimination', *British Medical Bulletin, 6,* 1534.

We saw in Chapter 13 that tactile and proprioceptive information is fed into the somatic sensory area in the post-central gyrus of the cortex. Careful analysis of this area with microelectrodes has shown that the neurons are organized into columns or cylinders.[1] These columns are orientated at right angles to the surface of the cortex. The neurons in each column are activated by stimulation of approximately the same peripheral receptive fields (Chapter 8). Moreover all the neurons of a column are responsive to the same type or mode of stimulation—temperature, pressure, etc. We have already noticed a possible histological basis for a 'physiological' column in section 13.2. It must be emphasized that so far evidence for columnar units of action in the cerebral cortex has been obtained solely by physiological techniques.

### 14.3 Auditory perception

Closely allied to the sense of touch is the sense of hearing. The basilar membrane (Chapter 8) of the cochlea may be considered as an exceedingly sensitive strip of skin. Indeed von Bekesy has reversed the analogy and demonstrated that most of the basilar membrane's properties can be shown to exist on a large scale, and in a relatively insensitive fashion, along the skin of, for example, the forearm.[2] The basilar membrane differs from the skin of our arms in being sensitive enough to respond to minute variations in the atmospheric pressure. Thus successive compressions and rarefactions in the atmosphere are made apparent to us, via our ears, as sound.

The means by which the cochlea of the ear detects sound waves in the atmosphere was outlined in Chapter 8. In Chapter 13 we saw that sensory information from the ears is ultimately analysed in the temporal lobes of the cerebral cortex. The auditory nerve does not, however, travel non-stop to this region of the cortex. In fact it halts at four intermediate junctions (Fig. 14.1). Fibres carrying information about the basilar membrane's states of vibration pass first to the cochlear nucleus in the roof of the medulla (section 10.4). From this nucleus the intelligence is relayed to the auditory cortex via the olivary nucleus, the inferior colliculus and the medial geniculate body.

[1] Mountcastle, W. B. (1957), 'Modality and topographic properties of single neurons in the cat's sensory cortex', *J. Neurophysiol.*, *20*, 408–434.

[2] von Bekesy, G. (1959), 'Similarities between hearing and skin sensations', *Psychol. Rev.*, *66*, 1–22.

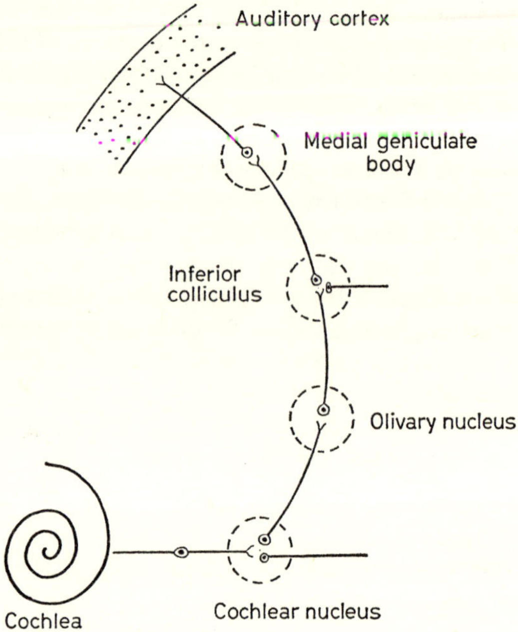


14.1 Schematic diagram to show the auditory pathway. Only the main route is shown. The figure indicates that fibres leave the cochlear nucleus and the inferior colliculus for the other side of the brain.

In recent years considerable progress in the analysis of the message at the various staging posts of Fig. 14.1 has been made. First of all several workers have examined the neuronal activity in the cochlea itself. Nomoto and his co-workers have been able to show that a type of lateral inhibition occurs among auditory nerve fibres.[1] In other words they succeeded in demonstrating that, in certain cases, the response of a nerve fibre to a pure tone was inhibited when a second, suitably chosen, pure tone was sounded. This inhibition is believed by these workers to occur in the cochlea and is similar in essentials to the lateral inhibition which, we saw, played so important a part in the physiology of retinae. The type of response obtained by Nomoto and his colleagues is shown in Fig. 14.2.

[1] Nomoto, M., Suga, N. and Katsuki, Y. (1964), 'Discharge pattern and inhibition of primary auditory nerve fibres in the monkey', *J. Neurophysiol.*, *27*, 768–787.

The existence of lateral inhibition in the cochlea is clearly of considerable physiological significance. It will be remembered from Chapter 8 that the ear discriminates between tones of different frequency by detecting the *place* at which the basilar membrane undergoes maximum disturbance. Sound, however, causes a very complex disturbance along the basilar membrane and in the absence of some such mechanism as lateral inhibition the place of maximum oscillation would be difficult to detect. The very fact that the human ear can be trained to distinguish between frequencies as similar as 1,000 c/s and 1,003 c/s implies some means of sharpening up the

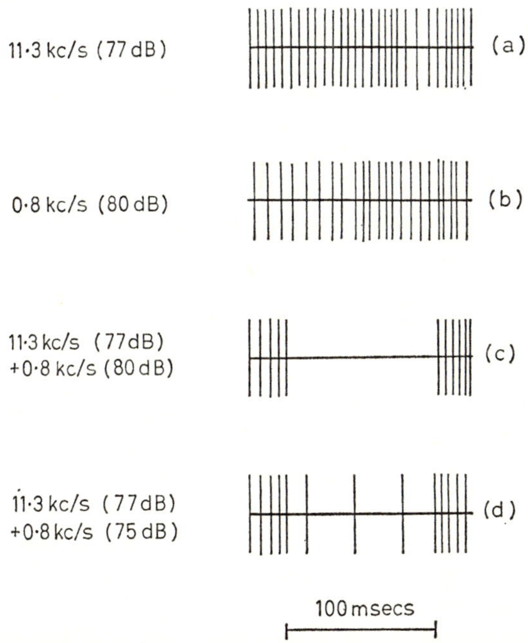


14.2 Response in a monkey's auditory nerve fibre to mixtures of pure tones. In (a) and (b) the response of the nerve fibre to pure tones of frequency 11·3 and 0·8 kc/s is shown. In (c) and (d) the response of the same nerve fibre to mixtures of these tones is depicted, the 0·8 kc/s tone being sounded for the 100 msec. period indicated in the figure. (dB = decibel). Simplified from Nomoto, M., Suga, N., and Katsuki, Y. (1964), 'Discharge pattern and inhibition of primary auditory nerve fibres in the monkey', *J. Neurophysiol.*, *27*, 768–787.

localization. This means, of course, is, as we saw in the case of the *Limulus* compound eye, very adequately provided by the mechanism of lateral inhibition.

When the auditory message is traced inwards we find that further processing occurs. Greenwood and Maruyama,[1] for instance, have shown that cells in the cochlear nucleus responsive to a pure note of a particular frequency are surrounded by an inhibitory area. At low intensity stimulation a smallish group of activated neurons is surrounded by a population of cells whose discharge is inhibited. As the intensity of the pure tone is increased the size of the inhibited population decreases. It is not difficult to see that this organization is well adapted to the recognition of auditory patterns. The various different components of a complex sound are mapped into various different regions of excitation in the cochlear nucleus; the size of these excited regions symbolizes the intensity of each component.

The cochlear nucleus is not, however, the ultimate destination of auditory information in the mammalian brain. As Fig 14.1 shows, nerve fibres from the cochlear nucleus pass onwards via at least three intermediate stages to the auditory cortex. A number of studies have been made of neurons in the auditory cortex itself. Many of these investigations have concentrated on establishing the response of cortical units to steady tones or sudden clicks. But as Whitfield and Evans have pointed out[2] these stimuli are, to say the least, rather artificial. An animal does not normally live in an auditory environment consisting of unexpected clicks and/or sustained pure tones! Quite the contrary: in its natural surroundings an animal is concerned to make sense of complicated sonic patterns continuously varying in pitch and intensity. In order to initiate work on the problem of auditory pattern recognition Whitfield and Evans examined the response of cells in the auditory cortex to frequency-modulated sound.

A frequency-modulated (FM) sound is one in which the frequency varies throughout the duration of the sound. In the simplest cases the frequency may continuously decrease or continuously increase. Whitfield and Evans showed that the response of cortical cells to FM sound

[1] Greenwood, D. D. and Maruyama, N. (1965), 'Excitatory and inhibitory response areas of the auditory neurons in the cochlear nucleus', *J. Neurophysiol.*, *28*, 863–892.

[2] Whitfield, I. C. and Evans, E. F. (1965), 'Responses of the auditory cortex neurons to stimuli of changing frequency', *J. Neurophysiol.*, *28*, 653–672.

could not be predicted in any simple manner from their response to pure tones of constant frequency. We shall see below that this finding is analogous to the outcome of some of the very interesting work on pattern recognition in the visual cortex.

It was shown that as many as 10% of all the cortical neurons responsive to FM sounds would not respond to steady tones at all. Furthermore it proved possible to distinguish three classes of these FM units. One class consisted of cells which responded only to sounds in which the frequency was increasing (frequency-up). A

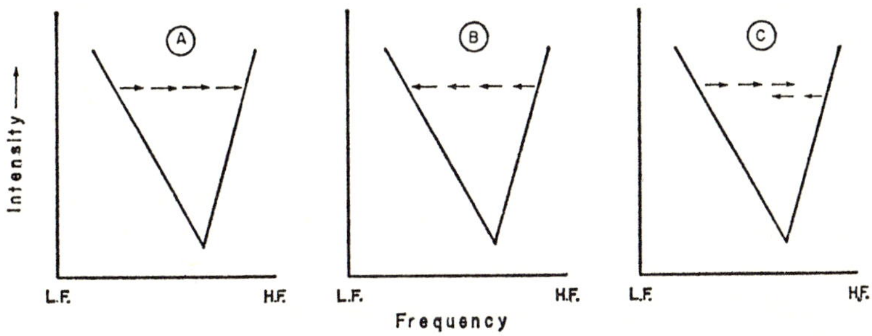


14.3 Responses of neurons in the auditory cortex of the cat to FM sound. The arrows in the figures indicate that in (A) a response was only obtained when the frequency of the tone was increasing throughout the frequency range, whilst in (B) the response occurred only when the frequency was decreasing. In (C) a response occurred to a downgoing frequency in the upper part of the frequency range and to an upgoing frequency in the lower part of the range. For further explanation see text. HF = high frequency, LF = low frequency. From Whitfield, I. C. and Evans, E. F. (1965), 'Responses of the auditory cortex neurons to stimuli of changing frequency', *J. Neurophysiol.*, *28*, 655–672.

second class responded only when the frequency was decreasing (frequency-down). A third class contained cells which, rather like the Duke of York's men, were neither wholly up nor wholly down, but responded to a downgoing FM in the upper part of their frequency range, and to an upgoing FM in the lower part of their range. The responses of these three classes of cortical neurons are shown in Fig. 14.3.

Whitfield and Evan's results thus suggest that for these auditory neurons both the movement (FM) of the stimulus and the orientation of this movement (whether up or down) are significant. This feature, as we have mentioned before, is reminiscent of units in the retina and the visual cortex.

The analysis of pattern recognition in the auditory cortex has been carried a stage further by Suga.[1] This investigator has examined the auditory cortex of echo-locating bats. Probably all mammals use their sense of hearing to some extent as a means of judging distance and direction. Who has not observed a domestic cat or dog prick up its ears to locate a strange sound? With the bats, however, the use of the ears as accurate distance receptors has reached an evolutionary peak.

There is nothing in the auditory world which corresponds to the sun. There is no great impartial source which bathes all objects in sound. Away from the centres of human civilization the world is predominantly a quiet place. Thus in order to use its ears as effective distance receptors an animal must fabricate sound itself. And this, of course, is precisely what we find that bats do. Various different sorts of 'orientation sound' are produced by the different orders of bats; the familiar insectivorous bats of Europe and North America emit a characteristically frequency-modulated 'chirp'. By attending to the echoes of these chirps bats are able to fly unscathed through darkened rooms hung with wires and to carry out the remarkable aerobatics necessary to catch moths, mayflies and mosquitoes on the wing.

The FM chirps of bats usually start at about 90,000 c/s and end, a couple of milliseconds later, at about 45,000 c/s. Why the orientation sounds of these bats should be frequency-modulated is not fully established. There are probably a number of advantages. One of these follows from the following physical fact. It is known that objects of about the same size as an impinging wave do not reflect so much as scatter the wave's energy. Only when an object in the path of a wave is large in comparison to the wavelength does accurate reflection occur. These physical characteristics are shown in Fig. 14. 4.

Now the wavelength of a sound wave is, of course, inversely proportional to its frequency. The higher the frequency the shorter the wavelength. Hence by emitting a series of frequencies—from 90 kc/s to 45 kc/s—the bat ensures that not only large but also small objects reflect an accurate echo. Furthermore if the bat can detect the range of frequencies giving an accurate reflection he might be able to estimate a minimum size for the object. Clearly all this information will be of considerable value in the animal's hunting behaviour. All this information, moreover, must be sorted out by the animal's auditory system.

[1] Suga, N. (1965), 'Functional properties of auditory neurons in the cortex of echo-locating bats', *J. Physiol.*, *181*, 671–700.

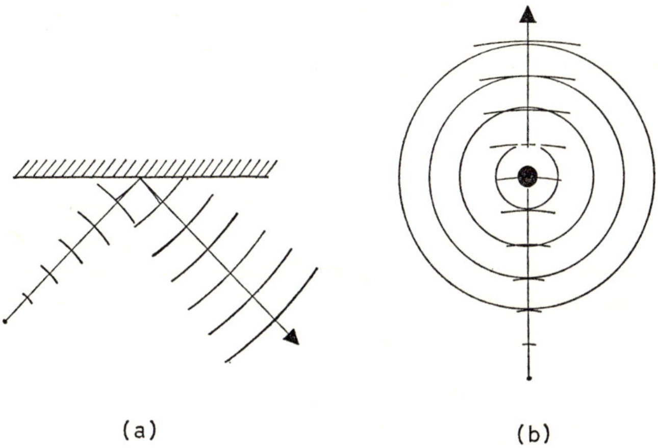


14.4 Reflections of waves. In (a) sound waves are reflected from a surface large in comparison with their wavelength. Here the familiar rule that the angle of reflection equals the angle of incidence obtains. In (b) the waves meet an object of somewhat smaller dimension than their own wavelength. In this case there is no single direction in which the reflected beam travels: instead the secondary wavelets radiate in all directions away from the obstacle.

Suga in his electrophysiological investigation of the bat's auditory cortex was able to distinguish six different types of cell. Each of these types of cell responded, to use the term introduced in section 8.6, to a different 'trigger' feature of the auditory environment. One type, for example, responded to FM tones no matter in which direction (up or down) the modulation occurred; another type showed a strong preferential response to one or other direction of modulation; yet another type responded to weak but not to strong FM tones; a fourth type of neuron was responsive only to pure tones and could not be activated by FM tones even though the FM sweep included the pure tone. We thus begin to see how the complex auditory pattern impinging on the bat's ear is sorted out into a map or model in the auditory cortex. We can speculate that when this map of activity 'fits' a pre-established pattern in the brain a certain behaviour pattern is initiated. Perhaps the bat makes the final complex manœuvre to catch the manœuvring moth.

The pre-established or inbuilt pattern mentioned in the previous paragraph may be inherited or it may be learnt or, of course, as is probably the case in bats, a bit of both. We shall have more to say of the possible physical bases of memory in Chapter 15. Before taking up this fascinating and controversial topic let us look at the intensively investigated field of visual pattern recognition.

### 14.4 Visual perception

Probably because of man's arboreal ancestry (see Chapter 10) sight plays a predominant part in forming the human perceptual world. Indeed, according to Dodwell,[1] over 90% of our information about the world arrives along our optic nerves. Thus it is not surprising to find that the topic of visual perception is one which has attracted many workers from many different fields.

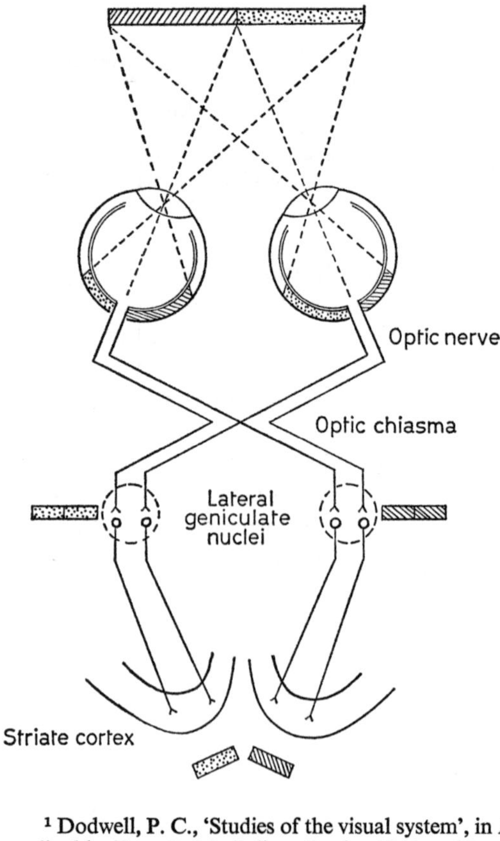


14.5 Pathway of fibres of the optic nerve from the retina to the striate cortex. The figure shows that the optic nerve fibres originating in the nasal half of the retina cross over at the optic chiasma beneath the brain. Fibres from the outside half of each retina do not, however, cross but run to the same side of the brain. The visual field is thus 'transmitted' to the visual cortex in two parts. This is shown in the figure by the stippled and cross-hatched bars.

[1] Dodwell, P. C., 'Studies of the visual system', in *New Horizons in Psychology*, edited by Foss, B. M., Pelican Books, 1966, p. 15.

We saw in Chapter 8 that information pertaining to the visual world is given a preliminary sorting out and classification in the retina. However this initial information-processing is only a foretaste of the more extensive operations of the brain itself. Some exciting and illuminating work has been done on this central computation in recent years.

First of all let us look at the anatomy of the mammalian visual system. This is shown in Fig. 14.5. It will be remembered from Chapter 8 that the photoreceptor cells of the retina synapse via bipolars and amacrines with the so-called ganglion cells. The axons springing from these cells form the optic nerve. The fibres of the optic nerve travel first to the lateral geniculate bodies (section 10.6). Here they synapse with other fibres which relay the visual information to the striate cortex of the occipital lobe. On the way to the lateral geniculate bodies the optic nerve fibres cross over, forming the optic chiasma. In fact, as Fig. 14.5 shows, not all the optic nerve fibres take part in this cross-over. Fibres proceeding from ganglion cells located in the outer edges of both eyes proceed to the ipsilateral side of the occipital lobe.

Now just as it has been possible to record activity in single retinal ganglion cells (Chapter 8), so it has proved possible to record from single cells in the striate cortex. Furthermore receptive fields of the same general type, though differing markedly in shape and other particulars, have been detected. Some most interesting work on this topic has been done by two American physiologists—Hubel and Wiesel—and the following outline is based mainly on their publications.

Fig. 14.6 shows the response of a single cell in the striate cortex of a cat to a small spot of light (about 0·25 mm. in diameter) impinging on the contralateral retina. The position of the spot of light on the retinal receptive field is shown on the left-hand side of the figure; the centre of the figure shows the response of the cortical cell; on the right-hand side a map of the cortical cell's receptive field, constructed to account for these observations, is shown.

Fig. 14.6 shows that the receptive field of this particular cortical cell appears to consist of a long narrow vertical strip from which *off* responses can be obtained, flanked on each side by areas from which *on* responses can be elicited. Hubel and Wiesel[1] define the region of

[1] Hubel, D. H. and Wiesel, T. N. (1959), 'Receptive fields of single neurons in the cat's striate cortex', *J. Physiol.*, *148*, 574–591.

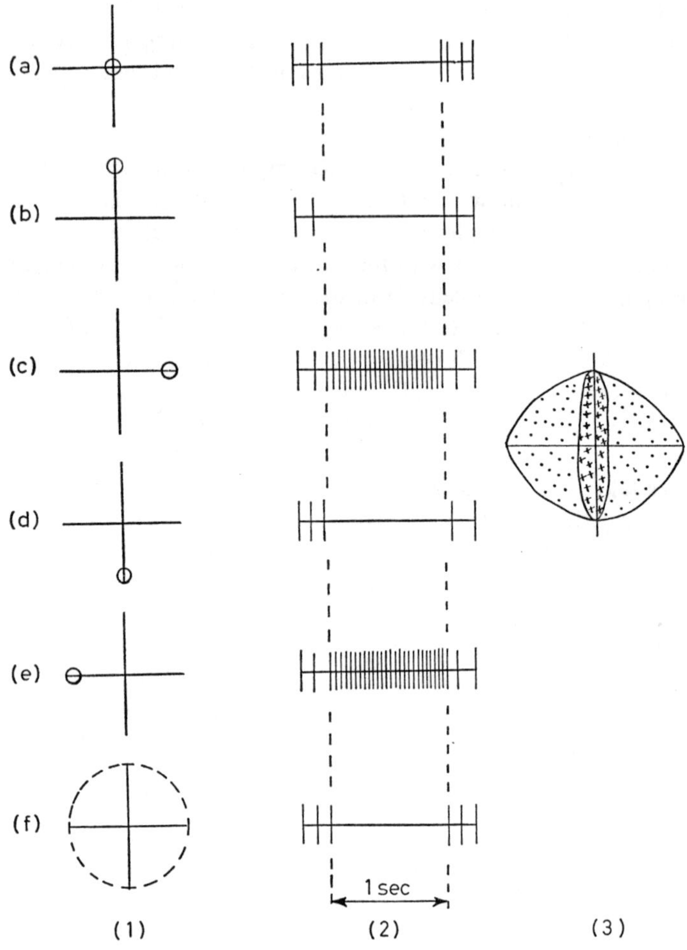


14.6 Receptive field of a cell in the striate cortex of a cat. The retina is illuminated, as the figure shows, by a small spot of light for a period of one second. The second column in the figure shows the response of the cortical cell, and the third column shows a diagram of the deduced receptive field. Illumination of the stippled area activates the cell, illumination of the area filled with small crosses inhibits the cell. Adapted from Hubel, D. H. and Wiesel, T. N. (1959), 'Receptive fields of single neurons in the cat's striate cortex', *J. Physiol.*, *148*, 574–591.

the receptive field causing *off* responses as an inhibitory area and the flanking, *on* response region, as excitatory.

Next it is important to notice that, just as in the case of retinal ganglion cells, inhibitory and excitatory influences summate algebraically at the level of the cortical neuron. If a large part of the excitatory area of the receptive field is stimulated then the response of the cortical cell is vigorous. If only a small part of the excitatory area is illuminated then the cortical response is correspondingly feeble. Furthermore excitatory and inhibitory[1] areas are mutually antagonistic. If both are simultaneously stimulated they cancel each other out at the level of the cortical cell. This is shown in experiment (f) of Fig. 14.6. Here a spot of light large enough to stimulate both inhibitory centre and excitatory surround is shown to have no effect on the cortical neuron. When this behaviour was observed it was also found that diffuse illumination of the entire retina had no observable effect on the cell.

Now it can be shown that the vast majority of ganglion cells in the feline retina have simple concentric receptive fields (Fig. 8.14). It is thus of considerable interest to find that this organization is not repeated in the cortex. The cortical cell of the above example, like some rabbit ganglion cells, 'sees' the world through a slit with a particular orientation. This slit may be inhibitory with an excitatory surround, as in Fig. 14.6 or, vice versa, it may be excitatory with inhibitory flanks. Whether the slit is excitatory or inhibitory it is, however, clear that when a patch of light with the correct orientation falls across the receptive field a maximum alteration in the cortical neuron's activity will be elicited. It will be remembered from the previous section of this chapter and from Chapter 8 that such a stimulus is called a trigger stimulus.

Fig. 14.7 shows an experiment carried out to test the above reasoning. The stimulus employed in this experiment was a slit-shaped patch of light. As this patch of light was rotated (1) the response of the cortical cell (2) was recorded. The receptive field of this cortical unit, worked out previously by the usual method of probing the retina with a spot of light, is shown at (3). Note that the receptive field of this cell has a central excitatory strip.

[1] In this context the terms 'excitatory' and 'inhibitory' do not necessarily imply that excitatory or inhibitory synapses are involved. It is likely that the nerve pathways are numerous and intricate and that the effects observed are the outcome of many synaptic interactions.

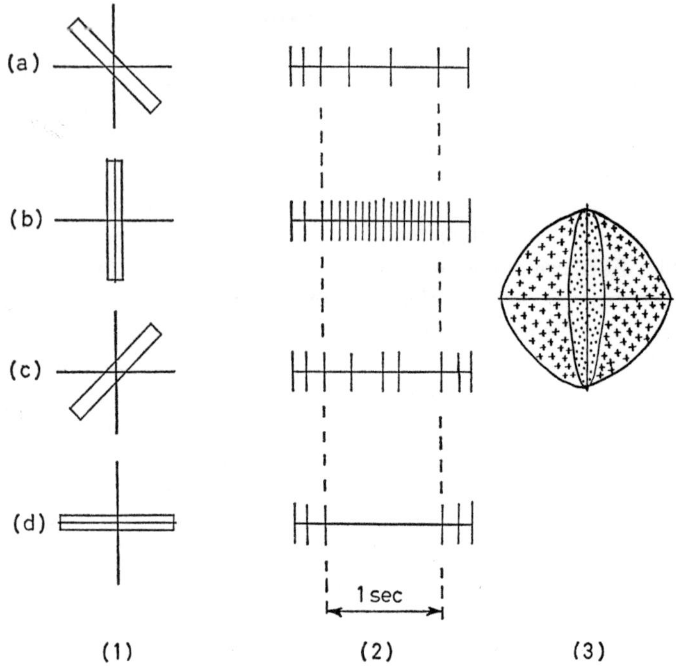


14.7 Response of a feline cortical cell to a slit-shaped patch of light. For explanation see text. Adapted from Hubel, D. H. and Wiesel, T. N. (1959), *loc. cit.*

Not only do such elongate receptive fields inform the cortical cells of the orientation of an illuminated edge or slit, but they also respond in a diagnostic manner to movement. Moreover the direction in which the movement takes place also has a considerable influence on the degree of activation of the cortical cell. Fig. 14.8 shows the effect on the cell of moving a slit of light vertically and horizontally across the receptive field of Fig. 14.7 (3).

In Fig. 14.8 (a) the slit is moved horizontally across the field. Clearly when it passes over the excitatory oblong a strong burst of activity results; otherwise the cortical unit is quiescent. In Fig. 14.8 (b) the slit is moved in a direction at right angles to the first. As (2) shows, no reaction is detectable in the cortex. Presumably this is because the extremities of the bright slit extend into the inhibitory flanks and thus cancel out any excitatory effect from the centre.

Hubel and Wiesel were able to show that other units located in the

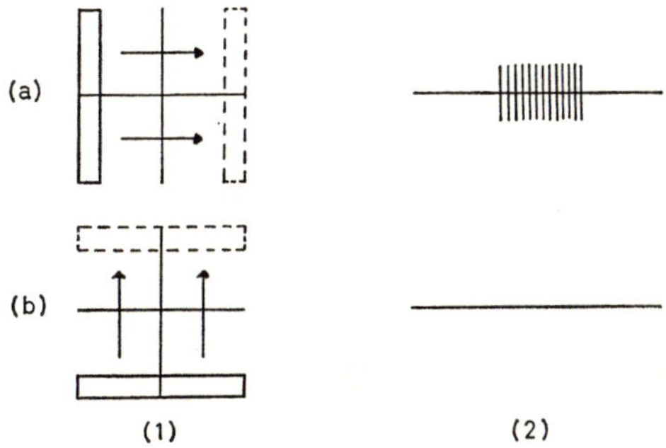


14.8 Response of the cortical cell of Fig. 14.7 to the movement of a slit of light (a) horizontally, (b) vertically across its receptive field. For explanation see text.

striate cortex were able to carry out a yet more sophisticated analysis of movement. They were able to show that in some cases movement of the slit in one direction could be distinguished from its movement in the reverse direction. This observation reminds us of the direction selector fields of the rabbit's retina (section 8.6). It will also be remembered from Chapter 8 that the physiological complexity of the rabbit's retina is more reminiscent of the feline cortex than of the feline retina. Hubel and Wiesel's observations on the direction selector units of the cat's cortex are summarized in Fig. 14.9.

Fig. 14.9 (3) shows that the electrophysiological findings can be explained if a certain type of receptive field is assumed. On either side of a central inhibitory strip are two excitatory areas. These areas

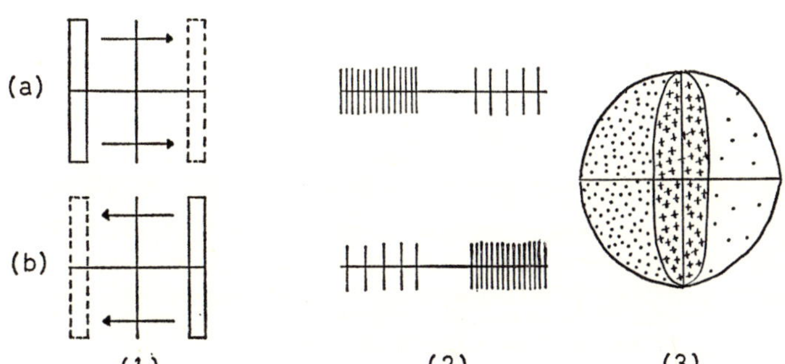


14.9 A direction selector field. The strengths of the excitatory parts of the field are indicated by intensity of stippling. For explanation see text.

differ, however, in their 'strength'. Stimulation of one gives rise to a far greater excitation of the cortical cell than a similar stimulation of the other. It is clear that a receptive field of this design allows a cortical cell to distinguish movement in one direction from movement in the reverse.

So far in our discussion of the receptive fields of neurons in the striate cortex we have emphasized that they can be mapped by probing the retina with a small circular spot of light. However, Hubel and Wiesel have subsequently demonstrated the existence of cells with more complicated fields.[1] In many cases these fields cannot be mapped by means of a spot of light. Instead cortical cells with these fields could only be demonstrated by noting their response to variously shaped moving and stationary forms. Such fields in consequence are called *complex* fields and classified apart from the *simple* fields so far described.

Complex fields are optimally stimulated by correctly orientated slits, edges and dark bars. In this respect, of course, they resemble many simple fields. Where, however, they differ from simple fields is that the stimulus is effective wherever it is placed in the field. This, it will be remembered, was not the case with simple fields; here the stimulus besides having an optimal orientation also had an optimal position in the field.

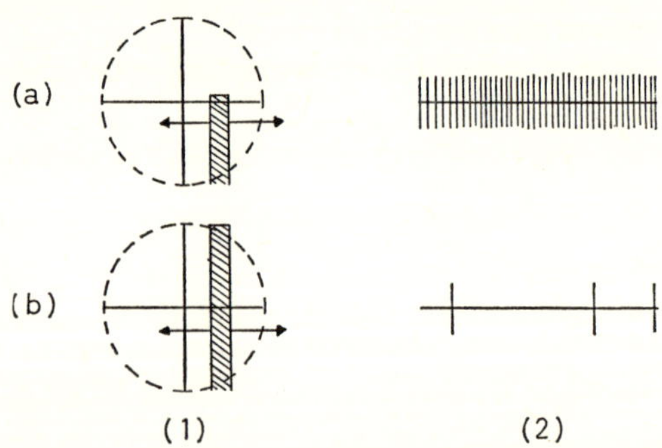


14.10 Cortical cell with a hypercomplex field. For explanation see text. Adapted from Hubel, D. H. and Wiesel, T. N. (1965), 'Receptive fields and functional architecture in two non-striate visual areas (18 and 19) of the cat', *J. Neurophysiol.*, *28*, 229–289.

[1] Hubel, D. H. and Wiesel, T. N. (1962), 'Receptive fields, binocular interaction and functional architecture in the cat's visual cortex', *J. Physiol.*, *160*, 106–154.

The electrophysiological analysis of cells in the visual cortex has not, however, culminated in the discovery of cells with complex fields. Hubel and Wiesel[1] have demonstrated a class of cells with still more specific trigger stimuli. These neurons respond maximally when the line or edge falling across the receptive field in the retina is 'stopped' at one or both ends (Fig. 14.10). If the stimulating edge extends right across the field only a sub-maximal response is elicited from the cortical cell.

The type of field illustrated in Fig. 14.10 has been called a hypercomplex field. It is also characteristic of cells possessing this type of field that they respond maximally to certain corners. This interesting property is shown in Fig. 14.11.

Finally a yet more sophisticated type of cell has been detected. Because the receptive fields of this type of cell seem to differ markedly

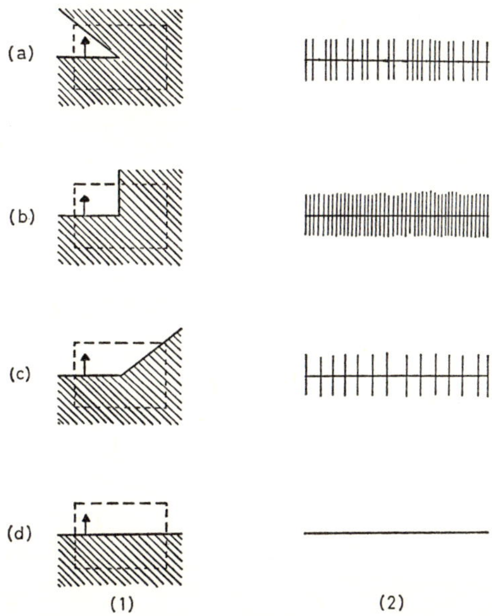


14.11 Cortical cell with a hypercomplex field. This cell responds optimally when certain corners are moved across its field. Adapted from Hubel, D. H. and Wiesel, T. N. (1965), *loc. cit.*

[1] Hubel, D. H. and Wiesel, T. N. (1965), 'Receptive fields and functional architecture in two non-striate visual areas (18 and 19) of the cat', *J. Neurophysiol.*, *28*, 229–289.

from the fields so far considered it is called a 'higher-order' hypercomplex cell. Thus the class of hypercomplex cells is subdivided into 'lower-order' types, which we considered in the previous two paragraphs, and 'higher-order' types which will be briefly discussed below.

Hubel and Wiesel have distinguished several different varieties of higher-order hypercomplex cell. Perhaps the most intriguing

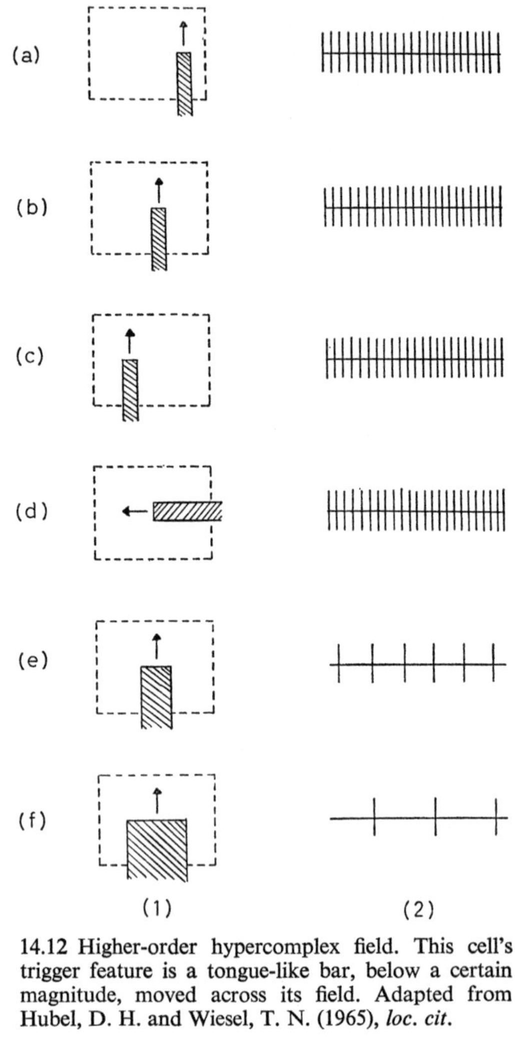


14.12 Higher-order hypercomplex field. This cell's trigger feature is a tongue-like bar, below a certain magnitude, moved across its field. Adapted from Hubel, D. H. and Wiesel, T. N. (1965), *loc. cit.*

variety possesses a receptive field in which the trigger feature of Fig. 14.11 is taken one stage further. Instead of responding maximally to a single right-angled shape moved over its receptive field the higher-order cell is most intensely activated by a tongue-like bar. This feature is shown in Fig. 14.12. The figure shows that the tongue may be presented to any part of the field and moved in two orthogonal directions. The figure shows, however, that the size of the tongue is critical. The cortical cell's response diminishes as the width of the tongue increases.

We see, therefore, in this series of electrophysiological analyses, cells which respond to ever more specific trigger features. There is a progress from straight lines presented with certain orientations in particular parts of a field to 'stopped' straight lines, to corners, to tongues, etc. which may fall across any part of the field. These are just a few of the patterns which specific cortical neurons can 'recognize'. Clearly the neurophysiologists are beginning to disentangle the cortical mechanisms responsible for visual perception.

### 14.5 Some hypothetical 'wiring diagrams' for visual perception

The precise neuroanatomical pathways responsible for the receptive fields of cells in the visual cortex are still unknown. However, by making use of the known properties of excitatory and inhibitory synapses Hubel and Wiesel have been able to show that, in principle, the fields of even higher-order hypercomplex cells are fully explicable.

We have already stressed that the ganglion cells of the feline retina have, in the main, concentric receptive fields. This type of field can also be detected for cells in the lateral geniculate body. It will be remembered that the axons of the retinal ganglion cells run to this body. It seems therefore that the nerve pathways responsible for the more sophisticated fields of cortical cells must occur central to the geniculate nuclei. What form might these pathways take?

Hubel and Wiesel[1] suggest that the slit-like field of the 'simple' cortical cell could arise if several geniculate neurons with *overlapping* concentric fields were 'wired' in such a way that they drove a single cortical neuron. This concept is schematized in Fig. 14.13.

If all the synapses in Fig. 14.13 are excitatory it follows that the cortical cell is maximally activated by a luminous slit with a width approximately equal to the diameters of the *on* centres of the retinal

[1] Hubel, D. H. and Wiesel, T. N. (1962), *loc .cit*

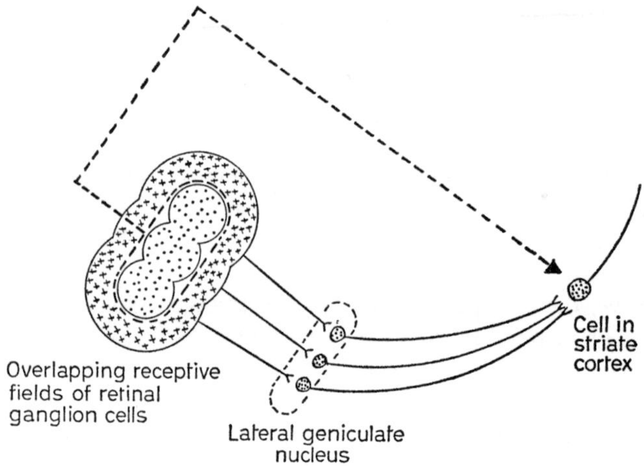


14.13 Hypothetical 'wiring diagram' for a cortical cell with a 'simple' receptive field. A large number of lateral geniculate cells (in this diagram only three are shown in order to simplify matters) have overlapping concentric fields whose *on*-centres form a straight line across the retina. All the geniculate cells project on to a single cortical cell and all the synapses are excitatory. The cortical cell will consequently have a field with an elongated *on* centre. This is indicated by the broken line in the figure. Adapted from Hubel, D. H. and Wiesel, T. N. (1962), *loc. cit.*

fields. This slit will be surrounded by an inhibitory penumbra. Clearly this type of field is identical to the simple fields of cortical neurons discussed earlier in this chapter.

Next it is possible to show how combinations of simple fields may be responsible for the characteristics of complex fields. For example, Fig. 14.14 shows the outputs from a number of cells with simple fields converging on another cortical cell. Each of the simple cells of Fig. 14.14 has a slit-like receptive field of the same orientation but located in a somewhat different part of the retina. If the simple receptive fields are spaced sufficiently close together it is clear that an edge with the correct orientation falling anywhere in the field will actuate the complex cortical cell. In the figure the complex field is outlined by a broken line.

Finally Hubel and Wiesel show how such comparatively simple 'wiring diagrams' can be developed so that they account for the properties of hypercomplex fields. They suggest, first, that the properties of a lower-order hypercomplex field would emerge if the outputs of two complex cells fed into the hypercomplex cell. This concept is

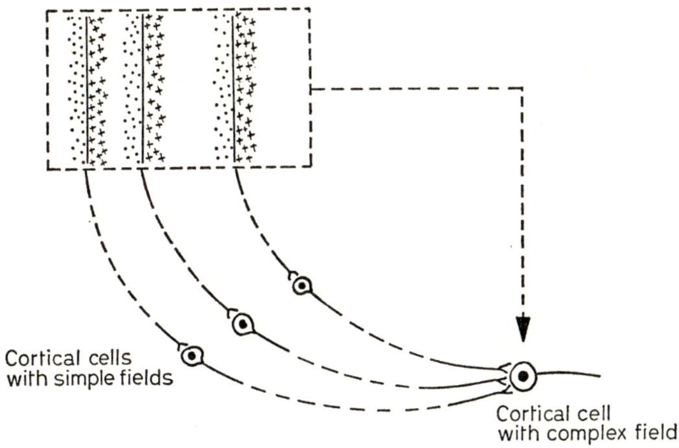


14.14 Hypothetical 'wiring diagram' for a cortical cell with a 'complex' receptive field. The figure shows a number of cortical cells with simple fields projecting on to a single higher-order cortical cell. Each simple field is organized in the form of a strip divided into excitatory and inhibitory areas. Within the space enclosed by the broken line a number of these fields (only three are shown in the interests of simplicity) are arranged. The excitatory area of one field may overlap the inhibitory area of its neighbour. This organization ensures that an edge of light possesssing the correct orientation (vertical) falling anywhere within the broken line will activate one or more of the simple field cells. This, in turn, leads to excitation of the higher-order cell. Adapted from Hubel, D. H. and Wiesel, T. N. (1962), *loc. sit.*

shown in Fig. 14.15. It is supposed that one complex field (outlined with broken lines) is connected to the hypercomplex cell via an inhibitory neuron, whilst the other is connected via an excitatory neuron.

It is clear from Fig. 14.15 that the 'stopped' edge 'A' will have a greater effect on the hypercomplex cell than the 'unstopped' edges 'B' and 'C'. Indeed the edge 'C' extending as it does into both inhibitory and excitatory domains exerts antagonistic effects on the hypercomplex cell. We may imagine that these antagonistic stimuli cancel each other out so that the hypercomplex cell remains in consequence quiescent. A similar explanation may be adduced for the hypercomplex cell's ability to 'see' certain corners (Fig. 14.11). We have only to endow the relevant receptive field with appropriate excitatory and inhibitory areas. One possible design is shown in Fig. 14.16.

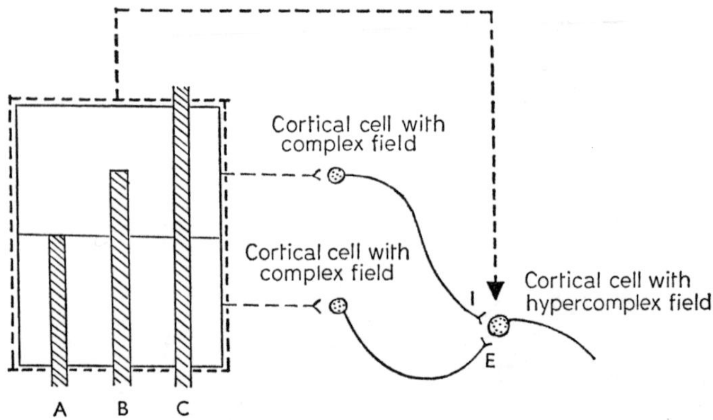


14.15 Hypothetical 'wiring diagram' for a cortical cell with a 'lower-order hypercomplex' field. Compare with Fig. 14.10. E = excitatory synapse, I = inhibitory synapse. Explanation in text. Adapted from Hubel, D. H. and Wiesel, T. N. (1965), *loc. cit.*

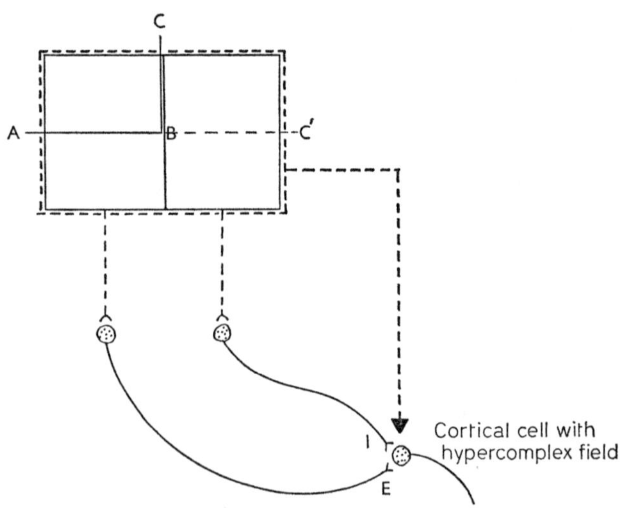


14.16 Hypothetical 'wiring diagram' to account for the observations depicted in Fig. 14.11. Movement of the corner ABC across the field will activate the hypercomplex cell whereas movement of the edge ABC[1] will not. E = excitatory synapse, I = inhibitory synapse. Adapted from Hubel, D. H. and Wiesel, T. N. (1965), *loc. cit.*

It is also easy to design a field for a hypercomplex cell whose trigger feature is a 'double stopped' edge. We have only to add a second inhibitory field below the excitatory field of Fig. 14.15. Finally the yet more specific trigger features of higher order hypercomplex cells may also be accounted for by suitable arrangements of inputs from complex cells.

To conclude this section it must again be emphasized that the wiring diagrams of Figs. 14.13, 14.14, 14.15, and 14.16 are, at present, entirely hypothetical. They have, however, the great virtue of showing how the rather sophisticated trigger features of cortical neurons may be accounted for, quite simply, by the known facts of neuron physiology. This, of course, is essential if we wish to sustain a physical theory of visual perception.

## 14.6 Columnar organization of the visual cortex

We stated above that the nerve pathways used to account for the different types of cortical receptive field were entirely hypothetical. This is not to say, however, that the visual cortex has not been examined by neuroanatomical methods. It has, and some very interesting findings have emerged. By examining the cortex under the microscope after electrophysiological recordings have been made it is possible to discover which cells the microelectrode has penetrated. In this way it can be shown that the cells of the striate cortex are arranged in functional columns. In some areas these functional columns are long and narrow having a diameter of about 0·5 mm., in other areas of the visual cortex they are more rotund. In all areas the long axes of the columns are perpendicular to the surface of the cortex. The functional organization of the visual cortex thus resembles that of the somaesthetic cortex (section 14.2).

There is evidence that the simple, complex and hypercomplex cells concerned with the processing of information picked up by one area of the retina are all located in the same cortical column. In other words the column turns out to be the 'unit of dynamic function' of the visual cortex.[1]

In some regions of the cortex the columns themselves appear to form orderly arrays. Thus rows of columns can be distinguished which contain cells whose receptive fields shift in orientation in a

[1] Hubel, D. H. and Wiesel, T. N. (1965), *loc. cit.*, p. 285.

regular manner from column to column.[1] This regularity is particularly apparent where the columns are long and thin. In regions of the cortex where the columns are more bulbous this regular organization is less easily shown.

Finally it must be emphasized, as we stressed in section 14.2, that the columns are only identifiable by a combination of electrophysiological and anatomical techniques. To date they have not been found by neuroanatomical techniques alone. It is clearly a fascinating task for the near future to establish the histological correlatives of this brilliant neurophysiology.

## 14.7 Is the organization inherited or acquired?

Another interesting question which may have already occurred to the reader is this: How far is the neuronal apparatus for the recognition of visual patterns inborn? Hubel and Wiesel have also investigated this aspect of the problem of visual perception. Working with very young kittens which had had no experience of patterned visual stimuli they were nevertheless able to show that the cells of the striate cortex had properties very similar, if not identical, to those found in the adult. In other words simple, complex and hypercomplex cells were demonstrable. They therefore concluded that the neuroanatomical connections for these cells were present at birth, or very soon thereafter.[2]

In a later investigation Hubel and Wiesel obtained a very interesting result. They were able to show that if a kitten was deprived of pattern vision for the first three months of its life very severe results ensued. It was found that such cats remained for the rest of their lives 'behaviourally' blind. The lenses and retinae of the eyes appear quite normal, but severe and apparently irreversible atrophy occurs in the lateral geniculate bodies and in the visual cortex. Thus it seems that the inbuilt neuronal connections which we saw appear to be present at birth are irretrievably lost if not reinforced during the first three months of the animal's life. This result reminds us of the somewhat similar findings in the human speech cortex (section 13.7). It will be remembered that the non-dominant hemisphere can only take over

[1] Hubel, D. H. and Wiesel, T. N. (1963), 'Shape and arrangement of columns in the cat's striate cortex', *J. Physiol.*, *165*, 559–568.

[2] Hubel, D. H. and Wiesel, T. N. (1963), 'Receptive fields of cells in the striate cortex of very young visually inexperienced kittens', *J. Neurophysiol.*, *26*, 994–1001.

this function if the dominant hemisphere is injured before the age of ten or so. The work on the cat visual cortex seems, however, at variance with some of the well known observations on humans who have gained their sight late in life.[1] These observations seem to show that some form of coherent pattern vision can be achieved in the visually naïve adult. However it has not always been established in these interesting cases that the individual concerned has been completely blind from birth.

## 14.8 Patterns of expectation

The preceding sections of this chapter have indicated the progress physiologists have made, and are making, towards an understanding of how the brain recognizes environmental patterns. We can see, in a general way, that particular patterns of environmental energy falling on the closely packed receptor cells of a major sense organ are sorted out in the sensory system so that unique groups of cortical neurons are activated. However it is clear that this can only be the initial step. Experimental psychologists have frequently pointed out that pattern recognition is a far more sophisticated phenomenon than the mere activation of specific groups of 'Hubel and Wiesel' cells.

For example it can be shown in a wide variety of animals that the recognition of a visual pattern does not depend on the *size* of the image falling on the retina. Animals resemble humans in being readily able to recognize a square whose dimensions are, say, twice or half those of the square originally presented. The area of the retina on which the image falls is also immaterial, as is its brightness. Now it will be remembered that the receptive fields of Hubel and Wiesel cells are localized in particular regions of the retina. It follows, therefore, that pattern recognition cannot be accounted for by supposing that it simply consists in the reactivation of specific, unique, groups of Hubel and Wiesel cells. It is likely that these cells are concerned in the initial processing of the visual image, an operation which leads to the abstraction of more and more general features of the pattern.

It is possible, and here we enter the realms of speculation, that the output from the Hubel and Wiesel cells is processed through still further matrices of neurons in the cerebrum. It is possible that these unknown nets abstract still more general features of the input

[1] von Senden, M., *Space and Sight*, Methuen and Co. Ltd., London, 1966.

pattern: features which are independent of retinal position, size, brightness, etc. Nets of these yet undiscovered 'pattern recognizer' cells would thus form the 'map' or 'model' of the animal's world.

In the lower animals where instinctive behaviour predominates it seems likely that many of these 'representations'[1] of the environment are inbuilt and perhaps permanently 'wired' to the groups of motor neurons responsible for fixed action patterns. In this way when the appropriate sign stimulus is presented, perhaps the orange belly of a gravid stickleback, the correct response, in this case the male 'zigzag dance', is automatically elicited. We may suppose that, in general, an animal explores its environment in a random fashion until one or other of the sign stimuli for one or other of its instinctive behaviours enters its perceptual field. This behaviour is triggered and, if all goes well, runs to its conclusion whereupon the animal is released so that it may continue its explorations.

In the higher vertebrates where learning becomes of more importance in behaviour the situation is more complicated. Instead of the neuronal connections between the 'representation' and the motor neuron pool being built into the nervous system they must be formed during the lifetime of the individual. What the physico-chemical nature of this change might be is not at the present time known. This intriguing problem, the problem of the physical basis of memory, is considered in the next chapter. The result of the learning process is, however, very much the same as that of the inbuilt, instinctive, behaviours discussed above. Each time the particular pattern of cerebral neurons representing a particular stimulus pattern is activated a particular (learnt) response is given. In the classical case of the Pavlovian conditioned reflex (section 15.2) each time the dog hears the bell ringing it salivates. The animal recognizes the bell as the sign of an imminent meal.

With humans the business of pattern recognition assumes even greater complexity. Even with us, however, what we *see* is frequently only a rather small part of what is there to be seen. We have noticed that the sign stimuli which trigger the instinctive behaviours of animals are frequently only a small part of the animal's perceptual environment. There is every reason to believe that the animal's sense organs can respond to a much wider perceptual field than the often rather simple, rather diagrammatic, sign stimuli which alone affect

[1] In the lower vertebrates and *a fortiori* in the invertebrates these representations are not necessarily located in the cerebral hemispheres.

its instinctive behaviour. Similarly, though of course to a much lesser extent, with human beings. Frequently we see only what we expect to see. What we perceive depends to some extent on our mental 'set', our pattern of expectations, and this in turn often depends on quite a complex background of education. Thus Fig. 14.17 may be seen by

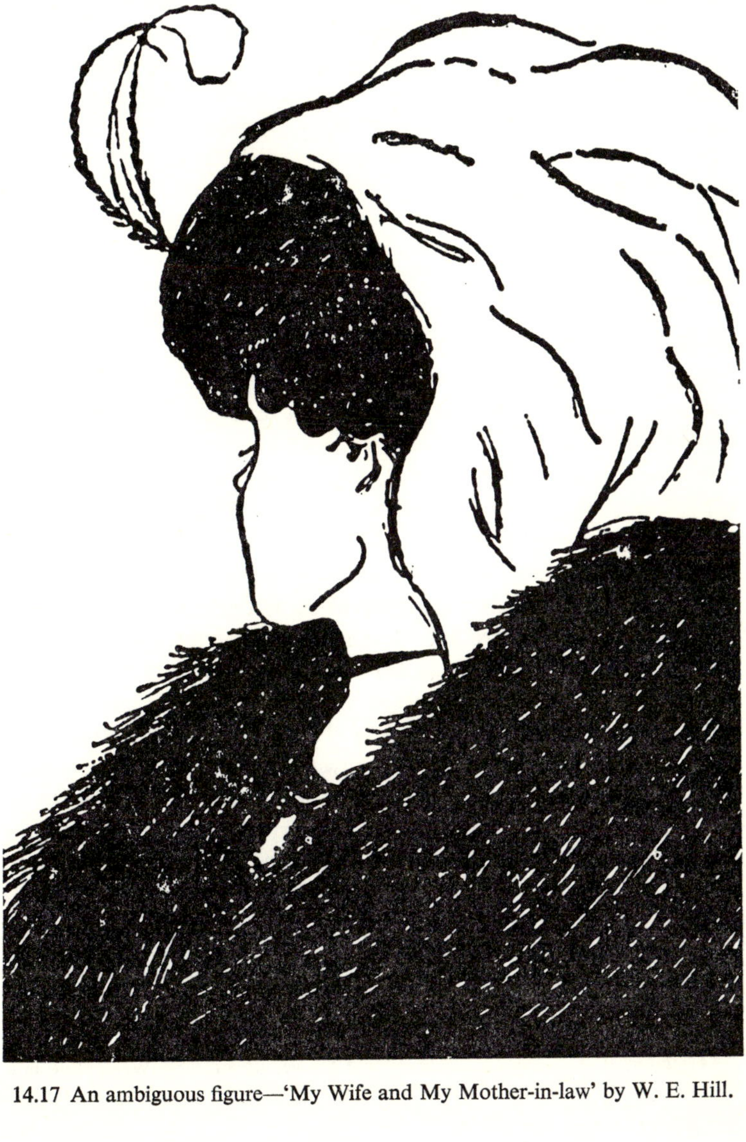

14.17 An ambiguous figure—'My Wife and My Mother-in-law' by W. E. Hill.

some as an old country woman and by others as a young lady of the Edwardian era. There is no 'right' or 'wrong' about this: the same retinal pattern can be 'seen' or interpreted in either way.

A somewhat similar comment may be made about several of the well-known visual illusions (see Plate XVIII). The brain 'reads into' the figure features which it 'expects' to find. One of the best known of these illusions is the Müller-Lyer figure. This is shown in Fig. 14.18.

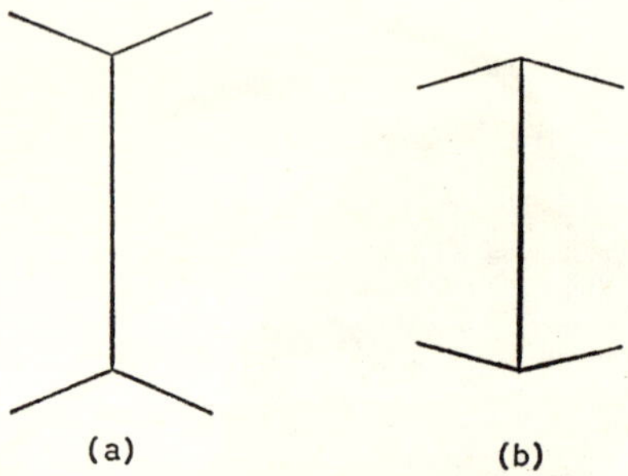


14.18 The Müller-Lyer illusion.

A casual inspection of Fig. 14.18 suggests that the vertical line in (a) is longer than it is in (b). Yet more careful examination of the figure shows us that both vertical lines are, in fact, exactly the same length. How are we to account for our original mistake? Gregory has presented convincing evidence to show that the illusion occurs because our 'minds' are accustomed to interpreting perspective in both nature and art.[1] Thus in (a) we might be looking at the inside corner of a room or box, whereas in (b) we might be looking at the nearest outside corner of a building. This is illustrated in Fig. 14.19.

If this were in fact the case, we know from our everyday experience of the three dimensions of space that the corner (a) is likely to be further away than the corner in (b). In everyday life our brains allow for this by 'scaling up' the more distant object. Gregory describes a neat experiment to demonstrate this fact. If the two hands are held in front of the face, one at the full stretch of the arm and the other close to the eyes, they will both appear approximately the same size. That they do not in fact throw equally sized images on to the retina can be easily shown by moving them together, laterally, so that they

[1] Gregory, R. L., *Eye and Brain*, World University Library, Weidenfeld and Nicolson, London, 1966, Chapter 9.

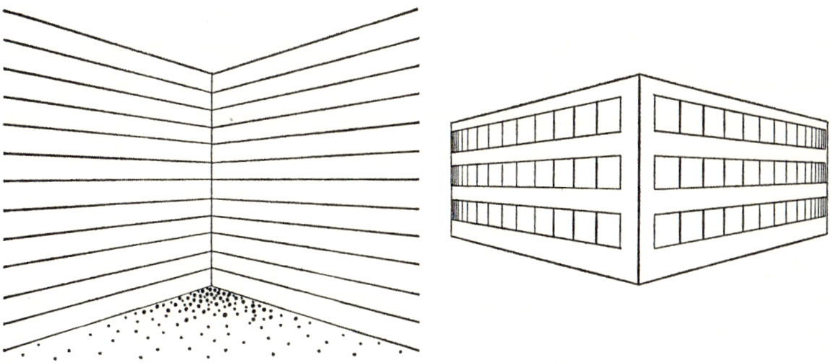

(a) (b)

14.19 An explanation for the Müller-Lyer illusion.

partially overlap. It is then clear that the nearer hand throws a far larger image on to the retina, an image which can completely cover that of the more distant hand.

We can generalize this perceptual expectancy still further. One interesting piece of experimental work consisted in presenting subjects with badly out of focus pictures of common objects.[1] The subject guesses the nature of the badly blurred picture. It is found that incorrect guesses impede the development of the correct perception as the picture is brought into focus.

Generalizing yet further we can begin to see that this expectancy can include quite sophisticated intellectual attitudes to the world around us. The Dutch historian Pieter Gehl, for example, carefully examined the treatment of the Emperor Napoleon by a large number of French historians.[2] He was able to show that there was an 'endless variety of interpretations of Napoleon, his career, his aims, his achievements'. As soon as something more than a mere catalogue of 'facts' is presented, as soon as 'sense' must be made of the 'raw data', then 'the personal element cannot be ruled out, that point of view which is determined by the circumstances of his time and his own preconceptions'. The importance of this intellectual 'set' is by no means confined to the arts. Many thinkers have suggested that it has a strong influence on how scientists 'see' the world. The movements

[1] Bruner, J. S. and Potter, M. C. (1964), 'Interference in visual recognition', *Science,* 144, 424–425.

[2] Pieter Gehl: *Napoleon: for and against*. Translated by Olive Renier, Penguin Books, Harmondsworth, 1965.

of the planets in the night sky may, for example, be accounted for by the complicated systems of epicycles devised by Ptolemy and his successors. On the other hand the observations may be fitted equally well by the heliocentric ellipses of Kepler and Galileo. N. R. Hanson asks whether, when day breaks, exponents of the Copernican and Ptolemaic systems 'see' the same thing. 'For Galileo and Kepler,' suggests Hanson,[1] 'the horizon drops; for Simplicius and Tycho the sun rises'. The same stimuli fall upon their retinae, but like the difference of opinion over the young lady and the old crone, there are two possible interpretations.

In the same way Darwin, T. H. Huxley and Bishop Wilberforce were presented with the same catalogue of observations: the biologists saw one pattern implicit in the facts, the theologian another. Perception is an active two-way process. Observation is frequently, to use Hanson's phrase, 'theory laden'. Our intellectual 'sets', our cultural and intellectual backgrounds, all influence the way we see things. Some of us, for instance, see communist or imperialist plots whilst others see only the antics of high-spirited students.

[1] Hanson, N. R., *Patterns of Discovery*, Cambridge University Press, 1961, p. 182.

## CHAPTER FIFTEEN

# Memory

### 15.1 Memory and recall

As humans we are to an extent bundles of memories. Someone who has lost this faculty simply does not know who he or she is. So central are our memories to our persons. In general, moreover, our memories are the hardest of all things to destroy. Shakespeare once more expresses our experience exactly when he makes Macbeth adjure his physician to

> 'Pluck from the memory a rooted sorrow,
> Raze out the written troubles of the brain'

only to be told that it is impossible.

Metaphorically we speak of 'reliving' the past. Of course what we are doing is scanning the traces the past has left behind. This is clear enough. The historian studies not the past but the relics of the past which have persisted into his own existential 'now'. Poring over old manuscripts, buildings, weapons he attempts the imaginative reconstruction of how things were. Similarly the organism, we must suppose, carries within itself the trace, the signature of events which occurred in its own past life.

Indeed this cannot be a strange concept to any biologist. The discipline of comparative anatomy teaches that the evolutionary past of each organism is represented in its present-day anatomy. The theory of Darwin allied to the rapidly developing science of genetics has taught us how this can be. We can see how the phylogenetic experience of the species comes to be built into the bodies of each of its members. The problem of individual memory, however, still awaits its Darwin. The Galapagos of the brain have yet to be visited, or if visited their lessons have yet to be learnt.

Hilgard, one of the great neuropsychologists of the recent past, writes as follows: 'It is a blot upon our scientific ingenuity that after so many years of search we know as little as we do about the physiological accompaniments of learning'.[1] In the thirty years since this sentence was first written a vast amount of painstaking work has been done, a great number of facts have been established, a whole new battery of techniques has been developed but the blot still remains. The Darwinian 'grinding' of an illuminating generalization from the flood of experimental findings has not so far been achieved. Indeed it seems that part of the difficulty lies in sheer uncertainty as to what sorts of question experimentalists ought to try to decide and what sorts of explanation theoreticians should try to devise.

In order to make a start on our review of the present understanding of the physical basis of memory let us try to define the problem somewhat. In the language of computer science what we are interested in is the way in which the living brain stores information. This information, moreover, is information presented to the brain during its life. It is not inborn or inbuilt. The problem of memory is thus a part of the problem of learning. It can be shown that the ability to store information, the ability to learn from experience, is, to a greater or lesser extent, a property of all nervous systems. Indeed this property is not restricted to nervous systems. It may be detected in other physiological systems. We are all familiar, for example, with the main facts of immunology. We all know that the body possesses a system of cells capable of manufacturing a specific antibody in response to a specific antigenic stimulus. This specificity is close and fatal to the antigen. It is also long-lasting. After infection by a particular antigen the body is for a considerable period of time immune to any further invasion. The antibody system has 'learnt' the pattern of that particular antigen.[2] And the lesson is not quickly forgotten. Memory, then, is not a phenomenon unique to the brain.

Unfortunately the immunological analogy set out above has one great drawback. At the time of writing the mechanism of immunological memory is not understood. Thus we are caught in the circularity of attempting to explain ignorance with ignorance. Nevertheless, daunting though the biochemical complexities of the immunological response may be, they are probably several orders of magnitude less complex than the neurological response. It is

[1] Hilgard, E. R., *Theories of Learning*, Appleton, New York, 1940.

[2] Mammals are believed to be capable of synthesizing over a million different antibodies. This powerful and highly specific response to antigenic stimulation has not been demonstrated in invertebrates.

probable that the mechanism of immunological memory will be understood in the foreseeable future: hopefully the mechanism which emerges may shed light on, or provide pointers to, the mechanism in the brain.

Let us next see if we can be a bit more precise about what we mean by the term 'memory' in the neurobiological context. Let us take as an initial definition: an enduring change in the behaviour of an animal in response to a stimulus. We can see that according to this definition it would be correct to include the immune response under the term 'memory'. However, the definition can, like most definitions in biology, be criticized. Perhaps the most telling criticism is that the definition conflates memory and recall. We probably all know of occasions in our own lives when we have 'forgotten' a name, or a number, but have, perhaps, remembered it again on awaking the next morning. This indicates, surely, that the memory 'trace' was all the time present somewhere in our nervous system but was for some reason inaccessible. Many striking instances of this distinction between memory and recall are documented in the literature. Perhaps some of the best known are cases where individuals under hypnosis recall details of their past, perhaps of their childhoods, of which their adult intelligences are apparently quite unaware. An even more thought-provoking instance is reported by Gerard[1] when he relates how 'details of a conversation by a surgeon and his assistant during a period of full anaesthesia have been subsequently reported by a patient under hypnosis'.

In essence the above analysis makes a distinction between structure and function. Memory, according to this account, is the structural change; recall is the 'location' of this structural change by the 'mind': a 'summoning up'.

Now that we are satisfied that we know what we mean by the term 'memory' let us look at some of the experimental situations in which it can be studied. Clearly these are situations in which the characteristics of learning and learnt behaviour are examined.

## 15.2 Learning in animals

Perhaps the most intensively investigated and precisely defined types of learning are the conditioned reflexes. We are, most of us, familiar

[1] Gerard, R. W. (1960), 'Neurophysiology: an integration (molecules, neurons and behaviour)', in *Handbook of Physiology: Section 1: Neurophysiology, Vol. 3*, American Physiological Society, p. 1946.

with the classical Pavlovian experiment where a dog learns to salivate on hearing a bell. In this type of learning experiment the environmental parameters can be very rigorously controlled. The investigator can thus have some confidence that the reaction he observes is a response to a precise stimulus, or stimulus pattern, and to nothing else.

Pavlov came to his studies on the physiology of the brain by way of an interest in digestive physiology. By placing meat powder on a dog's tongue he was, of course, able to elicit salivation. This was the result of a straightforward 'unconditioned' reflex built into the animal at birth. However, by coupling the presentation of the meat powder with the ringing of a bell Pavlov was able to show that, after a number of trials, salivation occurred in response to the bell alone. This is the conditioned reflex. Moreover Pavlov was able to quantify the strength of these reflexes by collecting and measuring the saliva secreted.

This, then, is the paradigmatic instance of conditioned reflexes. The so-called unconditioned stimulus (US)—the meat powder—becomes, over a number of trials, associated in the dog's central nervous system with the conditioned stimulus (CS)—the bell. The unconditioned response (UR)—salivation—thus comes to be elicited by the normally neutral CS. When training is complete salivation is induced by the sound of the bell alone: when this occurs Pavlov terms it a conditioned response (CR).

The four terms (US, UR, CS, CR) defined in the previous paragraph are of considerable importance in the study of conditioned reflexes. Pavlov believed that when he studied the properties of these reflexes he was in fact studying the properties of the cerebral cortex. However, reflexes of this type have now been induced, many times, in decorticate animals.[1] Hence conditioned reflexes of the Pavlovian type are not necessarily dependent on the presence of a cerebral cortex. However, the general Pavlovian concept of studying the higher functions of the central nervous system by means of conditioned reflexes, much as the chemist investigates the properties of molecules by examining, perhaps, the colours of solutions, remains valid. Pavlov's particular theories, however, involving flows of nervous energy have not received the neurophysiological confirmation that, to continue the analogy, the derided structural ideas of a

[1] Galambos, R. and Morgan, C. T. (1960), 'The neural basis of learning', in *Handbook of Physiology: Section 1: Neurophysiology, Vol. 3*, American Physiological Society, p. 1476.

chemist like van t'Hoff eventually received from the X-ray crystallographers.

In some ways rather different from the classical Pavlovian conditioning described above is the situation in which a painful (in a wide sense) stimulus is used as the US. In order to escape from his distasteful position the animal must make some appropriate response (CR). For example the US might be an electrical shock. In order to avoid this unwelcome stimulus the animal might have to make a suitable response—pressing a lever, perhaps, or raising a leg. This is the CR. The experiment consists in coupling a neutral stimulus (CS), such as a bell, with the electric shock. Intelligent animals are found to quickly learn to produce the CR on hearing the CS.

This type of conditioning differs in several important respects from the Pavlovian type. Most importantly the animal has to take an active part in the proceedings, not respond merely passively. This type of conditioned reflex has in consequence been called 'operant' or 'instrumental'. Galambos and Morgan suggest that the two types of conditioning be distinguished merely by labelling the first 'type 1' and the second 'type 2'.[1] We shall adhere to this terminology in the following discussion.

One of the important ways in which a type 2 CR differs from a type 1 CR lies in the former's much greater dependence on the integrity of the cerebral cortex. This, of course, only applies in the case of the higher vertebrates and, in particular, the mammals. Invertebrates which obviously do not possess a cerebral cortex are nevertheless well able to develop type 2 conditioned reflexes. It seems, however, that all central nervous systems capable of this type of reflex have certain architectural features in common. They all seem to possess, in one region or another, sheets of *apparently* randomly connected neurons.[2]

It is easy to see that type 2 CRs merge, as they increase in complexity, into simple and then advanced forms of trial-and-error learning. Thus a hungry animal confined in a box may have to experiment with levers or catches in order to get at its food. In this case hunger is the unpleasant US whilst the neutral CS, so far as the situation may be said to have one, is the sight of the appropriate lever or catch. Clearly such an experimental set-up may be altered in

[1] Galambos, R. and Morgan, C. T. (1960), *loc. cit.*, p. 1473.

[2] Adey, W. R. (1961), 'Brain mechanisms and the learning process', *Fed. Proc.*, *20*, 623–627.

many ways to test both the animal's sensory capacities as well as its learning abilities.

At a slightly higher level again are the maze-running problems. Here the animal, essentially by trial-and-error, learns to thread a simple or intricate maze in order to escape from its painful, usually hungry, condition.

Finally there are some interesting and important types of learning which seem rather less amenable to experimental analysis. One rather remarkable type has been discovered by close observation of the behaviour of very young animals. Ducklings, for example, immediately they leave the egg look for and follow the first large moving object in their near neighbourhood. This, of course, is normally the mother duck. But Konrad Lorenz has shown that the newly hatched birds will 'lock' on to humans and even on to loudly ticking alarm clocks concealed in boxes. It has been suggested that the nervous system of fledglings is for a short time immediately before and after hatching in a peculiar metastable state liable to 'lock' on to any one of a number of entities which fulfil certain broad conditions. This type of learning is consequently called 'imprinting'.

Another type of learning which is generally held to escape classification as an elaboration of either a type 1 or type 2 conditioned reflex is so-called 'insight learning'. A well known instance of this phenomenon is described by Kohler. He relates how a chimpanzee was long tantalized by a bunch of bananas just out of reach outside his cage. Suddenly the animal perceived that by fitting together two sticks with which he was provided he could reach the prize. This 'eureka' or 'aha' situation is said to involve a rearrangement of the perceptual environment so that a new pattern of, or relation between, sense data becomes apparent. Insight learning has also been regarded as 'virtual' or 'vicarious' trial-and-error learning. In other words the trial-and-error is all 'done in the head'. Insight learning is thus of great interest to us as human beings. For, we feel, it is this type which is closest to our own experiences of learning in educational situations.

Relevant though insight learning may be to the human condition it is not easy to study experimentally. The two types of conditioned reflex and their elaborations into trial-and-error and maze learning are much more amenable to precise analysis. With these forms of learning one can hope to determine when the process starts, how long it takes, how quickly it decays. By ablation and other techniques one can begin to study where in the brain learning is occurring. By electrical recording, injection of drugs, chemical analysis and microscopic investigation one can hope to discover its physical basis. All these questions are highly relevant to the process of learning—to the laying down of memory.

### 15.3 Where are the memory traces located in the brain?

Modern accounts of the localization of memory in the brain usually start with the work of Lashley. Lashley's work appears to show that particular memories are not localized in particular regions of the cerebral cortex but are diffused throughout this sheet of tissue. Lashley's experimental approach was to examine the ability of rats to retain the memory of a maze when varying quantities and parts of their cerebral cortices were removed. The conclusion he drew from a large number of experiments carried out over many years was that no single part of the cerebral cortex was specialized to store information. Excision of similar quantities of cortex from widely different regions seemed to have the same effect on the rat's memory. Lashley, in consequence, suggested that all parts of the cortex possessed the same potentiality for information storage. In other words the cortex possessed the property of equipotentiality with respect to memory. In addition to this property or, rather, following on from it, Lashley showed that memory deteriorated in direct proportion to the *quantity* of cortex removed. The greater the quantity removed, irrespective of its position in the cortex, the more defective was the animal's memory. This, Lashley believed, constituted a law of cortical mass action.

Lashley's ideas have been subjected to searching criticisms. Any animal having to run a maze must depend on sensory cues. It is these, presumably, that it learns. Denied the use of its sense organs an animal, clearly, cannot find its way. Yet, it can be argued, this is precisely what Lashley's experimental method does. The cerebral cortex we saw in Chapter 13 is the great end-organ and sorting office of the distance receptors. It is to this concourse that information about the external environment is directed. Ablation of the occipital lobe of the cortex blinds an animal, ablation of the temporal lobe deafens it. Thus it has been argued that Lashley's experiments really have nothing to do with learning and memory; they merely progressively deprive an animal of the sensory cues on which its performance inevitably depends.

Lashley went some way to meeting these criticisms by means of the following ingenious experiment. He taught *blinded* rats to run a maze and then showed that their memory was affected when portions of the visual cortex were removed. This experiment seems to overcome some of the objections raised in the previous paragraph. For removal of the visual cortex could hardly affect the senses of an already blind rat. However, even more convincing evidence for cerebral mass-action during learning has been obtained in more recent years by electrophysiological methods.

That electrical phenomena can be recorded from the surface of the living brain has been known since the late nineteenth century. Caton reported the first observations in the *British Medical Journal* in 1875. Caton used animals as the subjects of his experiments and recorded from the surface of the brain itself. When Caton retired from active research, investigation of brain potentials passed to physiologists in Eastern Europe and Russia. These workers were able to show that the brain developed spontaneous rhythmical variations in electrical potential. It was noted that these waves could be recorded from the surface of the skulls of experimental animals. However it was not until 1925 that Hans Berger, Professor of Neurology and Psychiatry in the University of Jena, first demonstrated the presence of these rhythmical brain waves in humans. It is his term which we still use when we refer to the study of these waves —electroencephalography (EEG).

In relaxed awake humans the EEG is present as a prominent sinusoidal oscillation with a frequency of from 8–13 c/s. This is called the alpha-rhythm. In addition to this rhythm a second, lower voltage, higher frequency (18–30 c/s) rhythm—the beta-rhythm—may be recorded. Experiments on animals suggest that the two rhythms are due to different populations of cerebral neurons.[1] The alpha- and beta-rhythms, however, are not the only oscillatory potentials detectable in the human brain: the human EEG in fact consists of a complex of many waves with shifting phase relationships and amplitudes.

Now how do these electrical phenomena help us in our attempt to localize the memory trace? The answer to this question is straightforward: it is found that when learning is occurring there are widespread electrical changes in the brain. To put it another way: the

[1] Brazier, M. A. B. (1953), *The Electrical Activity of the Nervous System*, Isaac Pitman and Sons Ltd., London.

process of memory formation is accompanied by electrical changes in many parts of the brain.

It is found, first of all, that any unusual sensory stimulus results in the disappearance of the alpha-rhythm. In fact this so-called alpha-blockade is the first indication of the orientation or 'what is it?' response of a mammal to a strange stimulus. The disappearance of this attentiveness as the animal becomes habituated to the new stimulus is accompanied by a return of the cerebral alpha-rhythm. The most well-known instance of alpha-blockade occurs when a mammal opens its eyes and attends to the visual scene (Fig. 15.1).

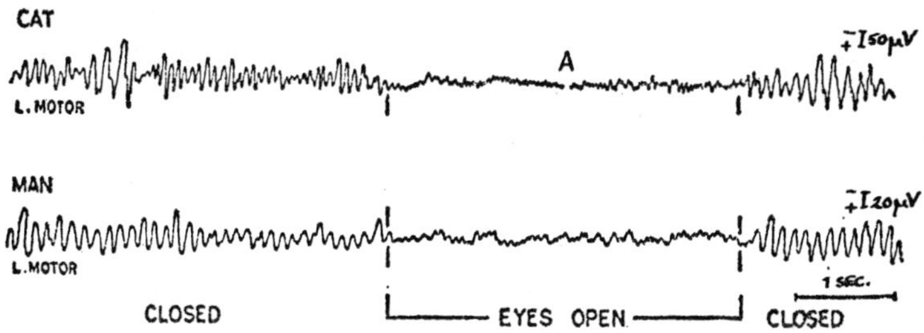


15.1 Effect of closing and opening the eyes on the alpha-rhythm of the cat. The effect is similar in man. From Rempel, B. and Gibbs, E. L. (1936), 'The Berger rhythm in cats', *Science*, *84*, 334–335.

Now when the early experiments on alpha-blockade were being done a rather interesting fact was noticed. It was shown that after a few trials an audible click heralding the illumination of the darkened cage itself elicited an alpha-blockade. In other words the click had become associated with the onset of illumination. The animal's attentiveness was raised to it on its own. There was no evidence of alpha-blockade in response to a click in the naïve animal.

In the nineteen-fifties techniques for implanting permanent electrodes into specifiable regions of the brain were developed. It then became feasible to examine these electrical correlatives of conditioning more closely. Morrell and Jasper[1] were able to confirm the EEG observations by showing that during the initial stages of conditioning a widespread desynchronization could be detected in all regions of the cortex. Clearly attention to the stimulus is a prerequisite of most

[1] Morrell, F. and Jasper, H. H. (1956), 'Electrographic studies of the formation of temporary connections in the brain', *Electroencephalog. and Clin. Neurophysiol.*, *8*, 201.

types of learning. However, once the reflex had been established alpha-blockade could be detected only in the projection area (section 13.4) of the unconditioned stimulus. Thus, to return to the example of the previous paragraph, it could be shown that, initially, alpha-blockade could be detected in most parts of the cortex in response to a click (the CS), whilst when the reflex had been fully established desynchronization could only be detected in the visual cortex.

In addition to experiments showing alpha-blockade many experiments have shown electrical correlatives of conditioning superimposed on the normal rhythmical EEG record. Fig. 15.2 shows an example of such an experiment carried out by Galambos.[1]

Fig. 15.2 (A) shows the electrical response detectable in various parts of the brain when a click is sounded once a second. The figure shows that little response can be picked up except in the auditory cortex. However, if each time the click occurs it is followed by a puff of air into the animal's face a totally different electrical picture is soon presented. This picture is shown in Fig. 15.2 (B). An electrical response can be detected in many different parts of the brain. This widespread response gradually disappears if the air puff is discontinued whilst the click still sounds. Clearly the electrical record closely follows the behavioural response characteristic of a type 1 conditioned reflex. Moreover, it is important to notice, the response is not restricted to the cerebral cortex: large areas of the brain participate.

Examples of experiments showing these widespread electrical correlatives of learning could easily be multiplied. Learning—memorizing—is a complex and active process. It is important, as we have already emphasized, to distinguish it from the trace of what is learnt. This may or may not be similarly widespread in the animal's central nervous system. 'Listening-in' to the processes whereby the brain learns cannot easily answer the question of where the brain *stores* the information it has learnt, or of the form in which the information is stored.

In mammals, as we have already seen in this book, there is much evidence that the memory trace is localized in the cerebral hemispheres. It will be recalled from Chapter 13 that stimulation of appropriate areas of the human cerebral cortex may elicit visual or auditory memories. Indeed it has been known since the times of

[1] Galambos, R. (1961), 'Neurophysiological studies on learning and motivation', *Fed. Proc., 20*, 603–608.

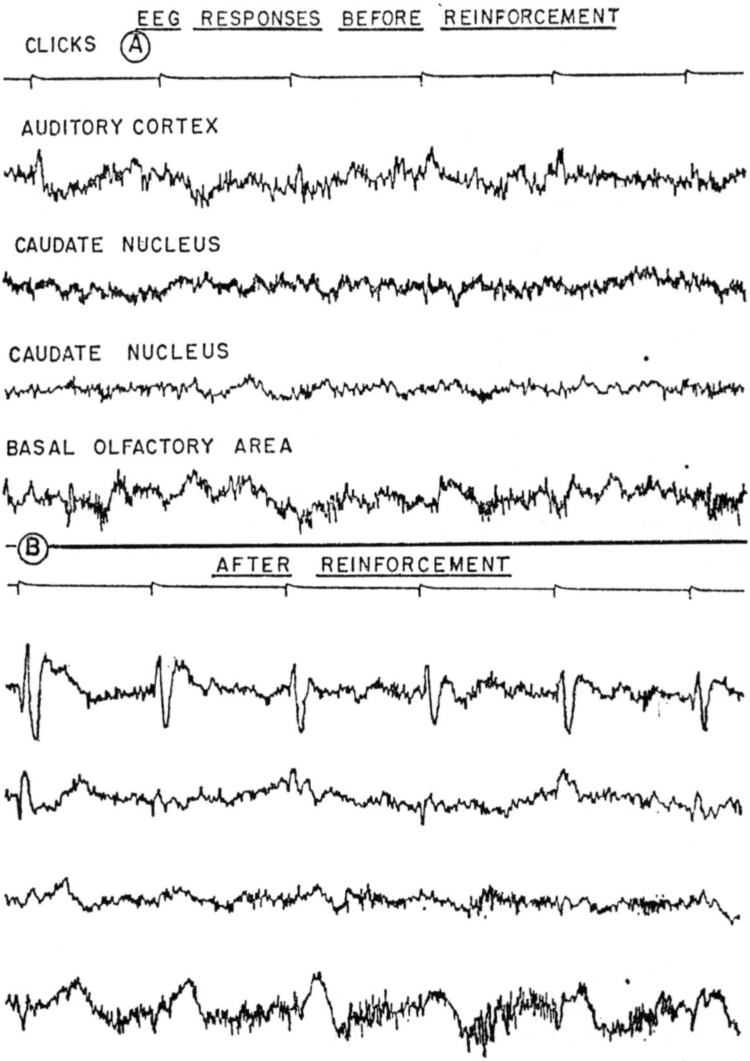


15.2 Electrical response to clicks before and after reinforcement. Electrodes are implanted into the cat's brain in the regions labelled in the upper part of the figure. In (A) the electrical response is recorded after a regular click had been sounded throughout the night. In (B) the response is recorded after the click had been coupled with a regular puff of air into the animal's face. Explanation in text. From Galambos, R. (1961), 'Neurophysiological studies on learning and motivation', *Fed. Proc.*, *20*, 605–608.

Broca and Wernicke in the nineteenth century that lesions of certain parts of the human cortex result in aphasias and/or apraxias. The subject either is unable to 'find' his words, or he is unable to understand words spoken to him. However these important observations tend to suffer from the defect stressed in earlier chapters. It is possible to criticise them on the grounds that the investigator may not be acting on the actual site, if such there be, of the function in question, but may be merely cutting connections to and from this putative centre.

Another approach to the location of memory traces within the brain emerges from experiments on 'split-brain' animals and humans. In these experiments the corpus callosum (Chapter 13) which normally connects the two cerebral hemispheres is sectioned. This operation has been carried out for many years on humans suffering from severe epilepsy. It has been found that the section is usually successful in preventing the spread of the seizure from one hemisphere to the other. Surprisingly, however, the subsequent behaviour of these split-brain individuals seemed quite normal. It was accordingly very difficult to ascribe a function to this prominent tract of fibres.

However in the early nineteen-fifties workers in Sperry's laboratory at Caltech began to show that section of the corpus callosum prevented one hemisphere sharing what it learnt with its neighbour. In a rather literal sense the right hand did not know what the left was doing. So far as learnt behaviour was concerned each hemisphere seemed to act quite independently of the other. The procedure adopted in these experiments was to cut the optic chiasma as well as the corpus callosum. This is shown diagrammatically in Fig. 15.3.

After the operation depicted in Fig. 15.3 information from the left and right eyes is confined to the left and right hemispheres respectively. Now let us consider what happens if we cover one eye with a patch and 'teach' a conditioned reflex through the other. Let us suppose, for example, that the animal learns to push a lever to obtain food when a visual stimulus is presented. So far so good, but what happens if the patch is removed from the eye and placed over the other? Does the animal respond in the correct way when the visual stimulus is presented? No. Far from it, the animal appears quite ignorant of what it had been so laboriously taught! The conditioned reflex has to be learnt again from scratch.

This observation, of course, is radically different from that made

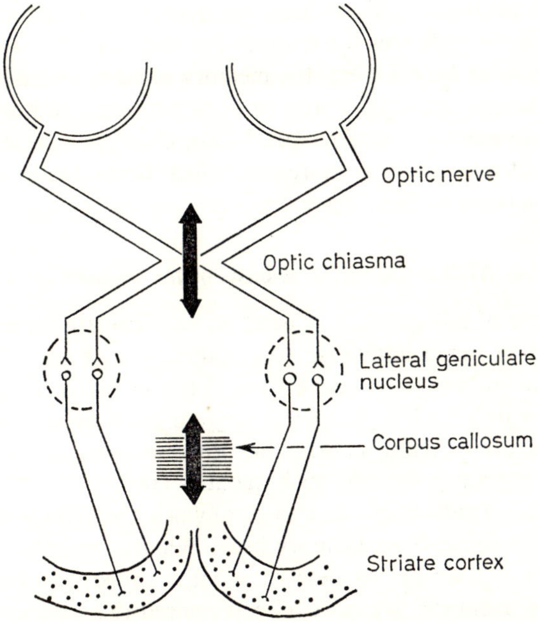


15.3 A 'split-brain' preparation is made by sectioning the optic chiasma and the corpus callosum. Information picked up by the lateral half of the left eye is thus confined to the left cerebral cortex and an analogous situation obtains for the right eye.

on an animal with an intact corpus callosum. A conditioned reflex taught through one eye can equally well be elicited through the other. As humans we all know that it is equally easy to recognize words through one eye as the other. Yet, as we saw in section 13.7, linguistic ability is largely restricted to one hemisphere.

Thus these experiments on split-brain animals seem to confirm our previous inclination to believe that visual memories, at least, are located in the cerebral cortex. By sectioning the corpus callosum they may be 'trapped' in one hemisphere. Similar types of experiment have shown that auditory and tactile memories may be trapped in a similar way.

The balance of evidence presented in this section therefore suggests that the 'engram' is, in mammals, laid down in the cerebral cortex. This concept fits in with our overall picture of the brain's machinery. We have come to regard the cerebral cortex, the 'roof-brain' in Sherrington's phrase, as the great analyser, the great storehouse of specific information, which may be activated or deactivated by deeper centres. Information fed into the cortex by the distance receptors may or may not 'fit' the memory patterns laid down there. In other words recognition may or may not occur. But what form might these memory patterns take? This, clearly, must be our next question. It is a question, moreover, which forms today one of the central concerns of brain research.

### 15.4 What is the physical basis of the memory trace?[1]

The essence of this question appears to be: How are the evanescent ion fluxes of nerve impulses, over and done with in a few milliseconds, to be converted into a trace that may last a lifetime? Vice versa, how may such a permanent engram be converted back into dynamic action potentials during the processes of recall? What form could an engram possessing such qualities take?

We have already taken care to distinguish the process of memorizing, of learning, from memory itself. What is probably the same distinction is often drawn between what is called 'short-term' and 'long-term' memory. We have all experienced this distinction when we have 'held' a telephone number, say, in our minds long enough to make the call, but forgotten it almost immediately after. On the other hand most of us retain a permanent record of, for example, the date of the battle of Hastings. Equally well known evidence for recognizing two types of memory is provided by retrograde amnesias. An individual who suffers severe concussion probably retains no memory of the events immediately preceding the blow. There is evidence, moreover, that the more severe the concussion the longer the period of retrograde amnaesia. In experimental animals similar effects may be obtained by methods involving electroconvulsive shock or anoxia. The conclusion to these observations seems clear. The processes, whatever they may be, of memory fixation take a little time, perhaps a few minutes; any attack on the integrity of the central nervous system during that period obstructs these processes. In consequence the 'short-term' memory is never fixed. More ancient memories remain, however, unaffected. The latter, as we mentioned at the outset of this chapter, are well-nigh impossible to erase.

[1] It is important to note that there may well be more than one way in which the brain can store information. It is only because of the necessity to keep things as simple as possible in a book of this nature that it is assumed in the following sections of this chapter that only one mechanism is operative.

A distinction between 'short-term' and 'long-term' memory, between memorizing and memory, also emerges from another very well known and much regretted observation. As we grow older our powers of memorizing begin to fade. Paradoxically, however, the vividness of those memories we have tends, if anything, to increase. We are all familiar with the pensioner who cannot remember what he did yesterday but seems to possess almost total recall of the events of half a century ago. It would seem that old age is accompanied by a progressive failure in the mechanisms which lead to memory fixation, whilst those which have been fixed in the past remain relatively unaffected.

These simple commonplace observations form the framework within which any discussion of the physical basis of memory must take place. We saw in section 15.3 that memorizing is accompanied by widespread and relatively long-lasting electrical activity in many parts of the brain. We may suppose that some at least of this activity reflects the process of memory fixation. A favourite hypothesis of the form taken by this dynamic phase of memory envisages circuits of neurons in which impulses 'reverberate'. A few minutes of such reverberation is long enough for several thousand impulses to pass around the circuits. There is plenty of scope in the histology of the cortex for such rings of neurons to exist. It may be, too, that deeper centres in the brain are able to set the level of such activity. There is certainly evidence[1] that such centres, in particular the amygdala, do influence the fixation of memories. If this is the case we seem to have a nice explanation for the common experience that emotional situations, which seem as we saw in Chapter 12 to have their physical bases in the deeper centres, usually leave the most ineradicable memories.

If the physical basis of 'short-term' memory is the activation of specific nerve circuits we can immediately see the neurophysiological reasons for the observations mentioned in the previous paragraphs. However, we can now no longer put off the sixty-four dollar question: How is this dynamic 'short-term' memory converted into 'long-term' memory? We have to suppose that the circulation of impulses in these putative circuits leaves behind some permanent residue, causes some permanent change.

Now what form could this change take? Presumably it must make

[1] See Gloor, P., 'Amygdala', in *Handbook of Physiology: Section 1, Neurophysiology*, Vol. 2, American Physiological Society, 1960.

these particular circuits distinguishably different from the billiards of other possible circuits in the cortex. Presumably it must alter the 'resistance' either upwards or downwards of these circuits to the transmission of impulses. It would follow that when the familiar conditioned stimulus is presented to the animal the cerebral activity would be significantly different from that attendant upon an unfamiliar sensory stimulus. The animal, in other words, would 'remember' the one stimulus but not the other.

Now as we saw in Chapters 5 and 6 the resistance of a neuronal circuit is a function of the synapses and, to a lesser extent, of the axon hillocks. The axons themselves, it will be remembered, conduct in an all-or-nothing fashion. Hence the easiest way to alter the resistance of a chain of neurons would be to alter the transmissibility of the synapses. However we have already mentioned that any cortical neuron may make up to 60,000 synaptic contacts with its neighbours. We have, as yet, no means of knowing which of these synapses are involved in a particular memory, or even if they are all functional. The problem of detecting changes in synaptic resistance in cortical circuits thus seems intractable.

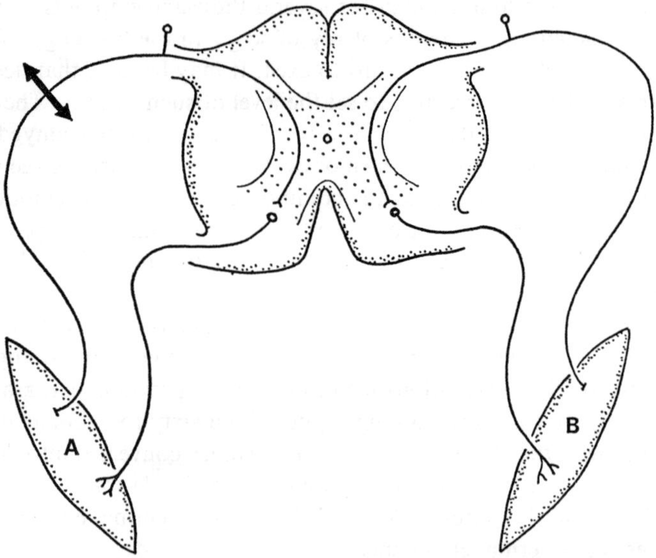


15.4 An experiment to determine whether synaptic resistance changes with use and disuse. The figure shows a T.S. of the spinal cord receiving spinal nerves from two muscles, A and B. The sensory nerve from muscle A is sectioned at the point indicated by the double-headed arrow.

Faced with an impasse of this sort the biologist's reflex is to seek simpler systems. One such simplified system is the monosynaptic reflex arc which controls mammalian skeletal muscle. It will be remembered that we discussed this system in section 6.3. Eccles and McIntyre investigated this system in 1953.[1] Their procedure was to cut the proprioceptor fibres from the muscles of one leg just before they entered the spinal cord. They reasoned that if synaptic resistance varied with use then the monosynaptic reflex on the cut side should, after a period of weeks, be slower, or have a higher threshold, than the reflex on the uncut, functional, leg. The principle of the experiment is shown in Fig. 15.4.

Eccles' expectations were confirmed. After several weeks it could be shown that the reflex elicited by stimulating the cut end of the proprioceptor fibre from muscle A was depressed compared with that elicited by stimulating the fibre from muscle B. Similar surgical procedures can be devised to ensure that the monosynaptic reflexes on one side are subjected to greatly increased use. Testing after several weeks shows that, in this case, the monosynaptic reflexes on the experimental side are considerably facilitated.[2]

However there is a snag. These experiments have been strongly criticized on the grounds that sectioning a nerve leads to histological changes even in the proximal parts of the nerve. It is therefore possible that the physiological effects observed by investigators using this technique are merely the result of the surgery. Clear proof of an alteration in synaptic resistance consequent upon use or disuse seems hard to come at by this technique.

An even simpler system for the study of reflex learning has been devised by insect physiologists. It has proved possible to isolate the thoracic ganglia of cockroaches from the rest of the central nervous system. These ganglia control the movements of the legs attached to the thoracic segments. It is, moreover, possible to recognise individual motor neurons in these ganglia. Now it can be shown that conditioned reflexes can be established in these isolated ganglia.[3] It is possible, for instance, to condition a leg to move in a characteristic manner. Clearly this opens up the possibility of studying learning in

[1] Eccles, J. C. and McIntyre, A. K. (1953), 'The effects of use and of inactivity on mammalian spinal reflexes', *J. Physiol., 121*, 492–516.

[2] Eccles, R. M. and Westerman, R. A. (1959), 'Enhanced synaptic function due to excessive use', *Nature, 184*, 460–461.

[3] Horridge, G. A. (1962), 'Learning of leg position by the ventral cord in headless insects', *Proc. Roy. Soc. B., 157*, 33–52.

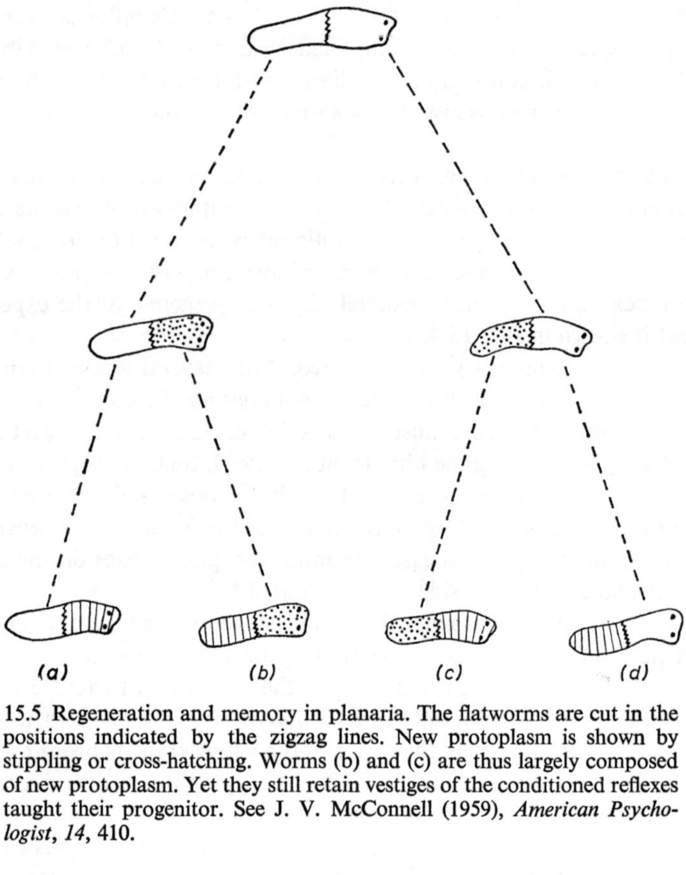


15.5 Regeneration and memory in planaria. The flatworms are cut in the positions indicated by the zigzag lines. New protoplasm is shown by stippling or cross-hatching. Worms (b) and (c) are thus largely composed of new protoplasm. Yet they still retain vestiges of the conditioned reflexes taught their progenitor. See J. V. McConnell (1959), *American Psychologist*, *14*, 410.

a nervous system many orders of magnitude smaller than that of the vertebrates. It may, furthermore, be possible by studying bilaterally matched pairs of motor neurons to determine the existence and nature of any structural changes accompanying learning.

A still simpler system for the study of learning and memory is provided by the diminutive free-living flatworms. These animals are common pond-living carnivores which have the distinction, after the coelenterata, of being the most primitive members of the metazoa. In 1959 some very seminal experiments were performed on these lowly creatures. It was shown by McConnell[1] that a conditioned

[1] McConnell, J., Jacobsen, R. and Maynard, D. M. (1959), 'Apparent retention of a conditioned reflex following total regeneration in the planarian', *Amer. Psychol.*, *14*, 410.

reflex established in one of these planaria could be detected in worms which had developed by regeneration from fragments of the original. Matters could be arranged (Fig. 15.5) so that these regenerate worms contained no part of the nervous system of the initial educated worm.

These experiments, which have been subsequently strongly criticized, swung the attention of neurobiologists towards a memory mechanism based on protein synthesis. For the process of regeneration is, essentially, a process of protein biosynthesis. This reorientation, of course, accorded well with the explosive development of molecular biology in the late fifties and early sixties. It was attractive to suppose that genetic and neurological memory depended on the same fundamental mechanisms. In consequence much ingenious research has been undertaken in an effort to obtain evidence for or against such a molecular theory of memory. This research does not, of course, supersede that directed towards detecting a synaptic change. In essence it takes this research a step further. For any biosynthetic effect would, on the face of it, express itself physiologically as a change in synaptic function.

### 15.5 Towards a molecular psychobiology

One of the pioneers in this comparatively new field of brain research was and is Holger Hyden. Working at the University of Goteborg Hyden has, over the last two decades, developed remarkably precise microminiaturized methods for analysing the nucleic acid content of nerve and glial cells. Let us look briefly at one of his now classical experiments.[1]

In the lateral vestibular nucleus (Deiters' nucleus) of the medulla are to be found certain very large neurons—Deiters' cells. These cells, like the rest of the vestibular nucleus, are primarily concerned with the animal's sense of balance. Hyden showed that it was possible to dissect these neurons out of the medulla and to analyse their RNA content. It proved possible to determine not only the total quantity of RNA but also the ratios of the four nucleotide bases. Hyden's initial experiments thus consisted of exposing Deiters' cells to a heavy traffic of nerve impulses and then comparing their RNA content with that of a control group of cells.

The method Hyden and his colleagues adopted was to present

[1] Hyden, H. and Egyhazi, E. (1962), 'Nuclear RNA changes of nerve cells during a learning experiment in rats', *P.N.A.S. (Wash.)*, *48*, 1366–1373.

young rats with the difficult task of walking a thin wire tightrope to reach their food platform. When this task had been successfully learnt he compared the RNA content of their Deiters' cells with those of control animals which had not had to learn this balancing act. For good measure Hyden also analysed the Deiters' cells of another group of rats which had been subjected to a passive form of equilibrial stress. This third group—the functional controls—were rotated in both vertical and horizontal planes.

Hyden's results showed that the RNA content of Deiters' cells from both experimental and functional control rats was significantly greater than the RNA content of Deiters' cells from the non-functional controls. Moreover he was able to show distinct differences between the base sequences of the experimental RNA and both control RNAs. Compared with both the controls the RNA from the experimental Deiters' cells contained more adenine and less uracil.

Similar experiments have now been carried out on planaria. It was shown that a clear change in the base composition of cerebral RNA occurred when these flatworms were conditioned. It was found that the quantity of adenine diminished and the quantity of guanine increased.[1] Furthermore Jacobsen, Fried and Horowitz have been able to extract RNA from conditioned planaria and to inject it into naïve flatworms. The latter planaria were then found to behave as if the conditioned response taught the first group had been transferred.[2]

Many other investigators have now demonstrated a relation between learning and the metabolism of proteins and nucleic acids in the brain. One of the most effective ways of investigating this relationship has depended on the intelligent use of certain drugs. These drugs may be used as molecular scalpels to interfere with the normal processes of protein biosynthesis.

Not least of the many important insights provided by modern work in molecular biology has been the discovery of where and how these drugs exert their effects. 8-azaguanine, for example, interferes with the synthesis of RNA as the cell 'mistakes' it for guanine. Actinomycin D, an antibiotic, inhibits the synthesis of mRNA on a

[1] Hyden, H. (1966), 'Introductory remarks to the session on memory processing', in *Neurosciences Research Symposium Summaries*, *1*, M.I.T. Press, Cambridge, Mass., p. 284.

[2] Jacobsen, A. L., Fried, C. and Horowitz, S. D. (1966), 'Planarians and memory', *Nature*, *204*, 599–601.

DNA template (see Chapter 3). Puromycin and acetoxycyclohexamide, on the other hand, prevent the translation of the information carried by mRNA into protein structure. The latter two inhibitors act, therefore, at the ribosomes. The sites at which these various inhibitors act are summarized in Fig. 15.6.

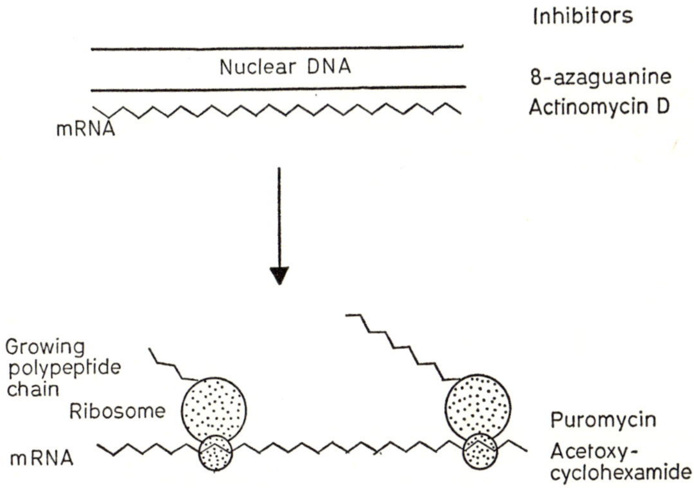


15.6 Sites of inhibitor action during protein synthesis. The inhibitors are listed on the right-hand side of the figure adjacent to the positions where they exert their effects.

All the drugs depicted in Fig. 15.6 have, at one time or another, been shown to have an effect on the learning ability of animals. To exemplify the type of experiment carried out we outline some of the interesting work on goldfish learning prosecuted in Agranoff's laboratory.[1]

Goldfish are quite intelligent as fish go and it is possible to establish type 2 conditioned reflexes. The procedure is shown in Fig. 15.7. The fish is placed in a tank partially divided into two compartments by an underwater barrier. The goldfish can cross this barrier by swimming very close to the surface. At each end of the tank is a light bulb, and in each compartment is a copper grid. When the grid in one compartment is electrified the fish escapes by swimming over the barrier.

[1] See Agranoff, B. W., Davis, R. E. and Brink, J. J. (1966), 'Chemical studies on memory fixation in goldfish', *Brain Res.*, *1*, 303–309.

It is not difficult with the set-up of Fig. 15.7 to establish a conditioned reflex such that the light acts as the conditioned and the electric shock as the unconditioned stimulus. After a number of pairings of CS and UCS the fish 'learns' to cross the barrier when the light is switched on.

Now if puromycin, acetoxycyclohexamide or actinomycin D are injected into the fish's cranium fixation of the reflex is greatly weakened. The drugs do not appear to interfere with the goldfish's initial ability to learn the correct behaviour but they do seem to prevent the laying down of a long-term memory. The drugs, furthermore, were found to be ineffective if they were not introduced within one hour

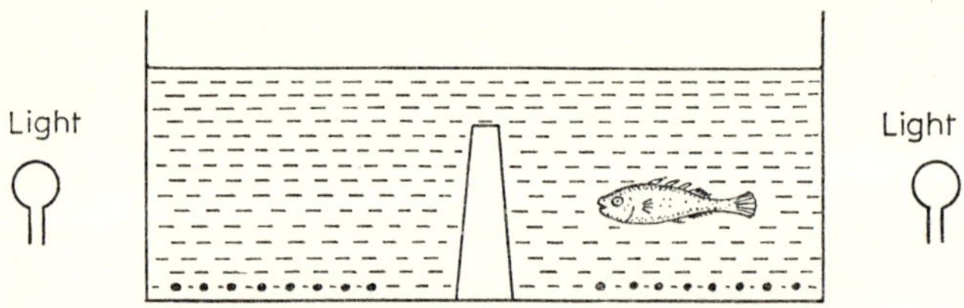


15.7 An apparatus for examining type 2 CRs in fish. Explanation in text. After Agranoff, B. W., Davis, R. E. and Brink, J. J. (1966), 'Chemical studies on memory fixation in goldfish', *Brain Research*, *1*, 303–309.

of the training period. The drugs thus have the same psychological effect as electroconvulsive shock. They separate short-term from long-term memory. Unlike electroconvulsive shock, however, their points of action are, as we have seen, precisely defined.

Agranoff's results thus suggest that memory fixation depends both on unimpaired mRNA synthesis and unimpaired translation into protein. Actinomycin D has also been employed by Hyden. It was shown[1] that the RNA differing in base composition which, as we saw, was characteristic of conditioned neurons, was being synthesized on nuclear DNA. It was, in other words, messenger-RNA.

### 15.6 Speculations

At present the facts of what we have called molecular psychobiology are not sufficiently well established to warrant the drawing of firm

[1] Hyden, H. and Egyhazi, E. (1964), 'Changes in RNA content and base composition in cortical neurons of rats in a learning experiment involving transfer of handedness', *P.N.A.S.* (*Wash.*), *52*, 1030–1035.

conclusions. It is, however, tempting to speculate. Bearing in mind the outline of molecular biology sketched in Chapter 3, we might search for a connection between neuronal activity and genetic switching. The work reviewed in the previous section suggests that mRNA is synthesized in active neurons. This conclusion is supported by some evidence obtained recently by Machlus and Gaito.[1] These workers have actually been able to isolate the mRNA produced in the brains of rats set a behavioural task and have shown that it is different from the mRNA obtainable from the brains of non-behaving animals. Our speculation thus begins to shape as follows. Perhaps the ionic fluxes characteristic of neuronal activity are geared to the system of genetic switches which all cells possess. How could this gearing be achieved? After all we saw in Chapter 5 that the ionic constitution of a neuron is hardly changed by the passage of an action potential along its membrane. Indeed only about a millionth part of the cell's potassium ions diffuse out. However let us remember that memories are not established by the passage of a single impulse. We have seen that memory fixation, or short-term memory, takes anything up to or above an hour to occur. If we suppose on the evidence presented in the preceding sections that memory fixation is a dynamic process, a process which quite possibly depends on the circulation of impulses in reverberatory circuits, then the intracellular ionic change may become appreciable. Suppose an impulse travels around the circuit in about 0·1 seconds. It will then complete about 35,000 circuits in an hour. If each time it passes about one millionth of the intracellular potassium escapes, then at the end of the hour the neuron will have lost about 3·5% of its potassium. This is appreciable. It is important, moreover, to bear in mind that the figures we have been considering relate to the squid giant axon. In smaller axons proportionately more ionic change will occur. Indeed there exist tiny axons, about 0·1$\mu$ in diameter, whose internal sodium ion concentration may be doubled after the passage of as few as ten action potentials. It is interesting to note that small neurons are particularly numerous in regions of the brain where learning is believed to occur.[2] It is also worthwhile considering whether these minute neurons might not bias the action of larger cells by forming

[1] Machlus, B. and Gaito, J., (1968), 'Detection of RNA species unique to a behavioural task', *Psychon. Sci.*, *10*, 253–254.

[2] Altman, J., in *The Neurosciences: A Study Programme*, edited by Quarton, G. C., Melnechuk, T., and Schmitt, F. O., Rockefeller University Press, New York, 1967, p. 743.

axo-axonic junctions (section 6.5) and thus exert an influence out of all proportion to their size.

We have considered the movement of potassium and sodium ions only because they provide a convenient example. Action potentials are, of course, also accompanied by the movements of other ions: $Ca^{2+}$, $Mg^{2+}$, $Cl^-$, etc. It seems likely that sustained activity in a small neuron will have a significant effect on the intracellular concentrations of any or all of these ions. Now it is known that proteins are very susceptible to their ionic environment. Many enzymes, for example, are activated by monovalent or divalent cations. Our speculation thus develops in the following way. It is conceivable that nerve cells possess repressor proteins (section 3.3) which are sensitive to the circumambient ionic concentration. When this concentration varies beyond certain critical limits their three-dimensional structure is altered. This structural change prevents them from doing their normal job of inhibiting an operator gene. The derepressed gene, in consequence, initiates the synthesis of an mRNA strand by the adjacent structural genes. This mRNA programmes, in turn, the manufacture of proteins by the neuron's ribosomes. Whether this series of events does in fact occur in nerve cells is at present quite unknown. It does, however, seem to fit many of the observations reviewed in the preceding sections of this chapter. Fig. 15.8 schematizes the main elements of the hypothesis.

In Fig. 15.8 it is supposed that it is the $mRNA_2$ which has been detected by Hyden and more recently by Machlus and Gaito. It is supposed that it is the synthesis of this mRNA which is inhibited by actinomycin D. Puromycin and acetoxycyclohexamide would interfere with the synthesis of the protein, P, by the ribosomes. It is known[1] that active neurons do synthesize protein at a rate considerably in excess of that found in resting cells.

Next let us consider the possible function of protein P. We have seen in Chapters 4, 5 and 6 that the critical points in the conduction of a nerve impulse are the initiation of the action potential at the axon hillock and the transmission to the next cell at the synapse. It is at these points that flexibility occurs. The passage of the impulse along the axon itself is an all-or-nothing, yes/no, event. Protein P might affect either or both of these points. It might make it more or less difficult for an action potential to be 'sparked off' at the hillock,

[1] Rose, S. P. R. (1967), 'Changes in visual cortex on first exposure of rats to light', *Nature*, *215*, 253–255.

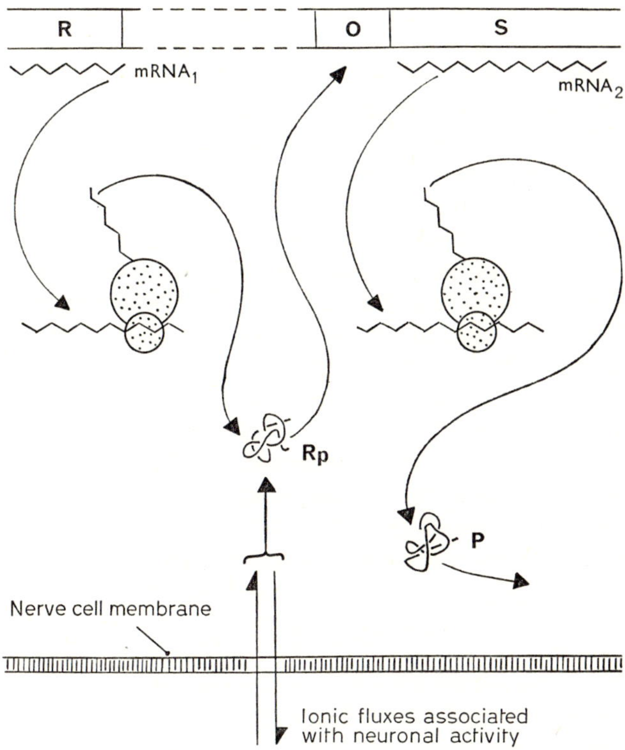


15.8 Diagram to illustrate a *hypothetical* molecular basis for memory. Compare with Fig. 3.2. O = operator gene, P = protein or polypeptide programmed by the structural gene, R = regulator gene, Rp = repressor protein, S = structural gene. Explanation in text.

or it might affect the ease of synaptic transmission. We saw in Chapter 4 that there is good evidence for vigorous axoplasmic streaming in nerve cells so there is no difficulty in imagining how a protein synthesized in the perikaryon might find its way to these relatively distant regions of the cell.

This molecular mechanism ensures that the nerve circuits excited in a learning situation have their resistance to impulse transmission permanently (in the context of milliseconds) altered. It would also account for the extinction of conditioned reflexes in the absence of reinforcement. For, in this case, the nerve circuits would not be reactivated and hence no more protein would be manufactured. We may suppose that, like all proteins, 'memory' proteins are subject to the usual metabolic processes of degradation.

We have suggested that the essence of memory fixation is the alteration of the resistance to impulse transmission of one or more neuronal circuits. Now this alteration may, of course, be either upwards or downwards: the resistance may be either increased or decreased. The simplest model is provided by a decrease in the resistance of the neuronal circuits involved. However, the alternative is also worth considering. Activation of the neuron may cause an inhibitory protein to be synthesized, or it may inhibit the production of an excitatory protein. In either case the widespread electrical activity in the brain during learning (section 15.3) might be the signature of the activation of a very large number of 'memory' circuits. In the vast majority of these inhibitor proteins might be produced or excitatory proteins suppressed. The biologically 'correct' circuits would in this way 'crystallize out' by the suppression of the inappropriate circuits. It has been said that 'we do not learn to catch the right bus so much as learn not to catch the wrong ones'.

## 15.7 'The hooked atoms'

We have suggested in the previous sections of this chapter that memories have a physical basis in the form of low resistance 'circuits' in the brain, particularly in the cerebral cortex. This, we have suggested, is the way the mammalian brain stores information derived from past experience; the cortex represents the animal's individual history in the form of a palimpsest of overlapping neuronal pathways. It may be that these hypothetical circuits include amongst their constituents groups of the pattern recognition cells we discussed in section 14.8. Thus when the pattern is familiar the impulses course smoothly from the pattern recognizers to the appropriate motor output. The child recognizes the glitter of the fire and withdraws its hand; the dog recognizes the tone of the ringing bell and salivates. On the other hand when the sensory input is unfamiliar no circuit of pattern recognizers is fitted: the impulses cannot flow through well worn channels and are, in consequence, more diffuse and widespread. Perhaps it is this difference in the physical state of the brain which appears subjectively as the difference between a feeling of familiarity—I've seen this before, I've been here before—and a feeling of unfamiliarity—I've never seen it before in my life, I'm a stranger here.

The mind/matter, subject/object, dichotomy is considered in more detail in Chapter 17. As human beings, however, we all know ourselves fully capable of 'summoning up remembrance of things past' more or less at will. It is true, as mentioned in section 15.4, that this is easier to do if the memory has some emotional connotation. In general, however, we do not have to wait for an outside stimulus to trigger our memories. The physical basis of these 'sessions of sweet silent thought' is an interesting and as yet unsolved problem in neurophysiology.

This 'summoning up' has certain features in common with the mechanism of selective attention which is considered in the next chapter (section 16.3). Both humans and animals are able to exclude biologically unimportant stimuli and concentrate their attention on important data. The great advance which marks off *H. sapiens* from the rest of the animals is, as we have mentioned more than once, the development of symbolic thought or, to use Pavlov's phrase, a 'second signalling system'. Neuronal activity may now represent, at one remove, the input from the sense organs. Thus it seems not improbable that the mechanisms of selective attention, which are so important in filtering the primary signals from the sense organs, may also influence the secondary signals which merely symbolize this primary information. The full development of this power of symbolization is, as we have stressed, found only in humans. It is probably an aspect of the development of self-awareness (section 16.8) which also seems to reach an evolutionary peak in mankind. Sometimes this consciousness of self fails. It is the mark of obsessional neurotics, as we shall see in the next chapter, that they are unable to gain access to crucial memories and are hence, according to Freud, unable to act rationally.

However, even in mentally normal humans much is stored in the memory which eludes the 'searchlight' of selective attention. This is perhaps especially the case in creative individuals.

In the creative imagination a constant rearrangement, reordering, turning-around of the representations of the perceptual world seems to occur. We can imagine, perhaps, that this play of free association occurring in the inattentive mind has a physical correlative in the form of activity in the overlapping circuits of the cortex. Conceivably activity in one circuit 'sparks off' activity in an overlapping circuit so that we become aware of 'images that yet fresh images beget'. With these new representations we 'see' the world in a novel light.

To use the terminology of the last chapter we achieve new patterns of expectancy.

Let there be no mistake: the creative mind does not spirit 'airy nothings' out of nowhere. Poincaré and others have made plain the central importance of what they call 'unconscious' cerebration.[1] Coleridge speaks of 'the hooks and eyes of memory' and J. L. Lowes in his great book on the poet[2] is emphatic that 'the pieces that compose the pattern are not new. In the world of the shaping spirit, save for its patterns, there is nothing new that was not old. For the work of creators is the mastery and transmutation and reordering into shapes of beauty of the given universe within us and without us'. Lowes demonstrates that 'The Ancient Mariner' and 'Xanadu' were the products of the mind of a 'literary cormorant' who had read enormously and who retained what he had read. This retention seems not always to be accessible to consciousness but forms 'a charged and electric background to a poet's mind'. From this background flash the images which reorganize our perceptions. Whilst on a starry night we, nowadays, perceive a myriad distant suns, Lorenzo perceived the paving stones of heaven.

[1] Henri Poincaré, *The Foundations of Science*, translated by G. B. Halsted, The Science Press, 1913.

[2] Lowes, J. L.: *The Road to Xanadu*, The Riverside Press, Cambridge, 1927.

# CHAPTER SIXTEEN

# Consciousness

'But for me it was enough if, in my own bed, my sleep was so heavy as completely to relax my consciousness; for then I lost all sense of the place in which I had gone to sleep, and when I awoke at midnight, not knowing where I was, I could not be sure, at first, who I was; I had only the most rudimentary sense of existence, such as may lurk and flicker in the depths of an animal's consciousness; I was more destitute of human qualities than the cave dweller; but then the memory, not yet of the place in which I was, but of the various other places where I had lived, and might now possibly be, would come like a rope let down from heaven to draw me up out of the abyss of not-being, from which I could never have escaped by myself: in a flash I would traverse and surmount centuries of civilisation, and out of a half-visualised succession of oil-lamps, followed by shirts with turned-down collars, would put together by degrees the component parts of my ego.'

MARCEL PROUST: *Swann's Way*, Vol. 1, p. 4,
translated by C. K. Scott-Moncrieff,
Chatto and Windus, London, 1964.

## 16.1 A behavioural definition of consciousness

The novelist's and the scientist's account of consciousness are going to be somewhat different. We have stressed throughout the last part of this book the deep distinction between our experience of ourselves and our knowledge of others. The novelist deals with himself, with his own experience and by implication, by a contra-solipsistic leap of faith, with the experiences of others. The scientist deals with the general case: he attempts by every means in his power to eliminate any personal idiosyncrasies which might make his observations unrepeatable. The scientist, *qua* scientist, tries to stand above the fray as an unbiased dispassionate observer. As a scientist he is not at all concerned with his own reactions to the observations, only with the magnitudes of the meter readings. Except in the microphysical world where the Heisenberg uncertainty relations become effective he believes that the act of observing has no effect on what is being observed. In the next chapter we shall consider some of the implications of this quasi God-like stance when the scientist comes to observe his own brain.

Here, however, we must first see if we can delineate the behavioural correlatives of consciousness. Only when this has been done can we hope to investigate it in others. One approach we can make is to cast the concept into its transitive form. We frequently speak of ourselves and others being conscious of this, or conscious of that. We might substitute 'aware' in this sentence. How do we know whether an individual is 'aware' of this or that? By observing whether he shows any signs of attending to it. We say, for example, that a person is very conscious of his duties when we see him paying meticulous attention to them.

Against this position it may, of course, be argued that an individual may be very conscious of some event and yet show no sign of attending to it. In polite society this may, for example, occur when a stranger commits some social solecism. The company may affect not to notice it. Yet, of course, it is merely an affectation. If asked afterwards they will laugh or shrug at the memory. Certainly there are behavioural tests which clearly indicate that the lack of attention was only a pretence: consciousness and attention are so far indistinguishable.

But what of our own private consciousness? The stream of consciousness so beloved of novelists of the last generation? Of the consciousness of self which Proust describes in the opening quotation? Does this also have a behavioural sign? We might be said to pay attention to the memories inscribed in our cerebral cortices. We are rapt in a daydream, or concentrating, perhaps, on a mathematical or logical problem. This situation is difficult for the behaviourist. For we might refuse to divulge the contents of our reverie. It would then be most difficult for another to say whether one is conscious of anything at all or whether one has, perhaps, lapsed into a coma. This difficulty arises in a particularly acute form in the case of the recessive hemisphere of a split-brain individual (section 15.3).

Questions about the nature and existential status of our private worlds are, however, postponed to Chapter 17. Here we shall neglect, for the moment, the difficulty outlined in the previous paragraph and work on the assumption that, to a first approximation, consciousness and attentiveness are identical. In the case of animals we might go one further step in this chain of equivalences and suggest that the behavioural sign of attentiveness is the presence of an orientating reflex. If, we shall argue, a stimulus is placed in an animal's perceptual 'space' and he 'takes no notice' of it, he shows no orientating reflex, then he is not conscious of that stimulus. By running through the gamut of possible stimuli we can, in principle, determine whether the organism is conscious of anything at all, or unconscious.

### 16.2 The 'what-is-it?' reflex

The orientating reflex is described in one of Pavlov's classic passages. 'There is a reflex,' he writes,[1] 'which is still insufficiently appreciated and which can be termed the investigatory reflex. I sometimes call it the "what-is-it?" reflex. It also belongs to the fundamental reflexes and is responsible for the fact that given the slightest change in the surrounding world both man and animals immediately orientate their respective receptor organs towards the agent evoking the change. The biological significance of this reflex is enormous. If the animal were not provided with this reaction, its life, one might say, would always hang by a thread.'

It is clear that the precise nature of this reflex will vary from one animal species to the next. It is, however, seldom difficult to recognize. In the higher animals, indeed, it grades into what Thorpe[2] has called 'anticipatory arousal'. Observation of animals in this state of expectation gives, according to Thorpe, 'an overwhelming impression of conscious and deliberate foresight'.

### 16.3 Neurological bases of the orientating reflex

Pavlov's account of the physiology underlying the 'what-is-it?' reflex is regarded by contemporary Western neurophysiologists as somewhat lacking in subtlety. And, of course, since the time of Pavlov's experimentation a very great deal of water has flowed beneath the neurophysiological bridge. Let us therefore start our account of the neurophysiological bases of the 'what-is-it?' reflex by describing a rather beautiful experiment carried out by Hernández-Péon, Scherrer and Jouvet in 1956.[3] These investigators implanted recording electrodes in the cochlear nucleus of a cat. Fig. 16.1 (a) shows the response detectable when a regular click is sounded.

[1] Pavlov, I. P., *Selected Works*, Foreign Languages Publishing House, Moscow, 1955, p. 184.

[2] Thorpe, W. H., in *Brain and Conscious Behaviour*, Springer-Verlag, 1966, p. 494.

[3] Hernández-Péon, R., Scherrer, H. and Jouvet, M. (1956): 'Modifications of electrical activity in the cochlear nucleus during "attention" in unanaesthetised cats', *Science, 123*, 331–332.

Fig. 16.1 (b) shows the effect of placing an interesting object in the animal's perceptual field. The response in the cochlear nucleus almost disappears. A similar inhibition occurs in response to a large number of 'compelling' stimuli: to painful stimuli, to interesting odours or, as in the figure, to interesting visual perceptions. When the object of attention is removed and the cat returns to its former semi-somnolent state the response in the cochlear nucleus returns (Fig. 16.1 (c) ).

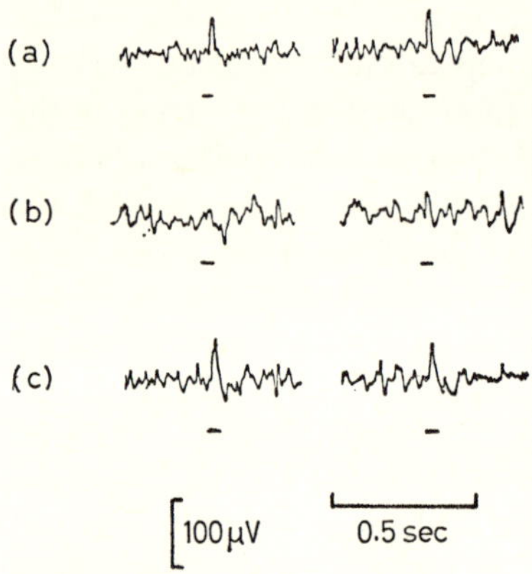


16.1 Electrical response in the cat's cochlear nucleus to a regularly sounded click. The click is represented by a bar beneath each trace. In (a) and (c) the cat is relaxed and somnolent, in (b) it is actively attending to an interesting visual object (a jar full of mice). Further explanation in text. From Hernández-Péon, R., Scherrer, H. and Jouvet, H. (1956), 'Modifications of electrical activity in cochlear nucleus during "attention" in unanaesthetised cats', *Science, 123,* 331–332.

This experiment provides a very clear demonstration of one of the physiological mechanisms underlying the 'what-is-it?' reflex. In order to concentrate attention on some item of biological importance other, biologically unimportant, stimuli are inhibited.

Similar central control of receptor sensitivity has been demonstrated on the much simpler system of the crustacean stretch receptor. Here, it will be remembered (section 7.3), a single neurosensory cell responds when the muscle is stretched. This neurosensory cell is, however, covered by the terminal ramifications of an efferent axon. Stimulation of the latter axon causes repolarization of the stretch receptor. In other words its response to stretch is inhibited. The 'bias' of the receptor is set centrally.

In both the examples quoted above the inhibition appears to occur in the sensory pathway. Experimental psychologists have also shown that, in the case of humans, a similar selection of incoming stimuli also probably occurs at the level of the cerebral cortex. For example we have all probably experienced the frustration of trying to attend to two conversations at once. This is the well-known cocktail party problem. It can be shown that the difficulty is not merely due to the physical interference of the two messages: it is not, in other words, a matter of one set of words drowning out the other, or part of the other, set of words. The explanation seems to be that, apart from a few exceptional individuals, the human brain can only attend to the sense of one conversation at a time.[1]

The moral we can draw from these experiments and the many other similar experiments which have been tried is that the organism is not merely a passive screen on to which stimuli, important and unimportant, rain. Rather it is an active selector amongst stimuli: clearly this is essential for an animal with a highly developed armamentary of sense organs for the brain would otherwise be inundated by so large a deluge of 'raw' information. This discrimination amongst stimuli is carried to an extreme in humans. We have a power of sustained concentration denied the rest of the animal kingdom. Bertrand Russell tells the story of how after concentrating on a mathematical problem he 'came to' realizing that he had 'forgotten' to breathe!

## 16.4 Consciousness and the EEG

The process of stimulus selection is a sure indicator of attention and thus, according to our equation, of consciousness. However, although it is a sufficient it is not a necessary sign of wakefulness. For as we pointed out in section 16.1 it is quite possible for humans, anyway, to feign lack of attention. The development of electroencephalography, however, allows another means of detecting the brain's state of consciousness. Figure 16.2 shows the effect of a loud hand-clap on the EEG record from a sleeping cat. On the left-hand side of the figure irregular slow waves characteristic of the sleeping brain are recorded. The vertical arrow marks the time at which the hands were clapped; to the right of this mark it can be seen that the EEG record has completely changed. In place of the large slowish waves are fast, low amplitude oscillations. This EEG change is accompanied by the cat rousing itself, opening its eyes and raising its head.

In Chapter 15 we discussed the effect of sensory stimuli on the human EEG. We saw that the alpha rhythm characteristic of the 'inattentive' brain is blocked by all types of sensory stimuli. Indeed alpha blockade also occurs when the subject attempts mental arithmetic, to visualize a scene or to recall a memory.

[1] See Broadbent, D. E. (1962), 'Attention and the Perception of Speech', *Scientific American* (April), 143–151.

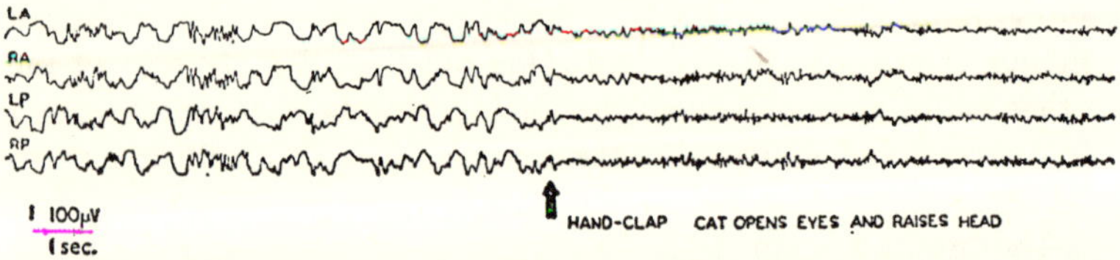


16.2 Arousal of a sleeping cat in response to a loud hand-clap. On the left of the arrow are slow irregular EEG waveforms characteristic of the sleeping brain; to the right is fast low amplitude activity. The four records are taken from four different parts of the cat's skull. The change in EEG record after the hand-clap is accompanied by the cat opening its eyes and raising its head. From Lindsley, D. B., Schreiner, L. H., Knowles, W. B. and Magoun, H. W. (1950), 'Brain stem lesions in the cat', *EEG Clin. Neurophysiol.*, *2*, 483–498.

Electroencephalography has thus proved a very useful method for determining the 'consciousness' of the brain. A person may feign sleep and deceive an observer depending only on behavioural signs. It is more difficult, however, to fox the electroencephalographer. If his sleep is genuine then his EEG will show certain characteristics (see Fig. 16.5), if it is feigned then these characteristics will be missing.

### 16.5 The reticular activating system

In the last two sections we have looked at some of the behavioural and physiological signs or accompaniments of consciousness. Let us now turn our attention to the question of whether this faculty of alertness, of attentiveness, has any known anatomical basis.

Considerable progress has been made towards answering this question in the last two decades. In 1949 Moruzzi and Magoun showed that stimulation of the reticular formation in the cat's brain stem caused behavioural arousal and alpha rhythm blockade. This was the first real indication that deep centres in the brain might control the level of cortical activity. Since this experiment a great deal of evidence has accumulated showing that, in general, this concept is valid.

Fig. 16.3 shows this concept in diagrammatic form. Because the theory holds that the cortex is kept 'awake' and active by impulses playing on it from the reticular formation the system is called the 'ascending reticular activation system', or ARAS. The figure shows two pathways running up the brain stem. The larger, more central, pathway is the ARAS, the smaller pathway running alongside consists of fibres belonging to the 'classical' sensory systems (Chapter 12).

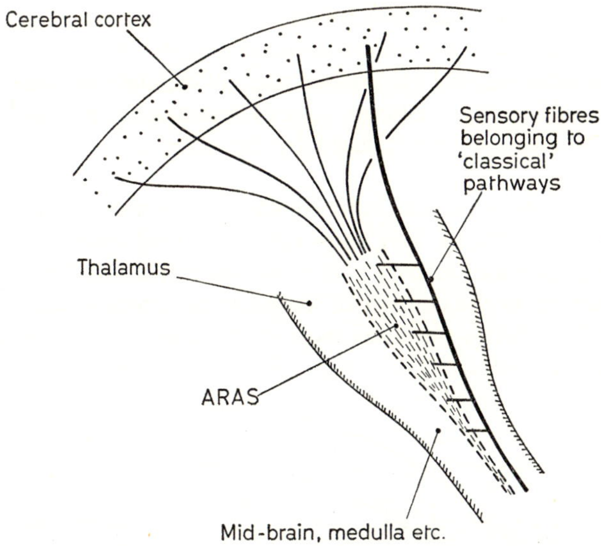


16.3 The ascending reticular activating system (ARAS). For explanation see text.

The figure shows that the ARAS branches in a diffuse manner to innervate wide areas of the cortex. Fig. 16.3 also shows that fibres belonging to all the sense modalities connect into the ARAS as it ascends the brain stem. These fibres are, of course, additional to those carrying sensory information as such to the projection areas on the cerebral cortex. It follows, however, that sensory stimuli of all types provoke electrical activity in the ARAS. Furthermore if all sensory input to the ARAS is eliminated consciousness—alertness—flickers out.[1]

It is interesting in this context to note the work of Gellhorn[2] and others which suggests that proprioceptive discharges from the body's musculature are of importance in setting the 'bias' of the ARAS. It is suggested that the posture of the body, whether triumphant or dejected, alters the proprioceptive discharge into the ARAS. Evidence is also presented to show that patterns of contraction of the facial musculature also alter the level of activation of the reticular system.

[1] Young, J. Z. (1963), *The Life of Mammals*, Oxford University Press, London, p. 473.

[2] Gellhorn, E. (1964), 'Motion and Emotion: the role of proprioception in the physiology and pathology of the emotions', *Psychol. Rev.*, *71*, 457–472.

Thus Shakespeare may have been incorrect in supposing that 'there's no art to find the mind's construction in the face'. By putting a cheerful face on it long enough we become, in fact, cheerful. Appearance evolves into reality. Gellhorn quotes Kretschmer's opinion that 'the inner attitude may be induced by the external posture and vice versa'.

Sensory fibres are not, however, the only influences affecting the ARAS. Physiologists have shown that electrical stimulation of the cortex itself causes activity in the reticular formation. This observation has led to the concept of 'corticofugal' fibres which feedback on to the ARAS controlling its level of excitation. This concept is shown in Fig. 16.4.

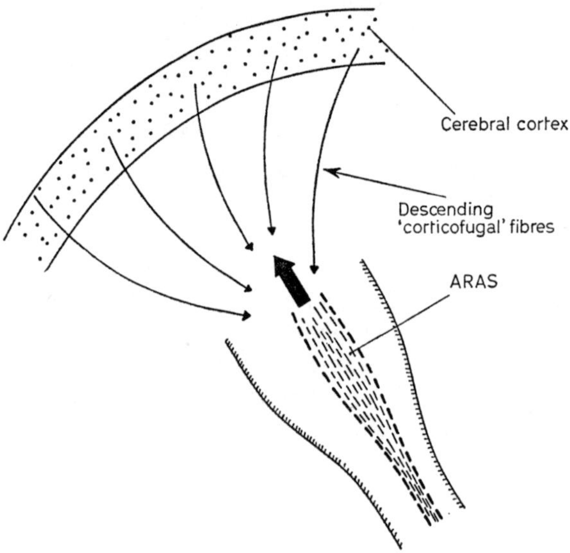


16.4 The concept of corticofugal feed-back on to the ARAS.

This is yet another instance of the complex interplay of 'feed-back' and 'feed-forward' loops which characterize so much of neurophysiology. It also indicates that 'higher' centres have some control over the level of alertness set by the ARAS. Perhaps we have all attempted to make use of this control when trying to keep awake whilst suffering from sensory deprivation due to a boring lecture or sermon.

## 16.6 The phenomenon of sleep

The nerve pathways between the cortex and nuclei in the brain stem are exceedingly intricate. The preceding section has merely outlined the wiring which is at present believed to be of most importance in maintaining a state of alertness. Perusal of any neurophysiology text will however assure the student that the situation is by no means so diagrammatic as our account may have suggested. Indeed, as is perhaps only to be expected, the neuroanatomical bases of consciousness are very far from being fully understood.[1]

Some further insights into the nature of the mechanisms responsible for attentiveness may, however, be obtained from a study of sleep. It is salutary to remember that about a third of our lives are spent in a state of unconsciousness. In some mammals, for example, the domestic cat, even larger portions of the life span may be spent asleep. In fact there seems to be a correlation between length of sleep and feeding habit. Predators tend to sleep for prolonged periods; herbivorous animals, on the other hand, make do with relatively short snatches.

Traditionally sleep is said to supervene when the organism can no longer sustain the effort of attentiveness. The brain lapses into quiescence. Proverbially, too, sleep has been likened to the inanition of death: 'The death of each day's life, sore labour's bath'. But the traditionalists and the poets may both be wrong. Sleep may be due to an active inhibition of consciousness; it may, moreover, be not merely a slackening of the brain's sinews but an alternative state of activity.

Let us briefly look at some of the evidence for these antitraditional possibilities. First it has been shown that section of the brain stem at the level of the pons can result in a nearly permanently wakeful animal.[2] Cats, which as we have seen are normally rather sleepy animals, can be induced to show a practically continuous waking EEG for several days after such an operation. This finding suggests that a centre exists in the brain stem, behind the section, which normally 'turns off' consciousness at regular intervals. In addition to this it is possible to demonstrate 'hypnogenic' areas in the brain stem. Injection of minute quantities of acetyl-choline into these regions induces sleep. This suggests that a 'multisynaptic sleep pathway' runs

[1] Routenberg, A. (1966), 'Neural mechanisms of sleep: changing views of reticular formation function', *Psychol. Rev.*, *73*, 481–499.

[2] Hernández-Péon, R. and Sterman, M. B. (1966), 'Brain Functions', *Ann. Rev. Psychol.*, *17*, 366–394 (p. 368).

up through all levels of the brain stem. The effect of acetyl-choline can be explained if we suppose that the synapses in this multisynaptic pathway are cholinergic. Lastly it has been possible to show by microelectrode investigations that many cortical neurons are rather more active during sleep than during consciousness.[1]

This approach to the phenomenon of sleep has certain heuristic consequences. It lifts some of the mystery from the phenomenon. We do not have to search so hard for an explanation for we might regard sleep as the 'normal' or 'basal' state of the brain and wakefulness as the oddity. We do not have to suggest that the state of sleep is essential for 'the stabilization of memory traces', for the 'recharging of synapses' or, more generally, for knitting up 'the ravell'd sleave of care'. We have only to 'explain' consciousness.

This approach might well please the animal behaviourist. For much ethological theory suggests that an animal acts so as to regain the *status quo ante*. In Chapter 12 we saw how many behavioural drives are designed to ensure that the main parameters of the internal environment remain constant. Clearly this approach may also be applied to the phenomena of sleep and attentiveness. We may say that consciousness is the animal's way of ensuring unconsciousness, in the same way as the chicken has been said to be the egg's way of reproducing itself. In other words wakefulness, attentiveness, supervene so that an animal may 'make its living'—may obtain food, drink and a mate, may escape predators and unpleasant environments. Having achieved these ends, having ensured that the *milieu intérieur* is as near optimal as possible, consciousness is no longer needed and the brain can be switched once more to its basal state.

### 16.7 The levels of sleep

The development of the EEG in the nineteen-thirties has proved of very great importance for the objective study of sleep. In Chapter 15 (section 15.3) we saw that the EEG records of drowsy and attentive human brains are distinctively different. Close study of the EEG records from sleeping brains shows that a number of different types of sleep may be distinguished.

Before the advent of the EEG the only means of objectively demonstrating the subjectively well known fact that sleep varies in

[1] Evarts, E. V. (1962), 'Activity of neurons in the visual cortex of the cat during sleep with low fast voltage EEG activity', *J. Neurophysiol.*, *25*, 812–816.

its 'depth' was to test the intensity of the sensory stimulus necessary to awake the sleeper. As Wilkinson[1] points out, we normally assess whether a person is asleep or awake by enquiring softly 'Are you asleep?' and if he replies, even if he replies 'Yes!', we take it he is awake. A more 'scientific' way of testing for sleep and depth of sleep is to determine the intensity with which a given note must be sounded to elicit arousal. By this means it is possible to show that the 'deepest' sleep in humans is attained within an hour or so of settling down and that this is followed by a gradual 'reascent' to consciousness. The EEG has, however, allowed investigators to explore the states of sleep in much greater detail.

Electroencephalographers recognize several different types of sleep. These types have been classified and named in different ways. The most usual classification is into four different stages although it is often very difficult to distinguish the EEG pattern of level 3 from that of level 4.

The characteristic EEG patterns are shown in Fig. 16.5. The awake, attentive, brain is characterized by rather irregular, high frequency, low amplitude oscillations. When the eyes are closed and the brain 'relaxes' into inattentiveness this irregular wave-form is replaced by the regular alpha rhythm. We discussed the characteristics of this rhythm in section 15.3. As drowsiness increases the alpha rhythm is itself replaced by lower voltage higher frequency waves.[2] This EEG pattern characterizes stage 1 sleep. As sleep becomes sounder the EEG pattern changes once again to one in which there are successive short bursts of waves with frequencies of about 14 cycles/second (sleep spindles). The brain is now in stage 2 sleep. Finally the deepest sleep of all, as judged by behavioural criteria—difficulty of arousal—is characterized by yet another EEG pattern. The waves characteristic of stage 3 and stage 4 sleep are of large amplitude and low frequency: usually from 1 to 3 cycles/second. The wave-form characteristic of stage 3 sleep is sometimes called the delta rhythm.

In both animals and humans these various stages of sleep can be shown to succeed each other in a rhythmical fashion. Bodily move-

[1] Wilkinson, R., in *New Horizons in Psychology*, Pelican Books, 1966: Chapter 13, 'Sleep and Dreams'.

[2] The terms 'relaxation', 'drowsiness', etc., are used in their psychological sense. As was pointed out in the previous section the overall physiological state of the brain may not become any less 'energetic'. It may be that activity merely shifts from one population of neurons to another as consciousness fades.

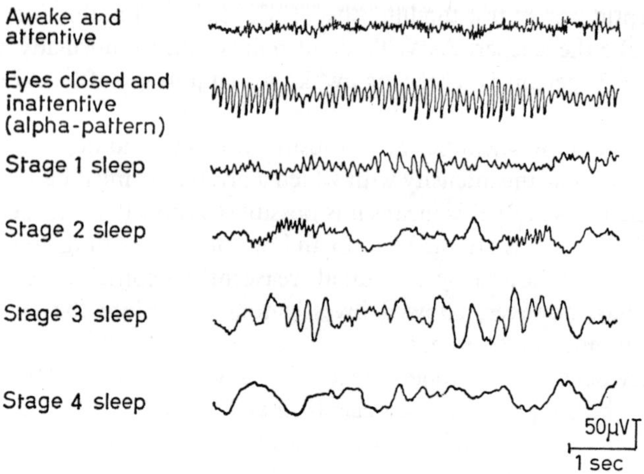


16.5 EEG correlatives of the depth of sleep. In general as sleep sets in the rapid electrical oscillation detectable in the waking brain is replaced by slower, larger amplitude oscillation. Superimposed on these more leisurely wave-forms there may, particularly in stage 2 sleep, be rapid oscillations. The latter are sometimes called sleep spindles. From Schadé, J. P. and Ford, D. H. (1965), *Basic Neurology*, Elsevier Publishing Company, Amsterdam, London, New York.

ments made during the period of sleep can also be correlated with the EEG records. This is shown in Fig. 16.6. In this figure the vertical lines at the bottom of the record register major bodily movements.

The correlation shown in Fig. 16.6 of stage 1 sleep and periods of rapid eye movement (REM) is of considerable interest. It is nowadays well known that individuals awoken during these REM periods report, in 80% of the cases, that they have been awoken in the middle of a dream. There is evidence to show that the REM periods are the physical sign of the dreamer 'looking around' at the visual events and scenery of his dream.[1] Oswald in his investigations has found that individuals who have been blind for many years do not have periods of rapid eye movement during their sleep, nor do they report visual dreams.

In addition to REM periods stage 1 sleep is also characterized by extreme flaccidity of many skeletal muscles. This is particularly marked in the neck muscles. Because of this somewhat paradoxical conjunction of muscular debility and a partially conscious brain,

[1] Oswald, J. (1964), 'Sleep accompanying dreaming', *Sci. Basis of Med. Prac.*, 102–124.

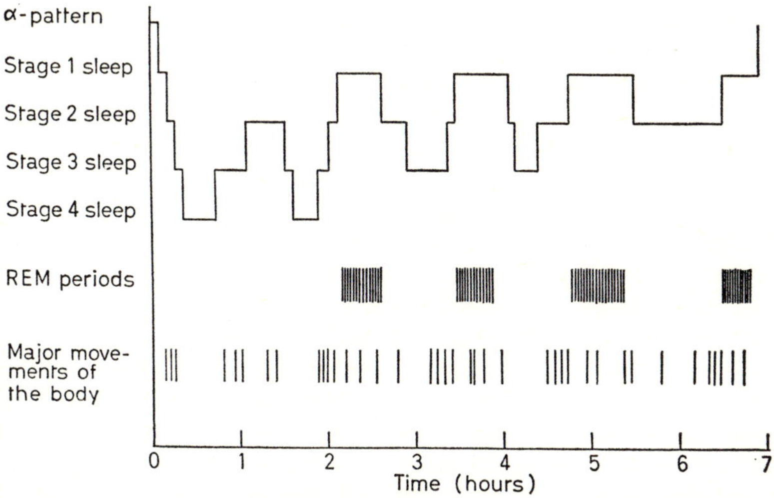


16.6 Cyclical changes in EEG pattern during sleep. The figure also shows the correlation between REM periods and stage 1 sleep; in addition it also indicates a possible relationship between stage 1 sleep and major bodily movements. Further explanation in text. Adapted from Dement, W. C. and Kleitman, N. (1957), 'Cyclical variations in EEG during sleep and their relation to eye-movements, body motility and dreaming', *EEG Clin. Neurophysiol.*, *9*, 673–690.

stage 1 sleep is sometimes referred to as 'paradoxical sleep'. Finally it is worth noting that Fig. 16.6 shows that REM periods are normally closely preceded by major bodily movements. It is possible that these movements send a shower of impulses coursing in on to the ARAS which, in turn, succeeds in partially reactivating the cortex.

It seems probable, however, that dreaming is of more neurophysiological significance than a mere accidental concomitant of the sleeper's postural readjustment. It has been shown, for example, that individuals awoken during REM periods on successive nights spend far longer than usual in this state when they are at last allowed to sleep undisturbed. To ensure that this finding was not the result merely of the sleeper's 'sub-conscious' expectation of being awoken a comparison was made with a control group. This second group of sleepers was awoken during stage 2 or stage 3 sleep. It could be shown that this latter group did not increase their REM sleep when finally left undisturbed to the same extent as the experimental group.

Similar experiments have been carried out on laboratory animals. These experiments depend on the fact, mentioned above, that REM periods are accompanied by a loss of tonus in the neck muscles. Thus if the animal is isolated on a small platform in the middle of an area of water every time it enters a REM period its head will sink until it touches the water. This ensures that the animal awakens. Somewhat surprisingly the animal shows few signs of distress. However, as in the case of humans, when finally allowed to sleep undisturbed a great deal more time than usual is spent in REM sleep.

Although REM sleeping thus seems to be of importance to the brain its precise neurophysiological function remains obscure. It is also important to bear in mind that recent work suggests that dreams are not restricted to REM periods. Individuals awoken from other stages of sleep frequently report some form of 'dream': this is normally less vivid than the dreams of REM sleep, often being reported as quiet ruminative thought. It is clear, therefore, that the realm of sleep and the biological meaning of dreams, remains nearly as mysterious and quite as fascinating as it was to the ancients and to Marcel Proust.

### 16.8 Consciousness and self-consciousness

We have based this chapter on the premiss that the behavioural sign of consciousness is attentiveness. An organism, we have said, which is inattentive to a stimulus placed in its 'perceptual space' is unconscious of it. In the preceding section we have seen that the brain according to this definition, and also according to electroencephalographic evidence, may exist in a continuum of states ranging from profound sleep (inattentiveness) to acute consciousness. We have also seen that neurobiologists are beginning to unravel the mechanisms which control the brain's position in this continuum. Before leaving the topic of consciousness, however, it will be worth while to glance briefly at another approach to its definition. This approach stems largely from the ideas of psychoanalysis originating with Sigmund Freud.

As is well known (see also section 12.1) Freud's major achievement was to demonstrate the prevalence of 'unconscious' motivation in human behaviour. Some of the most striking examples of such behaviour are displayed by obsessional neurotics. These individuals are plagued by compulsive behaviours which they cannot control and cannot understand. As a type example Freud relates[1] the case of a

[1] Freud, S., *Introductory Lectures on Psychoanalysis*, George Allen and Unwin Ltd., London, 1949, pp. 220 ff.

patient long separated from her husband. Her neurosis consisted in running out of her room into an antechamber, standing by a particular table which was covered by a deeply stained cloth and calling her maid, only to send her away again with a trivial order or with no order at all. This nonsensical ritual she repeated several times a day. Freud was able to make sense of this 'irrational' behaviour when he learnt of the patient's traumatic wedding night; of how her husband had run innumerable times from his room into hers in order to make the attempt but had each time failed; of how in the morning he had said, 'It's enough to disgrace one in the eyes of the maid who makes the beds', and seizing a convenient bottle of red ink had emptied it over the sheets.

Now from the behavioural standpoint we have adopted in this book how are we to distinguish obsessive behaviour such as this from the 'normal' non-obsessive kind? One obvious point of difference lies in the appropriateness or inappropriateness of the behaviour in the prevailing circumstances. As Freud puts it, 'It is as though these persons had not yet been able to deal adequately with the (past) situation, as if this task were still actually before them unaccomplished. . . . The young lady had not been able to "get over" the impracticability of her marriage'. Once the unconscious antecedents of the neurotic's symptoms are fully understood by the sufferer the symptoms vanish. This is in fact the crucial tenet of Freudian psychotherapy: as soon as the 'unconscious' motives have been brought fully into the patient's 'consciousness' the compulsive behaviour disappears and the patient's actions are thenceforward correctly adapted to the prevailing, the contemporary, situation.[1]

By defining unconscious motivation in this way Freudians imply that conscious motivation involves understanding the ends of one's behaviour: 'self-knowledge and self-control'. It is clear that this is a considerably narrower sense of the term 'consciousness' than we have been employing in the preceding sections of this chapter. For consciousness, in the broad sense where it is equated with attentiveness, may well exist in organisms which have no comprehension of the ends of their behaviour. There are many cases reported in the ethological literature of animals displaying behaviour quite inappropriate to their particular circumstances. For example, if the flying squirrel (*Glaucomys volans*) is hand-reared it will, if it is provided with nuts, go through all the motions of burying them and

[1] Freud, S., *loc. cit.*, p. 237.

then move away contentedly, even though the nuts are left quite exposed on the bottom of the wire cage.[1] Similarly the egg retrieval habits of many birds seem, in Freud's sense of the term, to be unconsciously motivated. If, for example, the oyster catcher is presented with a model egg much larger than normal it will forsake its own eggs for this fatuous 'supernormal' stimulus. In addition ethologists have reported many examples of 'displacement' activities in all groups of animals and these certainly seem to resemble the rituals of obsessional neurotics. In general instinctive activities appear to be triggered, as we noticed in section 12.9, by rather simple sign stimuli and the behaviour then unrolls in an automatic, compulsive, manner. However, following the behavioural definition of consciousness adopted in this chapter it is impossible to deny that, however automatic the behaviour, the animal is nevertheless conscious of, for it certainly orientates towards, the triggering sign stimulus.

There seems good evidence, therefore, that whilst going through the motions of instinctive behaviour an animal is not aware of the ends of its activity. Many authorities indeed suggest that this faculty depends on the development of those systems of symbolization which we call language. If this is in fact the case it implies that 'self-awareness' or 'self-consciousness' is a human 'invention'. However it does not seem necessary to be quite so restrictive. We may recall the fact that amongst higher animals learning of one sort or another comes to play an ever more important role in the control of behaviour. It may be that it is here that we can first discern the roots of that special type of consciousness we call 'self-consciousness'. For in learnt behaviour the end must always be significant. Even in the simple case of type 1 conditioned reflexes, if the animal does not after a number of trials achieve the desired end the reflex decays. With more complex forms of learning, especially 'vicarious trial-and-error' or 'insight' learning (section 15.2), it is hard to see how the object of the behaviour cannot but play a significant part in the animal's 'deliberations'. It does not seem impossible, therefore, that the origins of 'self-awareness', of consciousness in Freud's sense, are to be found bound up with the origins and development of learning mechanisms in higher animals.

Finally let us be clear. If consciousness in the narrow sense of 'self-consciousness' is restricted to animals which display well developed

[1] Thorpe, W. H., *Learning and Instinct in Animals*, Methuen and Co. Ltd., London, 1956, p. 19.

powers of learning, we should not overlook the fact that consciousness in the broad sense used in the preceding sections of this chapter is probably widely diffused throughout the animal kingdom. Sherrington reports how he once had the opportunity to watch under the microscope a flea 'biting'. He describes his observations in the following terms:

'The act whether reflex or not, seemed charged with the most violent emotion. Its Lilliput scale aside, the scene compared with that of the prowling lion in "Salambo". It was a glimpse suggesting a vast ocean of "affect" pervading the insect world'.[1]

[1] Sherrington, C. S., *Integrative Activity of the Nervous System*, Cambridge University Press, Second Edition, 1947, Introduction, p. 22.

# CHAPTER SEVENTEEN

# The Brain and the Mind

'It is a routine work of neurological bedside practice from certain symptoms to infer the site of cerebral lesion, i.e. to execute cerebral localisation. This localisation essentially includes such mental activities as speaking, writing or calculation. Only habituation and everyday practice can prevent us being startled at such a notion'.

Bray, E. (1964), 'Problems, possibilities and limitations of the localisation of psychic symptoms within the brain', *Cortex*, *1*, 91–92.

## 17.1 The horns of the dilemma

Immanuel Kant, we remember, derided those who supposed that the mind was localized in space: 'This problem (the localisation of the self-conscious mind in the brain) is not only insoluble but self-contradictory, because self-consciousness as an intellectual concept is free from local spatial relations'.[1]

Such has, indeed, long been the common view. The disjunction of mind and matter first clearly formulated by Galileo and Descartes in the seventeenth century has sunk deep into our view of things. With the explosive development of natural science in modern times matter has come more and more to occupy the thoughts and energies of man. This side of the Cartesian dichotomy has grown so that it quite overshadows the other side. Indeed influential philosophers have in recent years seen mind merely as an unnecessary ghost in the physiological machine. And it is the fate of ghosts to be exorcized.

Yet is this not something of a scandal? Certainly it is arguable that 'mind' has never been seen in the world, that 'consciousness' is a redundant hypothesis and hence should fall victim to Occam's razor. Yet is not the primary datum of our experience, your experience and my experience, simply this: that we are conscious beings?

[1] 'On Soemmering's paper', in *Kant* by G. Rabel, Oxford University Press, 1963, p. 281.

The celebrated mathematical philosopher K. P. Ramsey devoted his short life to an analysis of the world, 'all that is the case', into mathematically valid propositions. Yet behind the philosophizing, he admitted, was a man who saw the human frame in the foreground, and only through the human frame the cold glitter of the stars: 'My picture of the world,' he wrote, 'is drawn in perspective and not like a model to scale. The foreground is occupied by human beings and the stars are as small as threepenny bits. I don't really believe in astronomy, except as a complicated description of part of the course of human and possibly animal sensation . . .'[1]

It is not easy to fault Berkeley and his followers for believing, with Descartes, that the observer must come before the observed. 'Cogito ergo sum': there is something which doubts, that in itself cannot be doubted though all else may be dubious. Our senses are, as we all know, inclined to be faulty and subject to illusion.

Berkeley, of course, carries the argument further. He draws conclusions which we tend to find extreme: 'For can there be a nicer strain of abstraction than to distinguish the existence of sensible objects from their being perceived, so as to conceive of them existing unperceived? Light and colours, heat and cold, extension and figures —in a word the things we see and feel—what are they but so many sensations, notions or impressions of the sense? And is it possible to separate, even in thought, any of these from perception? . . . in a word all those bodies which comprise the mighty frame of the world, have not any subsistence without a mind, that their being (*esse*) is to be perceived or known'.[2]

This position appears to be the antithesis of the position adopted in the preceding sixteen chapters of this book. In Chapter 14 perception itself was treated entirely in physico-chemical terms. We might thus turn Berkeley's conclusion completely on its head and say that 'mind', 'consciousness', has no subsistence without matter, that perception cannot be conceived of except as the outcome of matter organized in a particular fashion. Are we not, therefore, ready for the third term in the Hegelian dialectic: thesis, antithesis: synthesis?

[1] Ramsey, K. P., in *Foundations of Mathematics*, Kegan Paul, Trench, Trubner and Co. Ltd., London, 1931, p. 291.

[2] Berkeley: *Principles of Human Knowledge*, Paragraphs V and VI. Everyman's Library, J. M. Dent and Sons, Ltd., London.

The advances of modern neurophysiology have both sharpened the Cartesian dilemma and at the same time tended to obscure it. For few of us realize this scandal in the depth of our culture: this schizophrenia. For, on the one hand we feel bound to assert that minds do in fact act upon bodies, and on the other that they do not so act.

On the one hand it is intolerable to assert that the words appearing on this sheet of paper are anything other than the outcome of my conscious intention. I would feel, for example, that it was a total misrepresentation of the fact if one were to allege that they were merely the result of automatic writing. Arthur Koestler tells an amusing anecdote to illustrate this point.[1] He describes an argument about human freedom at an Oxford high table. An irate Australian philosopher counters the deterministic opinions of an elderly Oxford don by threatening to punch him on the nose. The elderly gentleman is outraged that the Australian should so lose control of his actions and says so. 'My case is proved,' retorts the Australian.

Yet, on the other hand, it is intolerable to assert that minds do act on bodies. For we have seen in the previous chapters of this book that neurobiologists are well on the way towards a satisfactory physical theory of the living brain. There is just as little room for a 'strange', immaterial cause like 'mind' within the machinery of this liquid state computer as there is within the machinery of the solid state computers used to solve business problems by industrialists.

Thus we seem to be caught on the horns of a dilemma, a concealed snag in the otherwise outstandingly successful *weltanschauung* of the West. 'What is matter? never mind! What is mind? no matter!'

### 17.2 An escape from the dilemma: psychoneural unity

Is it possible to find a way out of this impasse? Is it possible to resolve this profound dualism into a unified world-view? Many eminent neurologists and neurophysiologists have thought not. Perhaps the most well known and authoritative support for dualism has come from Sir Charles Sherrington: 'That our being should consist of *two* fundamental elements offers, I suppose, no greater inherent improbability than that it should rest on one only'.[2]

At root, however, we cannot but feel, as Sherrington himself seems to have felt, that psycho-physical interactionism is a pro-

[1] Koestler, A., *The Ghost in the Machine*, Hutchinson, London, 1967, p. 214.

[2] Sherrington, C. S., *Integrative Activity of the Nervous System*, Cambridge University Press, 1947: Introduction, p. 22.

foundly unsatisfying theory. For we, all of us, in our everyday existence seem to experience the bond between 'mind' and 'matter'; we, all of us, know that 'mind' acts on 'matter' and 'matter' on 'mind'. As Sherrington, again, has put it, 'My mind does bend my arm, and (in so doing) it disturbs the sun'.[1] Yet it is a mystery which has baffled the acutest intellects to explain how an immaterial cause can affect the world of physics. The nature of the connection, the gearing, between mind and matter remains shrouded in complete darkness.

Clearly there is something very odd here, something crooked in our thinking. Perhaps we can begin to see where this crookedness comes in if we examine the recent history of an analogous problem: the animate/inanimate dichotomy. This problem—the relation of animate to inanimate creation—is, with the rise of molecular biology, being resolved. The mysterious *élan vital*, Sherrington's 'urge-to-live', has been given body. No longer is it a concept for philosophers to tangle over. It is receiving a precise physico-chemical explanation in molecular terms. In an earlier book[2] it was shown how the living cell—the so-called unit of life—has come to be regarded as a close-knit 'republic of molecules'. The properties of a cell, which no one can deny are the properties of a living organism, can be seen to emerge from certain concatenations of macromolecules dissolved in an electrolyte solution and surrounded by and interspersed with lipoprotein membranes. It can be seen, moreover, that, in principle, the origins of these molecular concatenations are explicable in terms of Darwinian natural selection. It therefore follows that, in principle, the peculiar properties of living systems are totally explicable in physico-chemical terms.

Now how does this compare with the recent history of neurophysiology? At first glance we may feel that the ferment of activity which marks the advance of modern neurophysiology is leading to a bodying-out of the concept of mind. For, in the biophysical analogy, no one is disposed to regard the cell as any less a living entity for being fundamentally a physico-chemical system. Molecular biologists would hardly be interested in studying, say, *E. coli*, at all if they were not convinced that they were studying something which is alive. The word 'living' is not dropping from the scientists' vocabulary, it is merely being more precisely defined. Similarly with mind.

[1] Sherrington, C. S., *Man on his Nature*, Penguin Books Ltd., Harmondsworth, Middlesex, 1955, p. 258.

[2] *Molecular Biology: a Structural Approach*, Faber and Faber, London, 1968.

Neurophysiological advances would seem to deepen and sharpen our formerly imprecise notions of mentality.

Yet we should be badly wrong. For, as we have been at pains to emphasize throughout this book, neurophysiology only helps us to account for the behaviour of others, and of ourselves in so far as we can observe ourselves 'from the outside': it does not illuminate the nature of our own individual experience. This can in no way be straightforwardly identified with certain highly organized concatenations of matter. The dichotomy between mind and brain, between experience and behaviour, is far more profound than that. When, in the example of Chapter 7, Jessica admires the night sky she is not aware of certain physico-chemical happenings in her occipital cortex. She sees 'the floor of heaven'. Yet the neurophysiologist would only be able to demonstrate certain action potentials, certain chemical events at synapses.

If, as Herbert Feigl points out in his comprehensive essay on the mind/brain problem,[1] any 'hard-boiled behaviourist' or 'crass materialist' refuses to accept the reality of these 'psychologisms' we have only to ask him, 'Don't you want anaesthesia if the surgeon is to operate on you? And, if so, what you want prevented is the occurrence of some (very!) raw feels of pain, is it not?'

Thus it seems that in some way both accounts must be valid. This is the position of psychoneural identity, or unity. Metaphorically the 'mental' and the 'physical' are the same thing looked at from different positions. Somewhat in the same way that NaCl and cooking salt are the same thing looked at from different intellectual backgrounds.

Let us see if we can make the meaning of this position somewhat clearer by considering, in the tradition of Galileo, a 'thought experiment'. In Chapter 13 we saw how neurosurgeons at the Montreal Neurological Institute had succeeded in evoking complex imagery and memory in the 'minds' of their patients by electrical stimulation of their cerebral cortices. Vice versa the patient may be presented with some sensory stimulus and the neurosurgeon may record the ensuing electrical events in his cortex. In both cases what is being done belongs entirely to the 'public' world. The surgeon stimulates and records the patient's response. Except that the patient can speak the situation is in no way different to that of animal experimentation.

[1] Feigl, H., 'The "Mental" and the "Physical" ', in *Minnesota Studies in the Philosophy of Science*, Vol. 2, pp. 370–498, Minnesota Press, 1958.

But, in theory, this need not be so. We can imagine that by a suitable arrangement of mirrors and automatic facilities the surgeon could investigate his own brain. This apparatus, or one similar in its essentials, has been called by Feigl and others an 'autocerebroscope'. Suppose that the autocerebroscope is so arranged that the surgeon is able to place an electrode into his own interpretative cortex. On turning on the appropriate voltage he might become aware of scenes from his past, perhaps even of the sky at night. Or, with the electrode placed in his post-central gyrus he might ask someone to pinch his toe. He could then at one and the same time feel the pain and observe the electrical events in his cortex on the screen of the cerebroscope. What are the relations between these autocerebroscopic observations and these 'feels'?

In both cases the neurosurgeon might describe his experiences under the autocerebroscope into the microphone of a tape-recorder. Later he could play back the tape and listen to his own descriptions. But, and this seems to be the crux of the matter, it *is* only a description he listens to, not a 'recreation' of the experience itself.

Similarly all our descriptions of brains and brain mechanisms, of behaviour (including the behaviour which we call speech) are, simply, descriptions. Optimists believe that in the future it will become possible to 'translate' from one set of descriptions to another. For example, reductionists believe that the many and varied activities of an animal's behaviour will one day be explicable in neurophysiological terms. But we can never substitute a description for the thing itself.

Feigl phrases this central perception in the following way: 'What is *had-in-experience* . . . is identical with the object of *knowledge by description* provided first by molar behaviour theory and this is in turn identical with what the science of neurophysiology *describes* (or, rather, will describe when sufficient progress has been achieved) as processes in the central nervous system, perhaps especially in the cerebral cortex.'[1]

We have said that our autocerebroscopist when listening to the play-back of his experience under the machine listens only to a description, not a 'recreation' of the experience itself. This is only *completely* true in our second example. It is, anyway, rather difficult to give an accurate description of exactly what it feels like to have

[1] Feigl, H. (1958), *loc. cit.*, p. 446.

one's toe pinched. In our first example a linguistically gifted autocerebroscopist might in fact go some way towards 'recreating' or evoking the original experience by an impassioned description. It is not difficult to imagine a neurophysiological mechanism for this evocation. We need only suppose that the pattern of sounds emanating from the tape-recorder actuates neuronal circuits similar to or identical with those activated by the original experience. This ability to 'map' experience into a linguistic form is, according to many authorities, what most distinguishes us from the rest of the animal kingdom. The mapping of emotional experience into language is also probably what Wordsworth had in mind when he defined poetry as 'emotion recollected in tranquillity'. It is the poet's job, according to Wordsworth,[1] to 'map' the emotive response to experience in such a way that the original emotional terrain can once more be recognized.

That this cartography is possible implies that although each one of us is unique, we nevertheless possess *structurally* similar emotional landscapes or, to use Hopkins' term, 'inscapes'. It is important to notice that it is only the structure, the organization, of the inscapes which is common; the individual features, as we have been at pains to emphasize, are unique. It is this which has made the mind/brain duality so intractable. The perceptual worlds of each one of us are built of experiental 'thises' which, to use Bertrand Russell's formulation, are 'egocentric particulars'. That this is a commonplace notion is emphasized by the popularity of the conundrum which asks what each of us experiences when he reports that he sees a colour such as 'red' or 'blue'. It is impossible to say; it is merely a feature of our education, in a wide sense of this term, that we all apply the same word to the same segment of the electromagnetic spectrum. To emphasize this commonplace let us consider another 'thought experiment'.

Suppose that the optic nerve of one individual is 'wired' into the occipital cortex of another. Would the second individual experience the visual world of the first? Would he at last know what 'red' looked like to the first? The answer, according to the theory advanced in this section, would be: no. The optic nerve of the first individual would transmit certain patterns of action potentials to the visual cortex of the second. It is the job of this cortex to interpret, if it can, these signals. It is the physical state of this cortex which is the

[1] William Wordsworth: *Preface to the 'Lyrical Ballads'*, Thomas Nelson and Sons Ltd., London, 1937.

material correlative of the psychic apprehension. If we transplanted the occipital cortex in addition to the optic nerve it then becomes difficult to say exactly *who* is experiencing the 'raw feel'.

It is hoped that this brief excursion into the future terrors of spare-part surgery serves to emphasize the uniqueness of our individual experience. For it is this uniqueness which makes the mind/brain problem unique. Metaphorically we experience our egocentric particulars 'internally' as our consciousness; externally, if we are provided with an autocerebroscope, we can observe them as action potentials in the brain.

The egocentric particular, the 'raw feel', is thus a singularity which may be looked at from two aspects. Only in ourselves, with the help of a so far uninvented autocerebroscope, can we know both aspects. In others, despite the help of the poets, musicians and other artists, we can only fully know the 'external aspect'.

'Much is unknowable.
No problem shall be faced
Until the problem is;
I, born to fog, to waste,
Walk through hypothesis,
An individual.'[1]

### 17.3 Evidence for the hypothesis of psychoneural unity

In this section we turn back from 'thought experiments' to the disciplines of the lab. Let us look briefly at some of the evidence which suggests that physiological ($\varphi$) and psychical ($\psi$) events are in fact the same 'happenings' viewed from different 'standpoints'. In fact we have already noticed in several places in this book, particularly in Chapter 13, that ($\varphi$–$\psi$) identity is an assumption implicit in much neurophysiology.

Now we stressed in section 17.2 that the autocerebroscope is an entirely imaginary piece of apparatus. It makes sense to use it in the argument just as it made sense for pre-war positivists to discuss the far side of the moon in arguments about the origins of lunar craters. For the construction of an autocerebroscope is in principle possible and may be accomplished in fact in the far-distant future. In the absence of this piece of apparatus it is, however, impossible to obtain

[1] From 'Human Condition', in *The Sense of Movement* by Thom Gunn, Faber and Faber Ltd., London, 1968.

copper-bottomed evidence for ($\varphi$–$\psi$) unity. All we can do with present-day electrophysiological hardware is to correlate behavioural phenomena with neurophysiological 'central states'. With animals we can correlate sensory stimuli or bodily movements with electrophysiological events in the nerves or brain. With humans we can add linguistic behaviour to the behavioural phenomena we observe and try to correlate this with physiological measurements. We are left, however, with the necessity to make the crucial assumption that the linguistic behaviour corresponds to the same psychical state ($\psi$) which we ourselves experience when using identical language.

Serious doubt of the validity of this assumption is, however, as Schopenhauer points out, only to be found amongst the inhabitants of a 'madhouse' where 'it needs not so much refutation as cure'.[1] Let us therefore make the usual assumption that the psychical states of others exist and are very much like our own.

Now one way in which we might approach the problem of adducing evidence for the hypothesis of psychoneural identity is by attempting to quantify our 'raw feels'. We might, for example, try to find out how the sensation of 'loudness' varies when the physical stimulus is varied. We might then try to find out whether the neurophysiological response to the same stimulus varies in the same way.

Over two dozen sensory experiences have been quantified by Stevens and his co-workers at Harvard.[2] Stevens divides perceptual continua into two classes: those of which we ask 'How much?' and those of which we ask, 'What kind?' and 'Where?' These divisions roughly correspond to the classical distinction between quantitative and qualitative continua. For example, the first type of perceptual continua, called by Stevens *prothetic* continua, could be represented by 'loudness', whilst the second type, *metathetic* continua, could be represented by pitch.

It was found that all the fourteen perceptual continua Stevens examined, ranging from loudness, through taste, visual area, numerousness to flash rate, could be described by a very simple formula. In a typical experiment the investigator would present the subject with a series of sensory stimuli, say different intensities of light or different strengths of electric shock, and ask him to assign to each sensation in the series a number from a short scale corres-

[1] Schopenhauer, A.: *The World as Will and Representation,* Vol. 1, p. 104, translated by E. F. J. Payne, Falcon's Wing Press, 1958.

[2] Stevens, S. S. (1957), 'On the psychophysical law', *Psychol. Rev., 64,* 153–181.

ponding to its apparent magnitude.[1] Taking the mean of a large number of subjects it turns out that in all the prothetic continua so far tested the sensory 'magnitude', $\psi$, and the physical magnitude of the stimulus, S, are related by the following simple formula:

$$\psi = k.S^n \qquad \ldots\ldots (17.1)$$

In equation 17.1 'k' is an arbitrary constant depending on the units used for measuring the physical stimulus and the exponent 'n' varies from one type of stimulus to another. For example 'n' is about 0·33 when brightness is being estimated and about 3·5 when the sensation is an electric shock. Figure 17.1 shows the form of the graph obtained when $\psi$ is plotted against S for these two perceptual continua.

Fig. 17.1 emphasizes that whereas the perceptual magnitude of

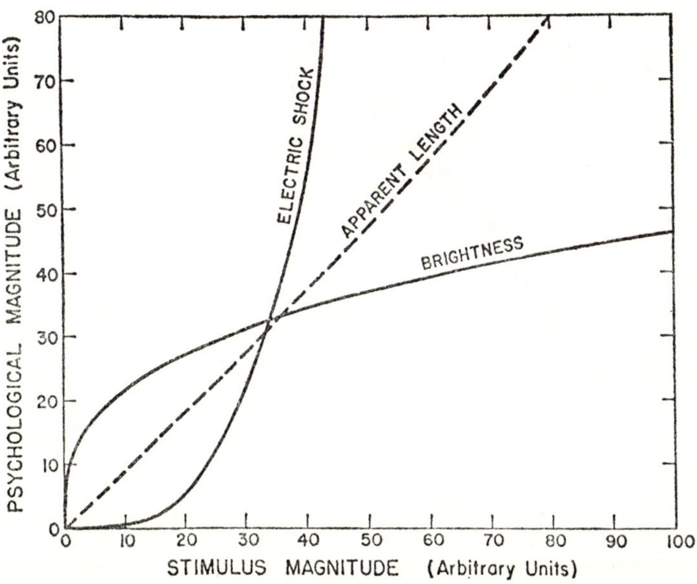


17.1 Psychophysical graph for three perceptual continua. Explanation in text. From Stevens, S. S. (1966), 'Quantifying the sensory experience', in *Mind, Matter and Method*, edited by Feyeraband, P. K. and Maxwell, G., University of Minesota Press, Minneapolis © Copyright 1966 University of Minnesota.

[1] Stevens has also shown that a similar relation can be obtained when the subject is not asked to report verbally the apparent magnitude of the stimulus but instead instructed to estimate the sensory magnitude by pressing a hand dynamometer with varying degrees of force.

an electric shock grows very much more rapidly than the physical stimulus the opposite is the case with the perception of brightness. Now it is not very easy to compare curves such as those shown in Fig. 17.1. This task is made very much easier if equation 17.1 is converted to a logarithmic form:

$$\log \psi = \log k + n \log S$$

$$\text{or,} \quad \log \psi = K + n \log S \qquad \ldots\ldots (17.2)$$

17.2 will be recognized as the equation to a straight line. Hence by plotting our psychophysical equation in the form of 17.2 the curves of Fig. 17.1 will be transformed into straight lines with slopes equal to the exponent 'n'. This transformation is shown in Fig. 17.2.

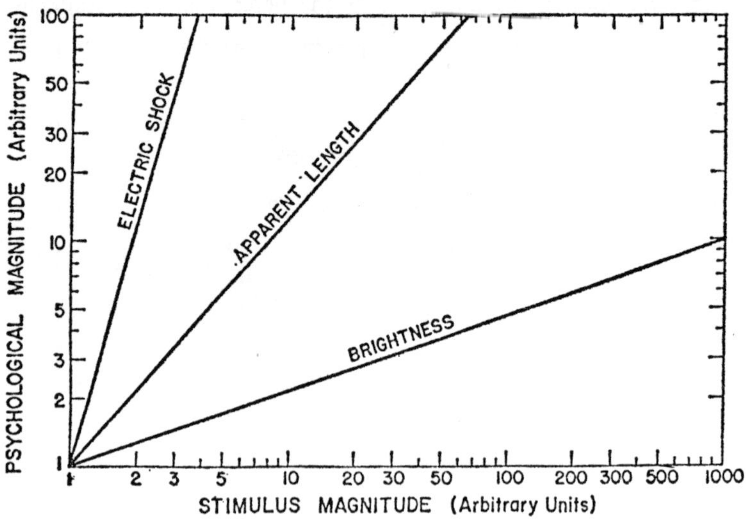


17.2 The three continua of Fig. 17.1 are here plotted on log-log co-ordinates. The slope of the line now corresponds to the exponent of the function which relates the physical and psychical continua. From Stevens, S. S. (1966), *loc. cit.*

The lines of Fig. 17.2 suggest that a very simple relation holds between the physical stimulus and the psychical experience. The next step in our argument must therefore be to see whether there is any evidence that a relationship of the same form holds between stimulus and neurophysiological response.

This question has been taken up by Mountcastle and Werner. These investigators have carried out a series of experiments in which the response of single mechanoreceptive nerve fibres from the hairy skin of monkeys and cats has been recorded.[1] The results of a large number of recordings show that the response of these fibres to variation in pressure on the skin follows a law of the same general type as the psychophysical law discussed above. In other words it was possible to show that where *R* is the impulse frequency in the fibre and *S*, as before, is the stimulus, the following relation obtains:

$$R = k.S^n \qquad \ldots\ldots (17.3)$$

The value for the exponent, *n*, is about 0·5; this value turns out to be closely similar to the value of *n* in the psychophysical equation describing human perception of skin indentation.

Now a mechanoreceptive nerve fibre is not, of course, the cerebral cortex. Before pressure information is delivered to the cortex it will have passed through several relays, passed across several synaptic junctions. Nonetheless it cannot but be profoundly suggestive to find that the same law governs the response of these sensory fibres as governs the psychical response of humans to a similar stimulus.

Next let us look at some rather different evidence which also seems to support the hypothesis of psychoneural unity. In Chapter 14 the electrophysiological work of Hubel and Wiesel on the mammalian visual cortex was described. We noticed that it was possible to detect the existence of neurons which responded optimally to certain 'trigger' features in the visual field. These features ranged from lines orientated at various angles to quite complicated geometrical forms. It is instructive to bear this work in mind whilst considering some of the important work which has been done in recent years on stabilized visual images.

It has been known for some years that the eye is never held completely stationary in its orbit when an object is fixated. Instead it is subjected to a high frequency tremor so that the image flicks from one set of retinal photoreceptors to another. In 1952 Ditchburn and his colleagues[2] devised an ingenious optical system, incorporating a contact lens on the eyeball, which ensures that the image of any object the observer fixates does, in fact, remain stationary on the retina. With this system the object periodically disappears followed

[1] Werner, G. and Mountcastle, V. B. (1965), 'Stimulus-response in cutaneous afferents', *J. Neurophysiol., 28*, 359–397.

[2] Ditchburn, R. W. and Ginsborg, B. L. (1952), 'Vision with a stabilised retinal image', *Nature, 170*, 36–37.

by intermittent reappearances. It is possible that this sensory phenomenon is due to successive bleaching and regeneration of the visual pigments in the photoreceptors on which the image falls.

Subsequent work,[1] however, has revealed a more complicated and a more interesting situation. It is found that when the stabilized image is of a fairly complicated object (Fig. 17.3) complete parts of the image disappear and reappear independently of each other. For example, entire straight lines (Fig. 17.3 (a)) tend to vanish and materialize as units and, in particular, circles seem to have a very high unitary value, tending to disappear and reappear *in toto* twice as often as any other figure tested.

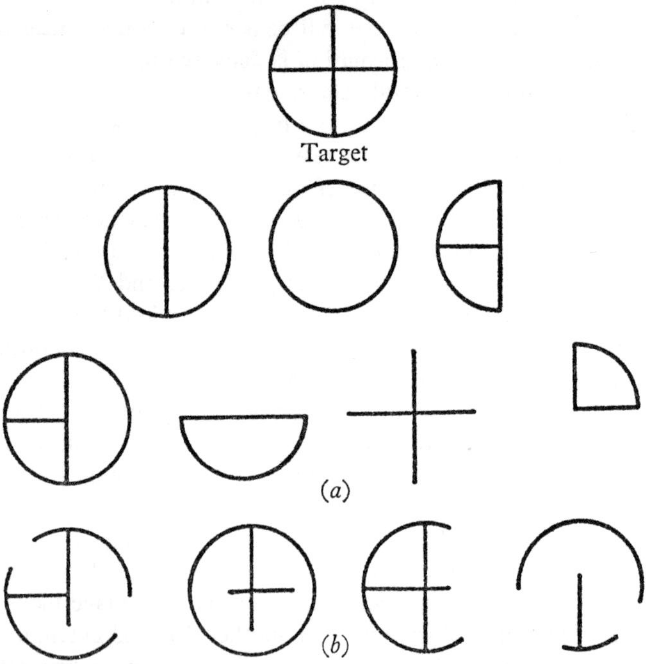


17.3 Examples of (a) 'structured' and (b) 'random' fragmentation effects seen when the target at top is viewed under stabilized conditions. From Evans, C. R. (1965), 'Some studies of pattern perception using a stabilised retinal image', *Brit. J. Psychol.*, *56*, 121–133.

[1] Pritchard, R. M., Heron, W. and Hebb, D. O., (1960), 'Visual perception approached by the method of stabilised images', *Can. J. Psychol.*, *14*, 67–77.

Evans, C. R. (1965), 'Some studies of pattern perception using a stabilised retinal image', *Brit. J. Psychol.*, *56*, 121–133.

It is difficult to believe that the latter occurrences are due to the satiation of retinal photoreceptors. It seems much more likely that cortical units like those investigated by Hubel and Wiesel are responsible. If this does indeed turn out to be the case we should have another instance where a sensory experience turns out to be the 'interior' view of a physiological occurrence.

### 17.4 The ethical consequences of the identity theory: 'free-will' or 'predestination'?

'*To the subject of knowing, who appears as an individual only through his identity with the body, this body is given in two entirely different ways. It is given in intelligent perception as representation, as object among objects. But it is also given in quite a different way, namely as what is known immediately to everyone and is denoted by the word* will. *Every true act of will is also at once and inevitably a movement of his body; he cannot actually act without at the same time being aware that it appears as a movement of the body. The act of will and the action of the body are not two different states objectively known, connected by the bond of causality; they do not stand in the relation of cause and effect, but are one and the same thing, though given in entirely different ways, first quite directly, and then in perception for the understanding.*'

Schopenhauer: *The World as Will and Representation*, Vol. 1, p. 100, translated by E. F. J. Payne, Falcon's Wing Press, 1958.

Feigl following Schopenhauer apostrophizes the mind/brain problem as the 'world-knot'. Its deep centrality was emphasized in sections 1 and 2 of this chapter. Not only does this problem cause profound difficulty on the sensory side (what is the status of a 'raw-feel'?), but it raises equally puzzling issues on the motor side. Not only does the Cartesian split induce the fantasy of a ghostly observer within the skull examining the input from the sense organs, much as a ship's captain might brood in the shelter of a chartroom over the patterns on a radar screen, but it also conjures up another ghostly figure (or is it the same one?) who initiates our bodily movements. We are so accustomed to following the chain of cause and effect in the physical world—from the murder bullet, to the gun, to the cartridge, to the firing mechanism, to the trigger, to the hand which pulls the trigger—that we begin to imagine a something or a someone within or behind the brain who sends out impulses down the nerves to, perhaps, the muscles of the hand. And yet, of course, on reflection we can see the deep absurdity of this idea or set of ideas. The 'buck' stops and starts with the brain, it is not passed down an infinite series of bureaucratic ghosts. Nor is there any ghostly 'I' which commands the finger muscle to contract. If we merely say or think, 'Move, muscle, move!' nothing happens—the finger remains limp on the trigger. In this connection we may remember the incisive story told of the first time a railway engine appeared at a remote country station. The local schoolmaster, taking his duties seriously, explained to the wondering villagers just how the great machine worked. At the end of his exposition, after having described the expansion of steam, the action of pistons, the arrangement of valves he paused for questions. Only one came: But where amongst all these pipes and boilers is there room for the horse?

Our acts, then, like our 'raw-feels' seem to be 'what is had-in-experience'. In others we can observe them 'externally' either by behavioural analysis or by electrophysiological techniques. In ourselves we can, in addition, observe them 'internally'. The terms 'internal' and 'external' are, of course, used metaphorically.

It is clear that this position is closely similar to the central thesis of Schopenhauer's philosophy: 'Every true, genuine, immediate act of will is also at once and directly a manifest act of the body.'[1]

Since Schopenhauer's day science, if not philosophy, has moved on. It might thus be argued that some of the experiments described in Chapter 11 allow us to separate the 'act of will' from the bodily movement. We may recall, for instance, the unfortunate amphibian which desiring to advance on a tasty morsel backed, because of certain operations on its motor nerves, remorselessly away (section 11.5). We can, however, translate Schopenhauer's 'act of body' into 'physical event in the brain'. This event can, in principle, be observed by means of the appropriate electrophysiological apparatus.

Let us now look at the consequences of this identity theory. If our volitions are (merely) the 'interior' aspect of certain physical happenings in our brains then we are at once presented with the problem of determinism. Indeed we appear to be faced by another dilemma. The major conviction of our own experience is that so far as our actions are concerned we are free. Few of those who are

[1] Schopenhauer, *loc. cit.*, p. 101.

not metaphysicians would disagree with Dr. Johnson's opinion: 'We are free and there's an end on't.'[1] I am convinced, for example, that I may freely choose between taking up my pen or putting it down, between finishing this sentence or not finishing it.

Yet the other horn of the dilemma is equally convincing. The brain, as we have tried to show throughout this book, is a piece of physico-chemical machinery. Mind-baffling in its complexity undoubtedly, but in principle no different from any other physical system. Now physical systems of magnitudes greater than those of subatomic particles may be described, in principle, by the laws of classical mechanics,[2] and these laws, as is well known, admit rigorous prediction. The best known statement of this position is due to Laplace: 'An intelligence acquainted with all the forces of nature, and with the positions at any given moment of the parts thereof, would include in one and the same formula the movements of the largest bodies and those of the smallest atoms'.[3] Such an intelligence given the state of the universe at time $t_1$ could, by use of the formula, calculate its state at any time, $t_2$, in the future. If this is even theoretically possible what then becomes of our intuition of freedom?

It is not difficult to see the homology between this dilemma and the dilemma set out in section 17.1. Its source is, of course, the same: the dichotomy between ourselves and others. Let us see if we can find a solution.

[1] Quoted by McIntyre, A. C. (1957), 'Determinism', *Mind,* LXVI, p. 40.

[2] It has been argued that the Heisenberg uncertainty relations which obtain in the subatomic world might, by a process of amplification, provide an answer to the determinist. However, apart from the philosophical blunder of confusing unpredictability of outcome with freedom of action there is no evidence in neurobiology to support this line of argument. The physical theory of the brain outlined in this book shows it to be an immensely complicated piece of machinery, but a piece of machinery firmly governed by the laws of the macroscopic world. It seems likely that the smallest unit of action is the packet of transmitter molecules released into the synaptic cleft, a packet, somewhat confusingly, called a *quantum* of transmitter substance. But a quantum of acetyl-choline or other transmitter consists of several hundred *molecules* whereas the physicist's quantum indeterminacy only becomes noticeable at the level of subatomic particles—many orders of magnitude smaller than a single molecule. But perhaps of even greater significance is the fact that the neuronal output from the brain which governs the animal's behaviour is the result of multitudinous cerebral operations proceeding in parallel. The whole design makes for stability, dependability, not eccentricity (see also section 12.2).

[3] Laplace, *Philosophical Essay on Probabilities,* 1840, translated by F. W. Truscott and F. L. Emory, in *Source Book in Astronomy,* edited by H. Shapley and H. E. Howarth, McGraw Hill, Inc., 1929, p. 169.

First of all let us be sure what the argument is all about. It is not about caprice. It is about the possibility of moral behaviour. It is about the validity of the words 'praiseworthy' or 'blameworthy' when they are used to qualify statements about human behaviour. It is about the idea of responsibility. Clearly, then, it is not a question which can in any way be shrugged off.

We have stressed that the argument is not about caprice. For this is the opposite of responsible behaviour. Only of fully intended, of fully deliberated, behaviour can we use the word 'responsible' or attach the notions of praise or blame. Of capricious behaviour, if the results are bad, we can always say, 'Well, he or she didn't really mean it'. In the same way we are not accustomed, in modern times at least,[1] to suppose that the behaviour of animals is 'praiseworthy' or 'blameworthy' and, again, we are likely to excuse the activities of the obsessional neurotic with the phrase, 'He didn't know what he was doing, he couldn't help it'. It is thus 'self-conscious' (section 16.8), 'rational', behaviour with which we are concerned.

Now here we meet with a paradox within our dilemma. For to a large extent responsible behaviour is, precisely, predictable behaviour. As R. E. Hobart points out, 'It is of the very best of men that we say, "I am sure of him".'[2] Thus at this level the clash between free-will and determinism is misconceived. The 'freest' man, the most responsible moral agent, is at the same time the most predictable.

Nonetheless, in spite of this insight, a problem seems to remain at a more profound level. For if, *pace* Laplace, our brains are like clockwork completely predictable then what sense is there in distinguishing 'the best of men'? It just so happens that this man is built like this whilst his neighbour, feckless and unreliable, just so happens to be built like that. The first is no 'better' than the second except in the sense that a more accurate watch is better than a less accurate watch. To neither can we impute praise or blame; in an ultimate sense neither is responsible for his actions. In short our fundamental intuition about ourselves is an illusion. If this is indeed the case something seems to happen to the so-called 'dignity' of man.

[1] It is interesting to notice that until comparatively recent times in Europe animals have often been assumed to be responsible moral agents. The *Encyclopaedia Britannica* mentions, for example, the case of a she-ass condemned to death in France in 1750 but afterwards pardoned because of excellent character references!

[2] Hobart, R. E. (1934), 'Free-will as involving determinism and inconceivable without it', *Mind, N.S., 43,* 1–27.

There seems to be one small chink in the prison-house of cause and effect. This chink can be traced, of course, to the self/not-self dichotomy we have been examining. Let us look again at our autocerebroscopist. Suppose his instrument tells him all he needs to know about his brain state, $\varphi_1$, at time $t_1$, the present. According to Laplace's principle he should then be able to predict his brain state, $\varphi_2$, at time $t_2$, in the future. Now according to the identity theory which we have been propounding it is possible to state, in general, $\varphi \equiv \psi$ (where $\varphi$ and $\psi$ have the meanings assigned in section 17.3). In other words the psychical state, $\psi$, *is* the brain state, $\varphi$, seen from another standpoint. Hence it looks as though our autocerebroscopist should be able to calculate, given adequate 'real time' computing facilities, what his brain state at any time in the future will be, and hence know in advance what choices he is going to make.

There seems, however, to be a snag in the determinist's argument. The location of this snag is analysed by MacKay in the twenty-first Eddington Memorial Lecture: *Freedom of Action in a Mechanistic Universe.*[1] The essence of the analysis is to bring out the obvious conundrum of how a knowledge of the future might affect our actions in the present. To be told one is to murder one's father might, one supposes, have a considerable effect on one's subsequent activities. To be told in complete detail exactly how one is to do it and of all the circumstances leading up to the fatal meeting would, one supposes, ensure that one never sets out on the road to Thebes. This is the essence of the problem of freedom of action. But it seems that our autocerebroscopist must, zombie-like, go through all the motions whether he wants to or no. Again we feel our minds beginning to swim a little: there must be a flaw in the argument.

The flaw is simply this: as soon as the autocerebroscopist *knows* his future brain state, $\varphi_2$, it affects his present psychical state, $\psi_1$, and hence by the principle of identity, his present brain state $\varphi_1$. This, after all is the essence of the identity theory. His present brain state, $\varphi_1$, is consequently changed to some other state, $\varphi_n$, which it *would not have achieved* if the knowledge of state $\varphi_2$ had not been available to it. Hence $\varphi_2$ will not necessarily follow.

Note, however, that an observer *who kept his knowledge to himself* could, according to our mechanistic brain theory, predict state $\varphi_2$ and hence $\psi_2$, given a knowledge of $\varphi_1$. But this is, after all, only

[1] Mackay, D. M., *Freedom of Action in a Mechanistic Universe*, Cambridge University Press, 1967.

what we mean when we say 'we are sure of him', he will not pocket the £1,000 note we left in the room with him.

Note, furthermore, that the possession of this knowledge would make no difference to the actions of an obsessional neurotic (section 16.8), nor, for that matter, to the instinctive behaviours of animals. For the neurotic would not, in so far as he is neurotic, take this intelligence into account in organizing his subsequent behaviour. The knowledge would make no difference to his mental state $\psi$. He is, as it were, 'beside himself': a mere spectator of his actions, and spectators, as we have seen, can predict. For as the knowledge of the predicted tragedy makes no difference to the protagonist's $\psi_1$ it, according to our hypothesis, has no effect on $\varphi_1$, and it follows that $\varphi_2$ can be predicted from the Laplacian formula.

Thus we might conclude this section and with it this book by suggesting that freedom of action and in consequence the possibility of a moral universe has entered the world with the evolution of self-awareness. What this morality might be, whether a *summum bonum* exists, and if it exists whether it is God, man or human society may be left to theologians and moral philosophers. All we have sought to establish here is that the physical brain theory adumbrated in this book does not eliminate the very possibility of human freedom: the possibility upon which all ethical systems are built.

# APPENDIX

# Evaluation of the Nernst Equation

It will be remembered that the equation may be written in the following form:

$$V_I = \frac{RT}{ZF} \ln \frac{[I]_o}{[I]_i}$$

where $V_I$=the electrical gradient across the membrane due to the distribution of the ion, I.

I = the ion under consideration.
R = 8·31 joules/mole/degree absolute.
T = 291°A (18°C).
Z = the valence of the ion, I.
F = 96,500 coulombs/mole (the Faraday).
ln x = 2·303 $\log_{10}$ x.

Hence for a univalent anion where Z = −1,

$$V_I = \frac{8{\cdot}31 \times 291 \times 2{\cdot}303}{-1 \times 96{,}500} \log_{10} \frac{[I]_o}{[I]_i} \text{ volts}$$

i.e.

$$V_I = -0{\cdot}058 \log_{10} \frac{[I]_o}{[I]_i} \text{ volts.}$$

Thus using the values for the concentrations of $Cl^-$, $K^+$ and $Na^+$ given on page 99, $V_{Cl}$, $V_K$ and $V_{Na}$ may be calculated:

$$\begin{aligned} V_{Cl} &= -0{\cdot}058 \log_{10} \frac{540}{40} \\ &= -0{\cdot}058 \log_{10} (13{\cdot}5) \\ &= -0{\cdot}058(1 + 0{\cdot}1303) \\ &= -0{\cdot}064 \text{ volts} \\ &= -64 \text{ mV.} \end{aligned}$$

$$
\begin{aligned}
V_K &= +0{\cdot}058 \log_{10} \frac{10}{400} \\
&= +0{\cdot}058 \log_{10} (0{\cdot}025) \\
&= +0{\cdot}058(-2 + 0{\cdot}3979) \\
&= -93 \text{ mV.} \\
V_{Na} &= +0{\cdot}058 \log_{10} \frac{460}{50} \\
&= +0{\cdot}058 \log_{10} (9{\cdot}2) \\
&= +0{\cdot}058(0 + 0{\cdot}9638) \\
&= +56 \text{ mV.}
\end{aligned}
$$

The reader may find that his insight into membrane biophysics is increased if he inserts different values of $Cl^-$, $K^+$ and $Na^+$ into the equation and discovers how the membrane potential is affected. Note that the equation only considers one ion at a time and is only valid when that ion is freely diffusible (see Chapter 2).

# Glossary

## 1. Units and symbols

A = Angstrom unit, i.e. $10^{-8}$ cms.

Coulomb = Electric current is conventionally measured in amperes. The quantity of electricity which flows along a conductor when one ampere of current flows for one second is defined as one coulomb.

$\triangle$ = Delta, a symbol denoting the difference between two quantities.

Dyne = The c.g.s. unit of force. A force of one dyne applied to a mass of one gram produces an acceleration of one centimetre per second per second.

Erg = The c.g.s. unit of work or energy. Work of value one erg is done when a force of one dyne (q.v.) acts through a distance of one centimetre.

ln = $\text{Log}_e$ or natural logarithm.

Mole = The molecular weight of a substance in grams. For example the molecular weight of NaCl is 58·44. It follows that 58·44 gms. is the mole or gm. molecular weight of this molecule.

Molar solution = If a mole (q.v.) of any substance is dissolved in one litre of a suitable solvent the resulting solution is said to be molar with respect to the solute.

mM = millimolar—a solution one thousandth the concentration of a molar solution (q.v.).

msec. = millisecond—one thousandth part of a second.

mV = millivolt—one thousandth part of a volt.

$\mu$ = micron, i.e. $10^{-4}$ cms.

$\mu_A^\alpha$ = chemical potential of a substance A in phase $\alpha$.

$\bar{\mu}_I^\alpha$ = electrochemical potential of a substance I in phase $\alpha$.

## 2. Terms

*Affect:* Mental disposition; emotional 'tone'; subjective feeling.

*Afferent:* A nerve (or blood vessel) conducting towards a centre. Afferent nerves conduct impulses from outlying parts of the body towards the C.N.S. (q.v.). Afferent nerves are also called sensory nerves.

*Amnesia:* Loss of memory.

*Anion:* A negatively charged ion, for example the chloride ion, $Cl^-$. The term derives from the fact that such ions, when in solution, move towards a positive electrode (anode).

*Aphasia:* A disorder of speech brought about by damage to the brain. Various types of aphasia are recognized. All are impairments of the ability to formulate and/or use symbols.

*Apraxia:* The inability to carry out a skilled movement. This inability is not due to paralysis, sensory defect or deficiency of the understanding.

*Atrophy:* Wasting away of an organ or tissue.

*Autonomic nervous system:* That part of the peripheral nervous system (q.v.) which controls those activities of the body which appear to occur automatically. Examples of such activities are the movements of the digestive tract, the beating of the heart, the secretion of sweat by the sudorific glands. The autonomic nervous system is customarily divided into two major parts: the sympathetic and the parasympathetic systems. Most of the organs innervated by the autonomic nervous system receive fibres from both divisions of the system. In general the two divisions exert antagonistic influences on the organ innervated. Thus whilst the sympathetic nerve to the heart accelerates its beat the parasympathetic nerve slows it. The consequence of this 'double innervation' is that the viscera are held in a state of 'dynamic equilibrium' between two opposing tendencies.

*Betz cells:* Large pyramidal cells located in the mammalian motor cortex. Their diameters range from $11\mu$ to $20\mu$.

*Billion:* In this book a billion is defined as one thousand million, i.e. $1 \times 10^9$.

*Cambrian:* A geological period stretching from 600 million B.C. to 500 million B.C.

*Catabolism:* The break-down of complex organic molecules into simpler units.

*Cation:* A positively charged ion, for example the potassium ion, $K^+$. The term derives from the fact that such ions, when in solution, move towards the negative electrode (cathode).

*Central nervous system (C.N.S.):* A mass of nervous tissue which co-ordinates the behaviour of an animal. In the vertebrates this consists of the brain and spinal cord, in the invertebrates it consists of solid cords of nervous tissue usually associated with larger masses called ganglia (q.v.).

*Cephalopoda:* A group of marine molluscs including the cuttle-fish, squids, octopods and nautili. These molluscs possess a definitely formed head with well developed eyes. Surrounding the head are arms or tentacles: hence the group's name.

*Chiasma:* Two lines placed across one another in the form of a letter 'X'. The optic chiasma is thus the cross-over position of the optic nerve fibres.

*Cilia:* Minute, usually motile, hair-like structures projecting from the surface of certain cells.

*Contralateral:* The opposite side. For example some optic nerve fibres from the *left* retina run to the *right* cerebral hemisphere.

*Coronal section:* The coronal suture separates the frontal bone from the more posterior parietal bones of the skull. A coronal section accordingly runs down in a left–right plane through body and brain.

*Dorsal:* Appertaining to the back of an animal.

*Efferent:* A nerve (or blood vessel) conducting away from a centre. Efferent nerves conduct impulses away from the C.N.S. (q.v.) towards the effector organs. Efferent nerves are also called motor nerves.

*Epilepsy:* A disease caused by sudden transient alterations in brain activity often preceded by certain psychic or neuromuscular symptoms and accompanied by alterations in consciousness.

*Epistemology:* The branch of philosophy which discusses the nature of knowledge and how it is obtained.

*Epithelium:* A sheet or tube of firmly coherent cells with little, if any, intercellular substance. Epithelial tissue lines body cavities and tubes and covers the surface of the body.

*Ganglion:* A concentration or mass of perikarya. Ganglia appear in the C.N.S. (q.v.) of invertebrates and just outside the C.N.S. of vertebrates. For example the dorsal (or posterior) root ganglia of spinal nerves house the perikarya of sensory neurons entering the spinal cord; sympathetic ganglia house the perikarya of the final motor neurons of the sympathetic system (q.v.).

*Gestalt:* Form, pattern, organization.

*Gyrus:* An eminence between two fissures, or sulci, on the surface of the cerebral cortex.

*Ipsilateral:* The same side. For example some of the optic nerve fibres from the *left* retina run to the *left* cerebral hemisphere.

*j.n.d.:* Just noticeable difference. This is a term used in psychophysics to denote the smallest discriminable change in the intensity of a sensory stimulus.

*Lateral line system:* A system of sense organs developed in aquatic vertebrates (fish and amphibia) which is sensitive to pressure changes, especially vibrational changes, in the surrounding water. The system consists of a number of pores or canals arranged in a line along the side of the body and in a more complicated pattern on the head.

*Mesozoic:* A geological era stretching from about 225 million B.C. to 135 million B.C.

*Metabolism:* The chemical processes occurring within a living organism.

*Monomer: see* Polymer.

*Motor neuron: see* Efferent neuron.

*Nerve, cranial:* In mammals there are twelve pairs of cranial nerves. They originate in the brain and innervate structures such as the eye, the facial muscles, the tongue, etc.

*Nerve, spinal:* A pair of spinal nerves emerge from each segment of the spinal cord. Each spinal nerve emerges from the cord in the form of two roots (Fig. 6.2). The dorsal, or posterior, root carries sensory fibres; the ventral, or anterior, root carries motor fibres. The perikarya of sensory neurons are housed just outside the cord in dorsal, or posterior, root ganglia (q.v.).

*Nerve trunk:* A cranial or spinal nerve, as seen in dissection, consists of many thousand nerve fibres running in parallel. Consequently such a structure is often said to be a nerve trunk. A transverse section of a nerve trunk is shown in Plate XII(b).

*Neuropil:* A reticulated network of neuronal processes making occasional synaptic contact with each other. The nature of this ravelled labyrinth was not clearly understood before the advent of the electron microscope. Electron microscopy shows that there is very little intercellular space in the brain. The subsequent change in our understanding of the structure of nervous tissue may be gathered by comparing Plate II(a) with Plate XVI(b).

*Neurosis:* There are several different types of neurosis. All are believed to be due to unresolved unconscious conflicts.

*Nucleus:* When used by students of the brain this term denotes a sharply bounded group of nerve cells surrounded by masses of white matter.

*Nudibranch:* A group of gastropod molluscs which, as their name suggests, lack a shell in the adult.

*Ordovician:* A geological period extending from 500 million B.C. to 440 million B.C.

*Parasympathetic system: see* Autonomic nervous system.

*Peripheral nervous system:* The nerves connecting the C.N.S. (q.v.) to the rest of the body.

*Phylum:* A major subdivision of the animal kingdom. A phylum consists of all the animals which share a common basic anatomical design. Thus the phylum Chordata contains forms as diverse as the lamprey and man; the phylum Mollusca forms as diverse as the limpet and the octopus.

*Polymer:* A molecule consisting of a chain of sub-units. The links in the chain, the sub-units, are called monomers.

*Pongid:* The Pongidae is the name of the family to which the great apes—gorilla, chimpanzee, orang-outan, gibbon—belong.

*Propioceptor:* A sense organ responsive to internal stimuli, for example tension or pressure in connective tissues, muscles or joints.

*Pyramidal tract:* An alternative name for the cortico-spinal tract. It consists of fibres originating in the cortex (not only the motor cortex) and running to the spinal cord.

*Sagittal section:* The sagittal suture separates the left and right parietal bones of the skull. Hence a sagittal section is one which runs down in the fore and aft plane through body and brain.

*Schizophrenia:* A condition usually characterized by delusions, hallucinations and a general loss of contact with the everyday world.

*Sclerosis, multiple:* A condition caused by random demyelination and destruction of axons in all parts of the C.N.S. (q.v.). The symptoms of the disease depend on which parts of the C.N.S. are affected.

*Sensory neuron: see* Afferent neuron.

*Set:* A readiness to respond to certain specific stimuli. In some ways the organism appears to be attuned to a particular aspect of its environment.

*Solvent, non-polar:* A non-polar solvent is one in which the constituent molecules bear no electrostatic charge. In other words, unlike water (Fig. 2.2), they are not electrically polarized. Examples of non-polar solvents are benzene, olive oil, etc.

*Spasticity:* A state of increased muscular tone (q.v.) accompanied by spasmodic (sometimes 'clasp-knife') reflexes. The condition is believed to be due to disease of the upper motor neuron so that its controlling influence is lost.

*Symbiont:* Two organisms living together to their *mutual* advantage are said to be symbionts.

*Sympathetic nervous system: see* Autonomic nervous system.

*Syncytium:* A tissue where, although there are numerous nuclei, there is no clear subdivision into cells.

*Tonus:* A state of continuous mild contraction of a muscle dependant on its integrity and on the integrity of its nerve connections.

*Transduction, sensory:* The 'bringing across' of energy from one form into another. Sensory cells, for example, are capable of 'transducing' an environmental energy flux into the energy of action potentials in sensory neurons.

*Ventral:* Appertaining to the lower surface of the body. The ventral surface of a four-footed animal faces the ground. In an upright biped such as man the original ventral surface faces forward and is hence renamed the anterior surface.

*Ventricle:* A cavity. The mammalian brain possesses four such cavities—two lateral ventricles in the cerebral hemispheres and a third and a fourth in the brain stem. All the cerebral ventricles communicate with each other and with the central canal of the spinal cord. In life all these cavities are filled with cerebrospinal fluid. The major part of this watery fluid is secreted by the walls of the lateral ventricles.

# Suggestions for Further Reading

The number of publications in the field of brain science is immense. Any short selection is bound to be influenced by personal bias and chance. Those listed below are merely a selection of those that I have read and found helpful.

An attempt has been made to include books at various interest levels. These levels are indicated by a system of asterisks. A single asterisk indicates a book which can be read with profit by the interested general reader. Two asterisks are set against those more suitable for undergraduate students of the subject, while three asterisks indicate a book written for the more advanced student. Clearly this tripartite division cannot be completely rigorous. Several of the books listed below overlap the categories.

Practically all the books include further references. The interested reader should thus be able to gain entry to the vast field of literature pertaining to the brain.

**General**

*McGaugh, J. L., N. M. Weinberger and R. E. Whalen, editors (1966): *Psychobiology*, W. H. Freeman & Company, San Francisco. This book consists of articles reprinted from *Scientific American.* It is thus written by authoritative authors at a fairly popular level. The illustrations are excellent.

*Patterson, S., editor (1969): *The Brain*, BBC Publications, London.
A collection of talks broadcast on the BBC Radio 3 programme. They provide excellent summaries of many aspects of the brain's functioning.

**Gardner, E. (1963): *Fundamentals of Neurology*, W. B. Saunders Company, Philadelphia and London.
An excellent clearly written introduction to the subject.

**Schadé, J. P. and D. H. Ford (1965): *Basic Neurology*, Elsevier Publishing Company, Amsterdam, New York & London. Another first-rate introduction. Slightly more advanced than *Fundamentals of Neurology*.

**Evans, C. R. and A. D. J. Robertson, editors (1966): *Brain Physiology and Psychology*, Butterworth & Co. (Publishers) Ltd., London.
This book consists of a collection of some of the seminal papers in the field of brain science.

***Quarton, G. C., T. Melnechuk and F. O. Schmitt, editors (1967): *The Neurosciences: a study programme*, The Rockefeller University Press, New York.
This large book consists of 'an integrated series of surveys of selected fields of obvious or demonstrable relevance to an understanding of brain function'. Not for beginners.

***Field, J., H. W. Magoun and V. E. Hall, editors (1960): *Handbook of Physiology*, Section 1: *Neurophysiology*: Vols. 1, 2 and 3. American Physiological Society, Washington. A comprehensive summary of neurophysiology as it existed at the beginning of the 1960s. Not recommended for beginners.

*Chapter 1* Fluxes of materials across membranes

**Spanner, D. C. (1964): *Introduction to Thermodynamics*, Academic Press, Inc., New York and London.

*Chapter 2* Ions and bioelectric potentials

**Katz, B. (1966): *Nerve, muscle, and synapse*, McGraw-Hill Book Company, New York. Chapter 4.

*Chapter 3* Proteins, nucleic acids and biomembranes

*Haynes, R. H. and P. C. Hanawalt, editors (1968): *The Molecular Basis of Life* (readings from *Scientific American*), W. H. Freeman & Company, San Francisco.

**Watson, J. B. (1965): *Molecular Biology of the Gene*, W. A. Benjamin, Inc., New York and Amsterdam.

**Haggis, G. H., D. Michie, A. R. Muir, K. B. Roberts and P. B. M. Walker (1964): *Introduction to Molecular Biology*, Longmans, Green and Co. Ltd., London.

*Chapter 4* Cells of the nervous system

*Hurry, S. (1965): *The Microstructure of the Cell*, John Murray (Publishers) Ltd., London.

**Sholl, D. A. (1956), *The Organisation of the Cerebral Cortex*, Methuen & Company Ltd., London.

***Ramón y Cajal, S. (1909–1911): *Histologie du système nerveux de l'homme et des vertébrés*, A. Maloine, Paris.

*Chapter 5* The nerve impulse

*Katz, B. (1961): 'How cells communicate', *Scientific American*, *205*, *3*, 209–220.

**Katz, B. (1966): *Nerve, muscle, and synapse*, McGraw-Hill Book Company, New York.

***Hodgkin, A. L. (1964): *The Conduction of the Nerve Impulse*, Liverpool University Press, Liverpool.

*Chapter 6* The synapse

*Eccles, J. C. (1965): 'The synapse', *Scientific American*, *212*, 1, 56–66.

*Gray, E. G. (1967): 'The synapse', *Science Journal*, *3*, 5, 66–72.

**Katz, B. (1966): *Nerve, muscle and synapse*, McGraw-Hill Book Company, New York.

***Eccles, J. C. (1964): *The Physiology of Synapses*, Springer-Verlag OHG, Berlin.

*Chapter 7* The sensory input

*Lowenstein, O. E. (1966): *The Senses*, Penguin Books Ltd., Harmondsworth.

*Adrian, E. D. (1947): *The Physical Background of Perception*, Clarendon Press, Oxford.

**Case, J. (1966): *Sensory Mechanisms*, Current Concepts in Biology series, Macmillan Company, New York.

***Davies, H. (1961): 'Some principles of sensory receptor action', *Physiol. Rev.*, *41*, 391–416.

***Cold Spring Harbor Symposia on Quantitative Biology (1965), Vol. XXX: *Sensory Receptors*. Cold Spring Harbor Laboratory of Quantitative Biology, New York.

*Chapter 8* Systems of receptor cells

*von Bekesy, G. (1957): 'The Ear', *Scientific American*, *197*, 2, 66–79.

*Miller, W. H., F. Ratliff and H. K. Hartline (1961): 'How cells receive stimuli', *Scientific American*, *205*, 3, 233–238.

**Lettvin, J. Y., H. R. Maturana, W. S. McCulloch and W. H. Pitts (1959): 'What the frog's eye tells the frog's brain', in *Brain*

*Physiology and Psychology*, edited by C. R. Evans and A. D. J. Robertson. Butterworth & Co. (Publishers) Ltd., London, 1966.

*Chapter 9* Crystals of neural activity

*Kennedy, D. (1967): 'Small systems of nerve cells', *Scientific American, 216*, 5, 44–52.

**Wiersma, C. A. G., editor (1967): *Invertebrate Nervous Systems: their significance for mammalian neurophysiology*. University of Chicago Press, Chicago.

**Roberts, T. D. M. (1966): *Basic Ideas in Neurophysiology*, Butterworth & Co. (Publishers) Ltd., London.

***Bullock, T. H. and G. A. Horridge (1965): *Structure and Function in the Nervous System of Invertebrates*, W. H. Freeman & Company, San Francisco.

*Chapter 10* The evolution of vertebrate brains

**Gardner, E. (1963): *Fundamentals of Neurology*, W. B. Saunders Company, Philadelphia and London.

**Hyman, L. H. (1942): *Comparative Vertebrate Anatomy*, University of Chicago Press, Chicago. Chapter XIV.

**Romer, A. S. (1950): *The Vertebrate Body*, W. B. Saunders Company, Philadelphia and London. Chapter XVI.

***Ariens-Kappers, C. U., G. C. Huber & E. C. Crosby (1960): *The Comparative Anatomy of the Nervous System of Vertebrates including Man*, Hefner Publishing Company, New York.

*Chapter 11* Patterns of neurons in the brain

*Sperry, R. W. (1959): 'The growth of nerve circuits', *Scientific American, 201*, 5, 68–75.

***Gaze, R. M. (1960): 'Regeneration of the optic nerve in Amphibia', *Int. Rev. of Neurobiology, 2*, 1–40.

***Weiss, P. (1967): 'Specificity in the neurosciences', in *Neurosciences Research Symposia Summaries I*, edited by F. O. Schmitt and T. Melnechuk, MIT Press, Cambridge, Massachusetts and London, England.

*Chapter 12* Motivation

*McGaugh, J. L., N. M. Weinberger and R. E. Whalen, editors (1966): *Psychobiology*, W. H. Freeman & Company, San Francisco. Section II, pp. 54–88.

*Tinbergen, N. (1951): *The Study of Instinct*, Clarendon Press, Oxford.

**Livingston, R. B. (1967): 'Brain circuitry relating to complex behavior', in *The Neurosciences*, edited by G. C. Quarton, T. Melnechuk and F. O. Schmitt, The Rockefeller University Press, New York, Pp. 499–515.

***Glass, D. C., editor (1967): *Neurophysiology and Emotion*, The Rockefeller University Press, New York.

*Chapter 13* The primate cerebral cortex

**Sholl, D. A. (1956): *The Organisation of the Cerebral Cortex*, Methuen & Co. Ltd., London.

**Penfield, W. G. (1958): *The Excitable Cortex in Conscious Man*, Liverpool University Press, Liverpool.

***Blinkov, S. M. and I. I. Glezer (1968): *The Human Brain in Figures and Tables: a quantitative handbook*, Plenum Press, New York.

*Chapter 14* Perception

*Abercrombie, M. L. J. (1960): *The Anatomy of Judgement: an investigation of the processes of perception and reasoning*, Hutchinson & Co. (Publishers) Ltd., London.

*Gregory, R. L. (1966): *Eye and Brain: the psychology of seeing*, Weidenfeld & Nicolson, London.

*Hubel, D. H. (1963): 'The visual cortex of the brain', *Scientific American*, *209*, 5, 54–62.

**von Senden, M. (1960): *Space and Sight: the perception of space and shape in the congenitally blind before and after operation*, translated by P. Heath. Methuen & Co. Ltd., London.

**Wyburn, G. M., R. W. Pickford and R. J. Hirst (1964): *Human Senses and Perception*, Oliver & Boyd, Ltd., London.

**Hanson, N. R. (1958): *Patterns of Discovery: an enquiry into the conceptual foundations of science*, Cambridge University Press, Cambridge.

*Chapter 15* Memory

*McGaugh, J. L., N. M. Weinberger & R. E. Whalen, editors (1966): *Psychobiology*, W. H. Freeman & Company, San Francisco. Section IV, pp. 118–168.

*Agranoff, B. W. (1967): 'Memory and protein synthesis', *Scientific American*, *216*, 6, 115–122.

*Russell, W. Ritchie (1959): *Brain, Memory and Learning*, Clarendon Press, Oxford.

**Young, J. Z. (1966): *The Memory System of the Brain*, Clarendon Press, Oxford.

***Lashley, K. S. (1960): *The neuropsychology of Lashley: selected papers*, edited by E. A. Beach. McGraw-Hill Book Company, New York.

**Lowes, J. L. (1927): *The Road to Xanadu: a study in the ways of the imagination*, Houghton Mifflin Company, Boston.

*Chapter 16* Consciousness

*Jouvet, M. (1967): 'The states of sleep', *Scientific American, 216, 2*, 62–72.

**Oswald, J. (1962): *Sleeping and Waking*, Elsevier Publishing Company, Amsterdam, New York and London.

**Freud, S. (1922): *Introductory Lectures on Psychoanalysis*, translated by J. Riviere, George Allen and Unwin Ltd., London.

***Eccles, J. C., editor (1966): *Brain and Conscious Experience*, Springer-Verlag OHG, Berlin.

*Chapter 17* The brain and the mind

*Brain, W. R. (1959): *The Nature of Experience*, Clarendon Press, Oxford.

*Sherrington, C. S. (1955): *Man on his nature*, Penguin Books Ltd., Harmondsworth.

**Stevens, S. S. (1966): 'Quantifying the sensory experience', in *Mind, Matter and Method*, edited by P. K. Feyerabend and G. Maxwell, University of Minnesota Press, Minneapolis.

**Ryle, G. (1949): *The Concept of Mind*, Hutchinson's University Library, London.

**Descartes, R. (1637): *A Discourse on Method*, Everyman's Library, J. M. Dent & Sons Ltd., London.

**McKay, D. (1967): *Freedom of Action in a Mechanistic Universe*, Cambridge University Press, Cambridge.

***Eccles, J. C. (1956): *The Neurophysiological Basis of Mind*, Clarendon Press, Oxford.

***Feigl, H. (1967): *The 'Mental' and the 'Physical'*, University of Minnesota Press, Minneapolis.

**Miscellaneous**

*Brains and computers*

*Sutherland, N. S. (1968): 'Machines like men', *Science Journal, 4*, 10, 44–59.

**von Neuman, J. (1958): *The Computer and the Brain*, Yale University Press.

**Wiener, N. (1948): *Cybernetics*, John Wiley & Sons Inc., New York and London.

**Anderson, A. R., editor (1964): *Minds and Machines*. Contemporary Perspectives in Philosophy series: Prentice-Hall, Englewood Cliffs, New Jersey.

*History*

**Field, J., H. W. Magoun and V. E. Hall, editors (1960): *Handbook of Physiology*, Section 1: *Neurophysiology*, Vol. 1, Chapter 1. American Physiological Society, Washington.

**Clarke, E. and C. D. O'Malley (1968): *The Human Brain and Spinal Cord: a historical study illustrated by writings from antiquity to the twentieth century*. University of California Press, Berkeley and Los Angeles.

*Technique*

**Whitfield, I. C. (1964): *Manual of Experimental Electrophysiology*, Pergamon Press, London.

***Bureš, J., M. Petran and J. Zachar (1960): *Electrophysiological Methods in Biological Research*, translated by P. Hahn. Czechoslovak Academy of Sciences, Prague.

# Index